ADVANCES IN Surgery

Editor-in-Chief
John L. Cameron, MD

ELSEVIER

PHILADELPHIA LONDON TORONTO MONTREAL SYDNEY TOKYO

ADVANCES IN
Surgery

VOLUMES 1 THROUGH 49 (OUT OF PRINT)

VOLUME 52

16. What Is the Best Pain Control After Major Hepatopancreatobiliary Surgery? *by Bradford J. Kim, Jose M. Soliz, Thomas A. Aloia, and Jean-Nicolas Vauthey*
17. Are Opioids Overprescribed Following Elective Surgery? *by Elizabeth B. Habermann*
18. Contemporary Management of Critical Limb Ischemia, *by Jonathan R. Thompson and Peter K. Henke*
19. The Use of Lavage for the Management of Diverticulitis, *by Cyrus Jahansouz and Mary R. Kwaan*

VOLUME 51

1. Can Neoadjuvant Therapy in Pancreatic Cancer Increase the Pool of Patients Eligible for Pancreaticoduodenectomy? *by Thilo Hackert, Alexis Ulrich, and Markus W. Büchler*
2. Can the Diagnosis of Appendicitis Be Made Without a Computed Tomography Scan? *by Yangyang R. Yu and Sohail R. Shah*
3. Sleeve Gastrectomy and Diabetes: Is Cure Possible? *by Amin Andalib and Ali Aminian*
4. Vascular Resections During the Whipple Procedure, *by Warren R. Maley and Charles J. Yeo*
5. Transplantation of the Patient with Human Immunodeficiency Virus, *by Kyle R. Jackson and Andrew Cameron*
6. What Is the Proper Use of Opioids in the Postoperative Patient? *by Thomas Peponis and Haytham M.A. Kaafarani*
7. How Do We Prevent Readmissions After Major Surgery? *by Tyler S. Wahl and Mary T. Hawn*
8. Can Surgery for Appendicitis Be Performed as an Outpatient Procedure? *by Richard Frazee*
9. Concurrent Surgery: What is Appropriate? *by David B. Hoyt and Peter Angelos*
10. Who Should Manage Patients with Adhesive Small Bowel Obstruction? *by Christopher T. Aquina and Fergal J. Fleming*
11. Do Patient-Reported Outcomes Correlate with Clinical Outcomes Following Surgery? *by Jennifer F. Waljee and Justin B. Dimick*

12. Minimally Invasive Gastric Surgery, *by Gabriel Herrera-Almario and Vivian E. Strong*
13. Is Axillary Lymph Node Dissection Necessary After a Positive Sentinel Lymph Node Biopsy? *by Lerna C. Ozcan and Armando E. Giuliano*
14. Do Patients Mandate Resection After a First Episode of Acute Diverticulitis of the Colon with a Complication? *by Ryan Francis Bendl and Roberto Bergamaschi*
15. Per-Oral Esophageal Myotomy: Is It a Safe and Durable Procedure for Achalasia? *by Eric S. Hungness and Juaquito M. Jorge*
16. Is Open Vascular Surgery or Endovascular Surgery the Better Option for Lower Extremity Arterial Occlusive Disease? *by Jeffrey J. Siracuse and Alik Farber*
17. The Use of Radiofrequency Detection to Mitigate the Risk of Retained Surgical Sponges, *by James M. Bardes and Kenji Inaba*
18. Professionalism in Surgery: Crucial Skills for Attendings and Residents, *by Mark S. Hochberg, Russell S. Berman, and H. Leon Pachter*

VOLUME 50

1. Management of Mixed-Type Intraductal Papillary Mucinous Neoplasm, *by Alexandra M. Roch and Christian Max Schmidt*
2. Minimally Invasive Esophagectomy: Is There an Advantage? *by Richard J. Battafarano*
3. Optimal Management of the Axilla: A Look at the Evidence, *by Eleftherios (Terry) P. Mamounas*
4. The Use of LINX for Gastroesophageal Reflux, *by Yulia Zak and David W. Rattner*
5. Bowel Preparation: Are Antibiotics Necessary for Colorectal Surgery? *by Alice Charlotte Adelaide Murray and Ravi P. Kiran*
6. Incarcerated/Strangulated Hernia: Open or Laparoscopic? *by James G. Bittner IV*
7. Strategies to Reduce Postoperative Urinary Tract Infections, *by Christina M. Papageorge and Gregory D. Kennedy*
8. The Aging Surgeon, *by Mark R. Katlic and JoAnn Coleman*
9. Maintenance of Certification, *by Mark A. Malangoni*
10. Treatment of Locally Advanced Pancreatic Ductal Adenocarcinoma, *by Andrew P. Loehrer, Christine V. Kinnier, and Cristina R. Ferrone*

Editor: John Vassallo
Developmental Editor: Laura Kavanaugh

Printed in the United States of America.

Editorial Office:
Elsevier
1600 John F. Kennedy Blvd,
Suite 1800
Philadelphia, PA 19103-2899

International Standard Serial Number: 0065-3411
International Standard Book Number: 978-0-323-72258-2

ADVANCES IN
Surgery

CONTRIBUTORS

ALEX ADDO, MD, MPH, Research Fellow, Department of Surgery, Anne Arundel Medical Center, Annapolis, Maryland

MARIA S. ALTIERI, MD, MS, Instructor of Surgery, Section of Minimally Invasive Surgery, Department of Surgery, Washington University School of Medicine, St Louis, Missouri

AMMAR ASBAN, MD, Department of Surgery, The University of Alabama at Birmingham, Birmingham, Alabama

ANDREA V. BARRIO, MD, Associate Attending Surgeon, Breast Service, Department of Surgery, Memorial Sloan Kettering Cancer Center, Assistant Professor of Surgery, Weill Medical College of Cornell University, New York, New York

KYLA M. BENNETT, MD, Assistant Professor, Department of Surgery, University of Wisconsin-Madison School of Medicine and Public Health, Madison, Wisconsin

L. MICHAEL BRUNT, MD, Professor of Surgery, Section of Minimally Invasive Surgery, Washington University School of Medicine, St Louis, Missouri

RACHEL L. CHORON, MD, Assistant Surgeon, Division of Acute Care Surgery, Department of Surgery, The Johns Hopkins Hospital, Baltimore, Maryland

ELIZABETH DAUER, MD, Assistant Professor of Clinical Surgery, Department of Surgery, Lewis Katz School of Medicine at Temple University, Philadelphia, Pennsylvania

GERARD M. DOHERTY, MD, Crowley Family Distinguished Chair, Department of Surgery, Brigham and Women's Hospital, Moseley Professor of Surgery, Harvard Medical School, Surgeon-in-Chief, Brigham Health and Dana-Farber Cancer Institute, Boston, Massachusetts

MATTHEW J. DOUGHERTY, MD, Clinical Professor, Surgery, Section of Vascular Surgery, Pennsylvania Hospital, University of Pennsylvania, Philadelphia, Pennsylvania

SOPHIE DREAM, MD, Department of Surgery, The University of Alabama at Birmingham, Birmingham, Alabama

NEETA J. ERINJERI, MD, Endocrine Surgeon, Endocrine Neoplasia Institute, Miami Cancer Institute, Miami, Florida

CRISTINA R. FERRONE, MD, FACS, Associate Professor, Department of Surgery, Massachusetts General Hospital, Boston, Massachusetts

ROBERT J. FITZGIBBONS Jr, MD, FACS, Harry E. Stuckenhoff Professor and Chairman, Department of Surgery, Creighton University School of Medicine, Omaha, Nebraska

KRISTALYN K. GALLAGHER, DO, FACOS, Department of Surgery, Division of Surgical Oncology, The University of North Carolina at Chapel Hill, Chapel Hill, North Carolina

AMY GOLDBERG, MD, Professor of Surgery, Chair, Department of Surgery, Lewis Katz School of Medicine at Temple University, Philadelphia, Pennsylvania

ROSS F. GOLDBERG, MD, Department of Surgery, Maricopa Integrated Health System, Associate Professor of Surgery, Creighton University School of Medicine, Phoenix, Arizona

DANIEL A. HASHIMOTO, MD, MS, Surgical Resident, Department of Surgery, Massachusetts General Hospital, Boston, Massachusetts

B. TODD HENIFORD, MD, FACS, Professor, Department of Surgery, Chief, Gastrointestinal and Minimally Invasive Surgery, Carolinas Medical Center, Charlotte, North Carolina

ANDREW T. HUBER, MD, Fellow, Division of Gastrointestinal and Minimally Invasive Surgery, Department of Surgery, Carolinas Medical Center, Charlotte, North Carolina

ASHLEY KREPLINE, MD, General Surgery Resident, Department of Surgery, Medical College of Wisconsin, Milwaukee, Wisconsin

BRENESSA LINDEMAN, MD, MEHP, Assistant Professor, Department of Surgery, The University of Alabama at Birmingham, Birmingham, Alabama

KRYSTAL C. MALONI, MD, Vascular Fellow, Pennsylvania Hospital, University of Pennsylvania, Philadelphia, Pennsylvania

WINTA T. MEHTSUN, MD, MPH, Surgical Resident, Department of Surgery, Massachusetts General Hospital, Boston, Massachusetts

DAVID W. OLLILA, MD, FACS, Department of Surgery, Division of Surgical Oncology, The University of North Carolina at Chapel Hill, Chapel Hill, North Carolina

JAVIER OTERO, MD, Fellow, Division of Gastrointestinal and Minimally Invasive Surgery, Department of Surgery, Carolinas Medical Center, Charlotte, North Carolina

ADRIAN E. PARK, MD, FRCSC, FACS, FCS(ECSA), Chairman, Department of Surgery, Anne Arundel Medical Center, Professor of Surgery, Johns Hopkins University School of Medicine, Annapolis, Maryland

RONAK B. PATEL, MD, Division of Vascular and Endovascular Surgery, Department of Surgery, Stony Brook University Hospital, Stony Brook, New York

RICHARD M. PETERSON, MD, MPH, FACS, FASMBS, Professor of Surgery, San Antonio, Texas

JOSEPH V. SAKRAN, MPH, MD, MPA, FACS, Assistant Professor, Department of Surgery, The Johns Hopkins University School of Medicine, Director, Emergency General Surgery, The Johns Hopkins Hospital, Baltimore, Maryland

JOHN E. SCARBOROUGH, MD, Associate Professor, Department of Surgery, University of Wisconsin-Madison School of Medicine and Public Health, Madison, Wisconsin

ALEXANDER D. SCHROEDER, MD, Senior Resident, Department of Surgery, Creighton University School of Medicine, Omaha, Nebraska

JOHN D. SCOTT, MD, FACS, FASMBS, Associate Professor of Surgery, Greenville, South Carolina

DON J. SELZER, MD, MS, FACS, FASMBS, Associate Professor of Surgery, Willis D. Gatch Scholar in Surgery, Chief, Division of General Surgery, Indiana University School of Medicine, Indianapolis, Indiana

SARABETH SPITZER, Medical Student, Stanford University School of Medicine, Stanford, California

DIMITRIOS STEFANIDIS, MD, PhD, FACS, FASMBS, Professor, Department of Surgery, Vice Chair of Education, Director, Minimally Invasive and Bariatric Surgery, Indiana University School of Medicine, Indianapolis, Indiana

APOSTOLOS K. TASSIOPOULOS, MD, FACS, Division of Vascular and Endovascular Surgery, Department of Surgery, Stony Brook University Hospital, Stony Brook, New York

DOUGLAS A. TROUTMAN, DO, Assistant Clinical Professor of Surgery, Section of Vascular Surgery, Pennsylvania Hospital, University of Pennsylvania, Philadelphia, Pennsylvania

SUSAN TSAI, MD, MHS, Associate Professor, Department of Surgery, Division of Surgical Oncology, Medical College of Wisconsin, Milwaukee, Wisconsin

DUSTIN J. TUBRE, MD, Senior Resident, Department of Surgery, Creighton University School of Medicine, Omaha, Nebraska

ROBERT UDELSMAN, MD, MBA, FACS, FACE, Director, Endocrine Neoplasia Institute, Miami Cancer Institute, Professor, Florida International University, Miami, Florida; Professor of Surgery Emeritus, Yale University School of Medicine, New Haven, Connecticut

KIMBERLY J. VAN ZEE, MS, MD, Attending Surgeon, Breast Service, Department of Surgery, Memorial Sloan Kettering Cancer Center, Professor of Surgery, Weill Medical College of Cornell University; New York, New York

ALLISON R. WILCOX, MD, Research Fellow, Department of Surgery, Dartmouth-Hitchcock Medical Center, Lebanon, New Hampshire

SANDRA L. WONG, MD, MS, William N and Bessie Allyn Professor and Chair, Department of Surgery, Dartmouth-Hitchcock Medical Center, Lebanon, New Hampshire; Dartmouth Geisel School of Medicine, Hanover, New Hampshire

H. REZA ZAHIRI, DO, FACS, Attending Surgeon, Department of Surgery, Anne Arundel Medical Center, Annapolis, Maryland

CONTENTS VOLUME 53 • 2019

Advances in Surgery 53 (2019) 1–19

ADVANCES IN SURGERY

Laparoscopic Hernia Repair

Javier Otero, MD, Andrew T. Huber, MD,
B. Todd Heniford, MD*

Division of Gastrointestinal and Minimally Invasive Surgery, Department of Surgery, Carolinas Medical Center, 1025 Morehead Medical Drive, Suite 300, Charlotte, NC 28204, USA

Keywords

• Ventral hernia repair • Laparoscopic hernia repair • Robotic hernia repair
• Abdominal wall reconstruction • Laparoscopy • Incisional hernia
• Laparoscopic ventral hernia repair

Key points

- Surgeons must assess several patient factors as well as their level of comfort with LVHR and ultimately opt for an approach that provides the best outcome combined with a low potential for risk.
- The mesh to defect ratio strongly affects recurrence rates. In general, the broader the mesh, the lower the chance for recurrence.
- Compared with open, LVHR has decreased risk of surgical site infection and may be an appropriate approach for patients with risk factors for wound-related complications that cannot be modified.
- Consideration may be given to primary fascial defect closure during LVHR, which may reduce rates of postoperative seromas and recurrence.
- Advancements in technology and traditional LVHR technique, such as extraperitoneal mesh placement and robotic approach, have allowed for more advanced repairs and may improve the shortcomings of a bridged LVHR.

INTRODUCTION

Ventral incisional hernias are a ubiquitous problem for general surgeons; approximately 22% of patients develop an abdominal musculo-fascial defect within 3 years of laparotomy [1]. Furthermore, 229,000 Americans a year report hernias as the primary cause of their disability, affecting their ability

Disclosure Statement: Dr B.T. Heniford has previous grants and honoraria from W.L. Gore, Allergan, and Stryker. The remainder of the authors have no relevant financial conflicts or disclosures.

*Corresponding author. *E-mail address:* todd.heniford@atriumhealth.org

https://doi.org/10.1016/j.yasu.2019.04.001
0065-3411/19/

to perform activities of daily living and instrumental activities of life [2]. Thus, ventral hernia repair (VHR) remains one of the most common operations performed by surgeons and is a procedure of significant importance for its ability to restore quality of life (QOL) [3]. Although the use of mesh has improved the outcomes compared with a tissue-based repair and has long been accepted as the preferred method to minimize recurrence, less agreement surrounds the ideal approach to repair [4–6].

As with the other areas of surgical practice, the advent of minimally invasive surgery (MIS) added a new technique to the surgical approach of VHR. Although the generalized benefits of MIS include improved QOL, shortened recovery, decreased pain, and improved cosmesis, MIS approaches to VHR have had mixed outcomes in these areas but continue to garner attention, popularity, and academic study [7–10]. Since laparoscopic ventral hernia repair (LVHR) was first described in 1993 by Leblanc and Booth in a feasibility study of 5 patients who underwent a bridged intraperitoneal onlay mesh (IPOM) repair [11], LVHR is now used in 22% to 31% of VHRs in the United States [12–14].

Traditional LVHR takes advantage of the key principles of hernia repair surgery, such as wide mesh overlap and underlay mesh positioning and tries to take advantage of the Law of LaPlace by distributing intraabdominal pressure across a large area of overlapping mesh. Proponents of LVHR note the advantages of shortened hospitalization, reduced rates of wound complications, and minimal soft-tissue dissection. Continued challenges of laparoscopic approach include lack of anatomic and physiologic reconstruction with bridged repair and increased and prolonged discomfort compared with open surgery [15]. However, modifications in technique are continuously presented in the literature and debated in an effort to improve on these weaknesses. For example, robotic surgery has been looked at as a possible tool to help surgeons facilitate a more functional hernia repair.

As described in our editorial of SAGES guidelines, the greatest problem that must be faced when discussing LVHR or, really, any VHR, is that many of the basic engineering fundamentals to perform a dependable, repeatable hernia repair have not been answered [16]. If the strength of the abdominal wall, the force generated in various levels of physical activity, the roles that body mass index or abdominal girth play in pressure generation within the abdomen, the impact of the size of an abdominal wall defect, the real and long-lasting strength of tissue in-growth of mesh, in general, and the various meshes in particular, against an intact peritoneum, the long-term impact of mesh-visceral adhesions are not known reliably, and how any and all of these blend together to have an impact on recurrence, QOL, and complications, then can a ventral hernia be treated effectively? How much is currently known about VHR pales in comparison with how much there is yet to understand. Truly, with the evidence that is available, how do we know how strong a mesh needs to be? How many sutures or tacks should be applied? Should fixation be with permanent or absorbable materials? Where should fixation be placed? What mesh should be chosen? How much overlap is appropriate and what role do the defect size and patient characteristics play in this decision? What physical activities should be limited after surgery and for how long? This article provides a summary of LVHR with a focus on technical considerations, special populations, outcomes, and innovations in methods as expressed in the literature.

INDICATION FOR LAPAROSCOPIC VENTRAL HERNIA REPAIR

As many as one-third of patients with incisional hernia are asymptomatic from their hernia [17]. Thus, the question of watchful waiting for such patients may be considered. Longitudinal studies have noted low rates of incarceration or need for emergent surgery with at least 2 to 5 years of observation [18,19]. However, a noticeable deterioration in physical function with worsening of pain and pain severity may be observed [19]. A multicenter randomized controlled German study (AWARE study) is currently recruiting to assess the effects of watchful waiting versus surgical repair on pain during normal activities for patients with asymptomatic and oligosymptomatic incisional hernias [20,21].

The consideration of surgical approach, namely open versus minimally invasive, should be addressed during consultations for appropriate ventral or incisional hernias (Table 1). Current recommendations for repair include symptomatic hernias, including those with pain or discomfort as well as patients with disability or reduced QOL as a result of their hernia. Further indications for surgical correction include prevention or treatment of complications, such as enlargement, skin problems, obstruction, incarcerations, and strangulation [22,23].

Historically, open VHR had been the standard approach for incarcerated hernias. However, the laparoscopic approach is being increasingly used for emergent VHRs with decreased infectious and wound-related morbidity [24]. The incidence of complications and recurrences in emergency cases are similar to elective cases. However, selection criteria for such emergent cases is important and the following should be considered [25]:

Table 1
Indications and contraindications of LVHR

Indications	Possible contraindications
Symptomatic relief	Medical contraindication for general anesthesia (eg, hemodynamic instability or coagulopathy)
Avoid/prevent future complications	Hostile/frozen abdomen
Treatment of acute complications	Gangrenous or perforated viscus
	Open abdominal wounds with active infection or enterocutaneous fistula
	Loss of domain
	Abdominal skin grafts
	Patients in need of skin or soft-tissue reconstruction

- Absence of marked bowel distention that would impede the working space
- Lack of peritonitis or other high-risk septic situations (eg, enterocutaneous fistula, bowel necrosis, or perforation)
- Hemodynamic stability
- A patient without any acutely moribund or severe medical comorbidities precluding pneumoperitoneum

Ultimately, a surgeon's level of comfort and expertise and training significantly dictate the options for laparoscopic hernia repair. SAGES guidelines for LVHR encourage surgeons to base their decision to perform LVHR on the anticipated complexity, resource availability, and surgeon experience with LVHR [22]. Several preoperative and intraoperative factors associated with increased complexity include incarceration, suprapubic location, recurrent hernias, and larger defects [26]. Further factors to consider include the potential for adhesion formation associated with intraperitoneal mesh. The LVHR approach with placement of an intraabdominal mesh may be ill suited for patients highly likely to require subsequent intraabdominal surgeries, such as young patients, or those with inflammatory bowel disease or certain malignancies with potential for future debulking procedures. Conversely, a minimally invasive approach is well suited for patients with comorbidities that make them high risk for wound complications, such as patients with diabetes, smokers, or obese patients [27–29].

SPECIAL CONSIDERATIONS

Obesity

Obesity is a major risk factor for postoperative complications in several surgical fields. In part due to the increased risk of postoperative complications and significantly increased intraabdominal pressure, obese patients are also predisposed to incisional hernia formation and hernia recurrence. VHR is not immune to this problem; several studies have demonstrated that obesity is a major risk factor for postoperative complications, recurrence, and reoperation after hernia repair [30–32]. Laparoscopic surgery has been found to be superior to an open approach in obese patients undergoing VHR in terms of mitigating wound complications [33]. One national study demonstrated that, compared with LVHR, open surgery increased the odds of a surgical site infection (SSI) for all obesity classifications by greater than 2-fold [34]. Such findings have been so compelling that current guidelines from the International Endohernia Society (IEHS) state that for obese patients with ventral or incisional hernias, a laparoscopic approach is preferred; however, this is an opinion from that group and many factors must be taken into account [23].

Recurrence rates continue to be a concern for obese patients regardless of the approach and range from 5% to 19% [35–38]; a 4-fold increase in recurrence in morbidly obese patients (BMI >40 kg/m^2) has been described [32]. Patients with BMI greater than 30 kg/m^2 and defects larger than 8 to 10 cm are at risk of higher recurrence [39]. As a result, some investigators propose additional steps, such as larger mesh size, additional fixation points, or defect closure to mitigate this increased risk, but none of these recommendations have been proven.

GENERAL STEPS OF THE LAPAROSCOPIC VENTRAL HERNIA REPAIR TECHNIQUE

Bowel Preparation

Preoperative mechanical bowel preparation may be useful in select cases. Proponents note that it may allow for bowel decompression and potentially a resultant increase in working space [40], but this has not been proven. Furthermore, decompressed bowel offers theoretic advantages of safer bowel handling during manipulation as well as decreased risk of enteric contamination in the event of an enterotomy. However, opponents of mechanical bowel preparations note the inconvenience to patients and a lack of evidence to demonstrate a difference in postoperative wound events [41].

Abdominal Access and Trocar Placement

The point of initial abdominal access should take into consideration hernia location as well as any previous abdominal procedures and associated scars that would suggest potential intraabdominal adhesions. Several techniques are available, including Veress needle insufflation, direct optical trocar insertion, open Hasson technique, or combination of these. Optimal port placement may vary by case, however, typical placement is away from the defect to allow mesh placement that does not interfere with or cover trocars, but in some cases initial trocars are placed in the hernia itself. Care should be taken not to place the trocars excessively lateral because that may only act to impede access to the anterior abdominal wall due to obstructions from the patient's thigh or the operative table.

Frequent port configurations included 2 or 3 trocars staggered and separated by approximately 8 cm (or a handbreadths) along one side of the abdomen with an additional trocar on the opposite side. Alternatively, a pair of trocars can be placed along each anterior axillary line. This configuration lends itself to convenient mesh fixation with the laparoscope and tacking device having easy access and visibility of a contralateral quadrant of the mesh. Although descriptions of LVHR with minimal port placement and ports only along 1 side are described, a concern is that only placing that camera on 1 side of the mesh may affect proper mesh positioning, potentially increasing the risk of recurrence [42].

Adhesiolysis

The most difficult and time-consuming portion of the procedure is often adhesiolysis. Frequently a window of access and plane free from adhesions can be found between the costal margin and iliac crest on 1 side of the peritoneum. External manual compression of the anterior abdominal wall alters the angle of attack and may facilitate dissection when needed. The boundaries of the hernia sac should be delineated and dissected to the margins for approximately

5 cm to allow for the overlapping mesh to lay flat. If there is no concern of bowel obstruction, then any additional adhesiolysis beyond the boundaries of where the mesh will lay may only add risk without benefit from a technical perspective.

Measuring the Defect

Accurate measurements are important to determine appropriate mesh size and overlap. Several techniques have been described, with most advocating intraperitoneal dimensions for improved accuracy. Such internal appraisals of defect size negate the effect of abdominal wall thickness and curvature in overestimating defect size. Indeed, extracorporeal measurements of hernia defects on average can overestimate defect size by 1.7 to 3.1 cm compared with intracorporeal measures [43,44]. Commonly described measuring techniques include

- Insertion of a thin plastic ruler that can be directly opposed to the abdominal wall [45].
- Spinal needles inserted transabdominally at the edge of the defect facilitate longitudinal and transverse dimensions [46].
- A silk suture on a Keith needle can be introduced transabdominally at one extent of the hernia defect and exited at the opposite end. Using the suture, the internal dimensions can be marked and subsequently measured.

Primary Fascial Defect Closure

A question that has arisen with the maturation of LVHR techniques is whether to close the hernia defect as opposed to bridging the fascia with the traditional IPOM approach. Many investigators have noted that, except in the most extreme cases, bridging of mesh is used infrequently during open VHR. Therefore, the bridging technique of LVHR has naturally been called into question. Common reasons cited for primary facial defect closure included reduced rates of seroma and recurrence and possible improved functionality and contour of the abdominal wall. A metanalysis of almost entirely retrospective studies comparing fascial and nonfascial defect closure outcomes reviewed 16 articles and concluded that seroma formation and recurrence were higher in the nonclosure group [47]. A more recent single-institution comparative study of 783 patients demonstrated similar findings, with patients who underwent defect closure had a statistically significant decrease in surgical site occurrences, seromas, and objective recurrences [48]. Despite this, these advantages remain controversial with some conflicting data showing no difference in seroma, SSIs, or surgical site recurrences requiring procedural interventions between bridged repairs and repairs with defect closure [49]. Thus, whereas the International Endohernia Society Guidelines (IEHS) for the treatment of LVHR recommend primary fascial closure of hernia defects of limited size, the SAGES guidelines as yet do not recommend the practice and suggest it should be based on the surgeon's discretion, citing a lack of high quality data to suggest rigorous validation [22,23].

Mesh Selection

The characteristics of an ideal mesh have been previously described and included a noncarcinogenic, chemically inert material capable of sterilization that is sufficiently mechanically strong. The material should be nontoxic to native tissue with minimal risk of allergic or inflammatory foreign body reaction. Further properties important for mesh positioned within the intraperitoneal cavity include resistance to infection, barrier to adhesions along the visceral surface, and adequate incorporation [50,51]. Early reports of LVHR frequently used uncoated permanent synthetic mesh, commonly polypropylene or expanded polytetrafluoroethylene. However, issues with uncoated polypropylene mesh within the peritoneal cavity became readily apparent, and included erosion, fistula, bowel obstruction, and infection [52–55]. Thus, barrier-coated mesh should be used for IPOM positioned LVHR to minimize the risk of visceral adhesions to the mesh and associated complications. A variety of absorbable barrier options are available to provide protection against adhesiogenesis, including oxygenized regenerated cellulose, omega-3-fatty acid, carboxymethylcellulose, and hyaluronic acid.

Mesh Size and Overlap

Adequate mesh overlap is accepted as a key component to successful LVHR. Although the optimal degree of overlap is not proven, some guidelines suggest a minimum size limit of 3 to 4 cm, and others simply recommend that the mesh be sized with "appropriate overlap" based on defect size, hernia location, and important clinical factors such as obesity [22,23]. In general, it seems that investigators have increased the degree of overlap as they have gained experience and the technical savvy to do so [32]. One recent meta-analysis of 8864 patients noted the risk of hernia recurrence decreased with increasing mesh overlap from 8.6% with less than 3 cm to 4.6% with 3 to 5 cm, and to a remarkable 1.4% with greater than 5 cm of overlap during laparoscopic repairs [42].

It is being increasingly understood that a blanket cutoff of mesh overlap for all defect sizes and hernia types fails to fully address the forces at play and technical nuances of IPOM LVHR. Understanding of the mesh to defect ratio is being increasingly appreciated as an important consideration when attempting to positively have an impact on recurrence after LVHR. During IPOM repairs, the intraabdominal pressure exerts an episodic, unopposed force at the central bridge portion of the mesh. This force is proportional to the area over which it is delivered (using the equation force = pressure × area) and therefore increases with increasing size of the defect. Similarly, this force is offset by the degree of mesh overlapped and incorporated into the surrounding abdominal wall [56]. This concept demonstrates the importance of maintaining an adequate mesh overlap, which may be somewhat proportional to the defect. As the defect size enlarges, the oversimplification of 3 to 5 cm of mesh overall may increasingly fail [57]. Recent data suggest that an adequate defect to mesh ratio of at least 13 is required to maintain acceptably low recurrence rates. Hauters and colleagues [58] demonstrated that with long-term 5 year follow-up a defect area to mesh area ratio of less than 13 was independently predictive of recurrence and ratios of less than 8, 9 to 12, 13 to 16, and greater than 16 provided recurrence rate of 70%, 35%, 9%, and 0%, respectively. However, for a 100 cm^2 defect, a 1300 cm^2 mesh would be impossible to insert laparoscopically in most patients.

Mesh Fixation

Adequate mesh fixation of any intraperitoneal mesh is also a fundamental and controversial component of LVHR. Transfascial fixation with permanent sutures is a common method used in IPOM LVHR [59]. Other methods of fixation include sutures, tacks, glue, staples, or a combination of these. However, the optimal method of fixation is debated in the literature, and no clear consensus has been reached. Many investigators have reported excellent outcomes with low recurrence using a combination of tacks and sutures [60,61]. Reports of equally adequate outcomes have also been demonstrated with fixation by way of tacks alone [62,63]. A recent systematic review and network meta-analysis comparing sutures, tacks, and combination methods of fixation during LVHR failed to demonstrate a statistically significant difference between the methods analyzed, but it did note that crude recurrence rates and surface under the cumulative ranking curve (SUCRA) analysis favored suture fixation and suggested that sutures had a 93% probability of being superior [64]. Alternatively, proponents of tacks have demonstrated good outcomes with a "double crown" approach with decreased rates of acute postoperative pain lasting up to 3 months with no difference in recurrence compared with transfascial suture fixation [65]. A comparison of suture and tacks is provided in Table 2.

The most common method for transfascial fixation incorporates 4 cardinal sutures. Sutures are preplaced at the periphery of the mesh and the tails left long to be brought through the abdominal wall with a suture passer. Once the mesh has been prepared, it may be rolled up and introduced by way of an 11 or 12 mm trocar. Similarly, tacks, whether in conjunction with sutures or in isolation, should be placed along the periphery of the mesh at approximately less than 1 cm intervals and within 5 mm of the edge to prevent bowel from incarcerating between the mesh and the anterior abdominal wall. External

Table 2
Comparison of suture versus tack fixation

Sutures		Tacks	
Pros	Cons	Pros	Cons
Lower cost compared with tacks	Possible increased pain	Shorter operating room time	Possible decreased pain
More robust fixation to anterior fascia		Fewer incisions/ improve cosmesis	Need for increased mesh overlap (≥5 cm)

manual pressure and "cupping" of the abdominal wall around the tacking device ensures a perpendicular angle between the abdominal wall and the tacker. Such an orientation may avoid skiving of the tack and facilitate secure fixation.

INNOVATIONS IN THE LAPAROSCOPIC VENTRAL HERNIA REPAIR TECHNIQUE

Transabdominal Preperitoneal Repair

Transabdominal preperitoneal hernia (TAPP) repair has long been used for laparoscopic inguinal hernia repair. The benefits of extraperitoneal mesh placement have been realized, and the same approach is now being used for VHR with both laparoscopic and robotic techniques described [66,67]. Traditional LVHR includes the placement of intraperitoneal mesh. Such mesh position can exhibit visceral adhesion formation, and rarely, fistula formation, bowel obstruction, and chronic pain. However, with preperitoneal mesh placement, the parietal peritoneum acts as a barrier between the mesh and visceral cavity and avoids the intense inflammatory reaction caused by direct contact of the mesh with the intraabdominal viscera. Other proposed benefits of preperitoneal mesh placement include homogeneous distribution of forces across the entire surface of the mesh. An experimental swine model comparison of IPOM versus TAPP polypropylene mesh placement demonstrated significantly fewer adhesions and less intraabdominal inflammatory response with a TAPP approach. Furthermore, significantly better mesh incorporation occurred with a TAPP repair as marked by more robust fibroblast proliferation and foreign body reaction [68].

Several investigators have demonstrated the feasibility and safety of TAPP approach. Prasad and colleagues [69] reported on a series of 68 patients with moderate-sized hernias (mean defect size = 31 cm^2) without major complications. The most common postoperative complications included 6% seroma, 4.4% postoperative urinary retention, 4.4% SSI, and 2.9% bowel injury. At a mean follow-up of 22.7 months, a 3% recurrence rate was noted. The same investigators also performed a prospective comparative study of IPOM versus TAPP and noted reduced cost of the TAPP approach due to no need for a barrier-coated mesh as well as decreased seroma rates and similar recurrence rate at midterm follow-up of 23 months. The investigators concluded that the TAPP approach reduces the risk of complications related to intraperitoneal mesh but acknowledge that further comparative multicentric prospective trial are warranted [70]. Further benefits of the TAPP approach noted by proponents include a supposed ability to forego mesh fixation because the preperitoneal pocket provides added fixation especially with the use of self-fixating mesh, leading to improved postoperative pain and QOL [71].

Laparoscopic Retrorectus Repair/Enhanced-View Totally Extraperitoneal Repair

Retrorectus hernia repair as popularized Rives and Stoppa more than 3 decades ago has been a popular approach for open VHR. Like the TAPP approach, it excludes the mesh from the visceral cavity with the added benefit of a myofascial release of the posterior rectus sheath, thus releasing tension from the midline closure. Adapted for laparoscopy in the early 2000s by Miserez and Penninckx as a complete extraperitoneal method with sublay polypropylene reinforcement, they demonstrated its feasibility in 15 patients without any major complications and a single early postoperative recurrence at 5.5 months [72]. Other investigators have since described adapted versions of the repair with a combined intraperitoneal and extraperitoneal approach and use of a laparoscopic stapling device to plicate the posterior rectus sheath [73]. The only comparative study of open and laparoscopic retrorectus repairs demonstrated comparable outcomes with no differences in postoperative complications or QOL between the 2 approaches [74].

Most recently, Belyansky and colleagues [75] have again popularized the method, with their totally extraperitoneal retrorectus repair using either a laparoscopic or robotic approach, termed enhanced-view totally extraperitoneal repair (eTEP). The approach focuses on access at the lateral edge of the retrorectus space with retromuscular dissection and crossing over to the contralateral space to connect the 2 areas. Dissection is initially started with a balloon dissector and then continued with a combination of blunt and sharp dissection. The hernia sac may be addressed by sharp dissection of the distal attachments and dorsal mobilization or by sharply incising the sac and performing laparoscopic adhesiolysis as needed. The investigators included the addition of a laparoscopic transversus abdominal release as needed, noting the following indications for a posterior component separation:

- Defects wider than 10 cm
- Retrorectus space narrower than 5 cm
- Poorly compliant abdominal wall
- Undo tension on the posterior rectus sheath closure

Defects were sutured closed with barber sutures. The investigators note that fixation was optional in their study with some foregoing any mesh fixation with a retrorectus mesh. A robotic method has also been described, both with excellent postoperative outcomes [75,76].

Robotic Ventral Hernia Repair

Compared with laparoscopic, robotic ventral hernia repair (RVHR) is relatively new, with the earliest reports appearing in 2003 [77]. Since that time, its adoption was initially slow, but it has gained popularity in recent years. As a result, many questions concerning outcomes, costs, and technique are now a major topic of research with early articles showing conflicting results. Armijo and colleagues [78] demonstrated worse outcomes with RVHR in regard to infectious outcomes and other minor complications compared with LVHR. Conversely, in a comparative review of more than 21,000 patients, RVHR showed superior outcomes in length of stay and SSI after adjusting for comorbidities [79]. What does hold constant throughout the literature is the increased hospital cost, charges to the patient, and operative time for RVHR [78–80]. Many proponents hypothesize that with increased market competition from anticipated competing surgical systems, the cost gap will decrease. Currently, potential benefits of robotic repair include

- Facilitate ease of hernia defect closure
- Ease of extraperitoneal placement of mesh
- Reduced mesh fixation or fixation by an internal running suture, potentially leading to decreased postoperative pain
- Improved length of stay

A theme that has been constant among surgeons adopting robotic techniques is their comfort in approaching cases in a minimally invasive fashion that they would have previously been uncomfortable performing laparoscopically.

OUTCOMES OF LAPAROSCOPIC VENTRAL HERNIA REPAIR

Recurrence

Recurrence rates after LVHR have been demonstrated to be acceptably low and comparable with open repair, ranging between 0% to 17% with mid- to long-term follow-up (Table 3). Recurrence, which is often considered the traditional mark of excellence of hernia repair, depends on a myriad of factors as previously discussed, including mesh overlap and methods of fixation, postoperative infection or other wound complications, and the possible additive effect of fascial closure [56–58,81]. Optimizing patients preoperatively has also been a focus of many studies. Smoking cessation, weight loss, reduction of steroid dosage, and optimization of chronic illnesses have been shown to improve outcomes.

Seroma

Seroma formation represents one of the most common postoperative complications after LVHR. One small prospective study demonstrated that at 7 days

Table 3
Recurrence following LVHR

Study	N	Recurrence	FDC	Mesh overlap (cm)	Follow-up (months)
Agarwal et al [105], 2009	29	0%	Yes	>4	34
Franklin et al [106], 2004	384	2.9%	No	3–5	47.1
Chelala et al [107],2016	1326	3.2%	Yes	>5	78
Muysoms et al [65], 2013	63	7.9%	—	—	24
Orenstein et al [108], 2011	47	0%	Yes	5–7	16.2
Berger et al [109], 2002	147	2.7%	No	3–5	15
Clapp et al [97], 2013	176	8.3	Yes	3–6	24
Rosen et al [110], 2003	96	17.7	No	≥3–4	30
Heniford et al [32], 2003	850	4.3	No	≥4	20

Abbreviation: FDC, fascial defect closure.

postoperatively, seromas can be identified in 100% of patients with ultrasonography. With that, only a small percentage of these were clinically relevant, and, fortunately, most resolved without intervention [82]. Thus, although well published, treatment and prevention of seromas remain circumstantial. From a prevention standpoint, the use of pressure dressings has been controversial. Other techniques, such as hernia sac excision, cauterizing the hernia sac, or decreasing the dead space, have been tried but failed to show any prudence in trials [70]. When required, aspiration is an acceptable first-line treatment, but when used repeatedly, it has been shown to increase the infection risk [83]. Persistent seromas may be treated using percutaneous drainage with or without injection with doxycycline. Further aggressive surgical options include operative drainage of the seroma cavity and argon beam ablation of the mesothelial layer.

Surgical Site Infections

Perhaps the greatest argument for LVHR is the significant decrease in SSI. Franklin and colleagues [84] documented rates for laparoscopic repair to be 1.1%, whereas open repairs had an infection rate of 10%. The theoretic explanation stems from the small incisions, less exposure to skin flora, a reduction in dissection and devitalization of tissues, and less exposed subcutaneous tissues. Several studies have looked at risk factors associated with SSI after LVHR to identify areas that can be improved to decrease future infections. In elderly patients, chronic obstructive pulmonary disease and low preoperative albumin level were seen as independent factors [85]. Smoking cessation has been a focal point of preventable risk factors, with smokers demonstrating an up to 5-fold increased risk for SSI [86]. Other notable patient-centered risk factors include hypoxia, obesity, peripheral vascular disease, and history of infection [87–89]. Surgery-related risk factors include operative time greater than 3 to 4 hours, hypothermia, lack of glycemic control, and, in trauma patients, blood transfusions [87,90,91]. Mesh implantation did not influence infection rates but obviously carries greater consequences with infection.

Enterotomies

VHRs are associated with the risk of enterotomy. In addition to the potential for resultant infectious complications, enterotomies have a significant effect on the course of the repair, namely the use of mesh (synthetic versus nonsynthetic) or even tissue repair alone. Rates of enterotomy during adhesiolysis for LVHR range from 0.5% to 6% [26,36,92] This complication can lead to a significantly increased mortality rate [23].

When injuries do occur, they can be managed in a number of ways [32]:

- Conversion to open laparotomy and completion of the hernia repair without mesh placement or with the use of nonpermanent synthetic or biologic mesh
- Laparoscopic repair of the enterotomy and completion of adhesiolysis with a planned return in 3 to 7 days for LVHR
- In select cases, when little contamination has occurred, completion of LVHR with mesh can be performed with acceptable results [93,94].

Although the use of synthetic mesh in contaminated fields has been reported in the literature with favorable outcomes, the investigators do not advocate the insertion of a permanent synthetic implant in the face of contamination. Decisions regarding optimal management of an intraoperative enterotomy should be addressed on a case by case basis [95].

Pseudorecurrence

Apart from true hernia recurrence, 1 long-term shortcoming of standard bridged IPOM repairs is the slow eventration of mesh through the hernia defect leading to pseudorecurrence. The incidence of clinical pseudorecurrence, defined as the subjective sense of a bulge without any objective evidence of recurrence or seroma formation, may occur in up to 20% of LVHRs [96–98]. With regard to the patient's interpretation of their hernia repair, this may be associated with poor cosmesis [99]. In cases with significant symptoms from pseudorecurrence after LVHR, surgeons should consider repeat repair [23].

Quality of Life

Mesh fixation during LVHR seems to be an important source of postoperative pain and therefore a significant driver of QOL for up to 6 months postoperatively [100]. One large international prospective QOL study comparing laparoscopic and open ventral hernia found increased rates of symptomatic pain and activity limitation in the acute postoperative period, noting that the laparoscopic approach was independently associated with impaired QOL within the first month of surgery [15]. Many believe that the transfascial sutures may be a significant contributor to the development of acute postoperative pain experienced by many after LVHR, leading some to advocate local injection of sutures site as an effective treatment option for acute postoperative pain [101]. Efforts to compare fixation methods and identify a method associated with improved QOL have failed to definitively identify any approach that provides decreased pain or improved QOL when comparing absorbable or permanent tacks, transfascial sutures, fibrin glue, or a combination of these [63,102]. Once past the acute recovery phase, QOL after LVHR compared with open repair is comparable [103,104].

SUMMARY

Laparoscopic, and more generally minimally invasive, VHR has been established as a viable, safe, and effective method of hernia repair. To this point, clear benefits have been established with regard to fewer infectious wound complications, which make it an appropriate option for those with risk factors for wound complications that cannot be modified preoperatively. However, risk associated with intraperitoneal mesh placement and adhesiolysis require meticulous technique and patient selection to maintain acceptable outcomes. Important efforts by surgical innovators to improve on these shortcomings optimistically hope to effect meaningful change in areas such as postoperative pain, recurrence, and mesh-related complications. Inevitably these efforts will continue to refine the process of LVHR.

References

[1] Fink C, Baumann P, Wente MN, et al. Incisional hernia rate 3 years after midline laparotomy. Br J Surg 2014;101(2):51–4.

[2] Brault MW, Hootman J, Helmick CG, et al. Prevalence and most common causes of disability among adults – United States, 2005. MMWR Morb Mortal Wkly Rep 2009;58(16):421–6. Available at: https://www.cdc.gov/mmwr/preview/mmwrhtml/mm5816a2.htm. Accessed October 16, 2018.

[3] Poulose BK, Shelton J, Phillips S, et al. Epidemiology and cost of ventral hernia repair: making the case for hernia research. Hernia 2012;16(2):179–83.

[4] Arroyo a, García P, Pérez F, et al. Randomized clinical trial comparing suture and mesh repair of umbilical hernia in adults. Br J Surg 2001;88(10):1321–3.

[5] Mathes T, Walgenbach M, Siegel R. Suture versus mesh repair in primary and incisional ventral hernias: a systematic review and meta-analysis. World J Surg 2016;40(4): 826–35.

[6] Finan KR, Kilgore ML, Hawn MT. Open suture versus mesh repair of primary incisional hernias: a cost-utility analysis. Hernia 2009;13(2):173–82.

[7] Velanovich V. Laparoscopic vs open surgery. Surg Endosc 2000;14(1):16–21.

[8] Antoniou SA, Antoniou GA, Antoniou AI, et al. Past, present, and future of minimally invasive abdominal surgery. JSLS 2015;19(3) [pii:e2015.00052].

[9] Olmi S, Scaini A, Cesana GC, et al. Laparoscopic versus open incisional hernia repair. Surg Endosc 2007;21(4):555–9.

[10] Misiakos EP, Machairas A, Patapis P, et al. Laparoscopic ventral hernia repair: pros and cons compared with open hernia repair. JSLS 2008;12(2):117–25.

[11] LeBlanc KA, Booth WV. Laparoscopic repair of incisional abdominal hernias using expanded polytetrafluoroethylene: preliminary findings. Surg Laparosc Endosc 1993;3(1):39–41.

[12] Ecker BL, Kuo LEY, Simmons KD, et al. Laparoscopic versus open ventral hernia repair: longitudinal outcomes and cost analysis using statewide claims data. Surg Endosc 2016;30(3):906–15.

[13] Colavita PD, Tsirline VB, Walters AL, et al. Laparoscopic versus open hernia repair: outcomes and sociodemographic utilization results from the nationwide inpatient sample. Surg Endosc 2013;27(1):109–17.

[14] Aher CV, Kubasiak JC, Daly SC, et al. The utilization of laparoscopy in ventral hernia repair: an update of outcomes analysis using ACS-NSQIP data. Surg Endosc 2015;29(5):1099–104.

[15] Colavita PD, Tsirline VB, Belyansky I, et al. Prospective, long-term comparison of quality of life in laparoscopic versus open ventral hernia repair. Ann Surg 2012;256(5):713–4.

[16] Heniford BT. SAGES guidelines for laparoscopic ventral hernia repair. Surg Endosc 2016;30(8):3161–2.

[17] Verhelst J, Timmermans L, Van De Velde M, et al. Watchful waiting in incisional hernia: is it safe? Surgery 2015;157(2):297–303.

[18] Kokotovic D, Sjølander H, Gögenur I, et al. Watchful waiting as a treatment strategy for patients with a ventral hernia appears to be safe. Hernia 2016;20(2):281–7.

[19] Bellows CF, Robinson C, Fitzgibbons RJ, et al. Watchful waiting for ventral hernias: a longitudinal study. Am Surg 2014;80(3):245–52. Available at: http://www.ncbi.nlm.nih.gov/pubmed/24666865. Accessed December 12, 2017.

[20] Lauscher JC, Leonhardt M, Martus P, et al. Beobachtung vs. operation oligosymptomatischer narbenhernien: aktueller stand der AWARE-studie. Chirurg 2016;87(1):47–55.

[21] Lauscher JC, Martus P, Stroux A, et al. Development of a clinical trial to determine whether watchful waiting is an acceptable alternative to surgical repair for patients with

oligosymptomatic incisional hernia: study protocol for a randomized controlled trial. Trials 2012;13(1):14.
[22] Earle D, Roth JS, Saber A, et al. SAGES guidelines for laparoscopic ventral hernia repair. Surg Endosc 2016;30(8):3163–83.
[23] Bittner R, Bingener-Casey J, Dietz U, et al. Guidelines for laparoscopic treatment of ventral and incisional abdominal wall hernias (International Endohernia Society ([IEHS]) - Part 1. Surg Endosc 2014;28(1):2–29.
[24] Pechman DM, Cao L, Fong C, et al. Laparoscopic versus open emergent ventral hernia repair: utilization and outcomes analysis using the ACSNSQIP database. Surg Endosc Other Interv Tech 2018;32(12):4999–5005.
[25] Silecchia G, Campanile FC, Sanchez L, et al. Laparoscopic ventral/incisional hernia repair: updated guidelines from the EAES and EHS endorsed Consensus Development Conference. Surg Endosc 2015;29(9):2463–84.
[26] Jenkins ED, Yom VH, Melman L, et al. Clinical predictors of operative complexity in laparoscopic ventral hernia repair: a prospective study. Surg Endosc 2010;24(8):1872–7.
[27] Ross SW, Oommen B, Walters AL, et al. Smoking and ventral hernia repair: quantifying the national burden of tobacco abuse. J Am Coll Surg 2014;219(4):e97.
[28] Sorensen LT, Karlsmark T, Gottrup F. Abstinence from smoking reduces incisional wound infection: a randomized controlled trial. Ann Surg 2003;238(1):1–5.
[29] Huntington C, Gamble J, Blair L, et al. Quantification of the effect of diabetes mellitus on ventral hernia repair: results from two national registries. Am Surg 2016;82(8): 661–71. Available at: https://www.ncbi.nlm.nih.gov/pubmed/27657579.
[30] Bittner R, Bingener-Casey J, Dietz U, et al. Guidelines for laparoscopic treatment of ventral and incisional abdominal wall hernias (International Endohernia Society [IEHS])—Part 2. Surg Endosc 2014;28(2):353–79.
[31] Arita NA, Nguyen MT, Nguyen DH, et al. Laparoscopic repair reduces incidence of surgical site infections for all ventral hernias. Surg Endosc 2015;29(7):1769–80.
[32] Heniford BT, Park A, Ramshaw BJ, et al. Laparoscopic repair of ventral hernias: nine years' experience with 850 consecutive hernias. Ann Surg 2003;238(3):391–9 [discussion: 399–400].
[33] Pierce RA, Spitler JA, Frisella MM, et al. Pooled data analysis of laparoscopic vs. open ventral hernia repair: 14 years of patient data accrual. Surg Endosc 2007;21(3):378–86.
[34] Regner JL, Mrdutt MM, Munoz-Maldonado Y. Tailoring surgical approach for elective ventral hernia repair based on obesity and National Surgical Quality Improvement Program outcomes. Am J Surg 2015;210(6):1024–30.
[35] Ching SS, Sarela AI, Dexter SPL, et al. Comparison of early outcomes for laparoscopic ventral hernia repair between nonobese and morbidly obese patient populations. Surg Endosc 2008;22(10):2244–50.
[36] Tsereteli Z, Pryor BA, Heniford BT, et al. Laparoscopic ventral hernia repair (LVHR) in morbidly obese patients. Hernia 2008;12(3):233–8.
[37] Novitsky YW, Cobb WS, Kercher KW, et al. Laparoscopic ventral hernia repair in obese patients: a new standard of care. Arch Surg 2006;141(1):57–61.
[38] Raftopoulos I, Courcoulas AP. Outcome of laparoscopic ventral hernia repair in morbidly obese patients with a body mass index exceeding 35 kg/m2. Surg Endosc 2007;21(12): 2293–7.
[39] Moreno-Egea A, Carrillo-Alcaraz A, Aguayo-Albasini JL. Is the outcome of laparoscopic incisional hernia repair affected by defect size? A prospective study. Am J Surg 2012;203(1):87–94.
[40] Vlot J, Slieker JC, Wijnen R, et al. Optimizing working-space in laparoscopy: measuring the effect of mechanical bowel preparation in a porcine model. Surg Endosc 2013;27(6):1980–5.

[41] Krpata DM, Haskins IN, Phillips S, et al. Does preoperative bowel preparation reduce surgical site infections during elective ventral hernia repair? J Am Coll Surg 2017;224(2):204–11.
[42] LeBlanc K. Proper mesh overlap is a key determinant in hernia recurrence following laparoscopic ventral and incisional hernia repair. Hernia 2016;20(1):85–99.
[43] Carbonell A. A gold standard for measuring defects during ventral hernia repair. Presented at Hernia Repair, Hollywood (FL), March 7–11, 2007.
[44] Jin J, Rosen MJ. Laparoscopic versus open ventral hernia repair. Surg Clin North Am 2008;88(5):1083–100.
[45] Costanza MJ, Heniford BT, Arca MJ, et al. Laparoscopic repair of recurrent ventral hernias. Am Surg 1998;64(12):1121–5 [discussion: 1126–7]. Available at: http://europepmc.org/abstract/MED/21355179/reload=2.
[46] Cobb WS, Kercher KW, Matthews BD, et al. Laparoscopic ventral hernia repair: a single center experience. Hernia 2006;10(3):236–42.
[47] Tandon A, Pathak S, Lyons NJ, et al. Meta-analysis of closure of the fascial defect during laparoscopic incisional and ventral hernia repair. Br J Surg 2016;103(12):1598–607.
[48] Martin-del-Campo LA, Miller HJ, Elliott HL, et al. Laparoscopic ventral hernia repair with and without defect closure: comparative analysis of a single-institution experience with 783 patients. Hernia 2018;22(6):1061–5.
[49] Papageorge CM, Funk LM, Poulose BK, et al. Primary fascial closure during laparoscopic ventral hernia repair does not reduce 30-day wound complications. Surg Endosc 2017;31(11):4551–7.
[50] Shankaran V, Weber DJ, Reed RL, et al. A review of available prosthetics for ventral hernia repair. Ann Surg 2011;253(1):16–26.
[51] Vorst AL. Evolution and advances in laparoscopic ventral and incisional hernia repair. World J Gastrointest Surg 2015;7(11):293.
[52] Kokotovic D, Bisgaard T, Helgstrand F. Long-term recurrence and complications associated with elective incisional hernia repair. JAMA 2016;316(15):1575–82.
[53] Jenkins ED, Yom V, Melman L, et al. Prospective evaluation of adhesion characteristics to intraperitoneal mesh and adhesiolysis-related complications during laparoscopic re-exploration after prior ventral hernia repair. Surg Endosc 2010;24(12):3002–7.
[54] Snyder CW, Graham LA, Gray SH, et al. Effect of mesh type and position on subsequent abdominal operations after incisional hernia repair. J Am Coll Surg 2011;212(4):496–502.
[55] Paton BL, Novitsky YW, Zerey M, et al. Management of infections of polytetrafluoroethylene-based mesh. Surg Infect (Larchmt) 2007;8(3):337–41.
[56] Warren JA, Love M. Incisional hernia repair: minimally invasive approaches. Surg Clin North Am 2018;98(3):537–59.
[57] Tulloh B, de Beaux A. Defects and donuts: the importance of the mesh:defect area ratio. Hernia 2016;20(6):893–5.
[58] Hauters P, Desmet J, Gherardi D, et al. Assessment of predictive factors for recurrence in laparoscopic ventral hernia repair using a bridging technique. Surg Endosc 2017;31(9):3656–63.
[59] LeBlanc KA. Laparoscopic incisional hernia repair: are transfascial sutures necessary? A review of the literature. Surg Endosc 2007;21(4):508–13.
[60] Heniford BT, Ramshaw BJ. Laparoscopic ventral herma repair: a report of 100 consecutive cases. Surg Endosc 2000;14(5):419–23.
[61] Sharma A, Mehrotra M, Khullar R, et al. Laparoscopic ventral/incisional hernia repair: a single centre experience of 1,242 patients over a period of 13 years. Hernia 2011;15(2):131–9.
[62] Baker JJ, Öberg S, Andresen K, et al. Adding sutures to tack fixation of mesh does not lower the re-operation rate after laparoscopic ventral hernia repair: a nationwide cohort study. Langenbecks Arch Surg 2018;403(4):521–7.

[63] Harsløf S, Krum-Møller P, Sommer T, et al. Effect of fixation devices on postoperative pain after laparoscopic ventral hernia repair: a randomized clinical trial of permanent tacks, absorbable tacks, and synthetic glue. Langenbecks Arch Surg 2018;403(4):529–37.
[64] Baker JJ, Öberg S, Andresen K, et al. Systematic review and network meta-analysis of methods of mesh fixation during laparoscopic ventral hernia repair. Br J Surg 2018;105(1):37–47.
[65] Muysoms F, Vander Mijnsbrugge G, Pletinckx P, et al. Randomized clinical trial of mesh fixation with "double crown" versus "sutures and tackers" in laparoscopic ventral hernia repair. Hernia 2013;17(5):603–12.
[66] Hilling DE, Koppert LB, Keijzer R, et al. Laparoscopic correction of umbilical hernias using a transabdominal preperitoneal approach: results of a pilot study. Surg Endosc 2009;23(8):1740–4.
[67] Sugiyama G, Chivukula S, Chung PJ, et al. Robot-assisted transabdominal preperitoneal ventral hernia repair. JSLS 2015;19(4) [pii:e2015.00092].
[68] Díaz-Pizarro Graf JI, Moreno Portillo M, Cárdenas Lailson LE, et al. Laparoscopic transabdominal preperitoneal approach to place a polypropylene mesh on the abdominal wall: an experimental swine model of a technique that can be used for incisional hernia repair. Surg Endosc 2005;19(7):990–5.
[69] Prasad P, Tantia O, Patle NM, et al. Laparoscopic transabdominal preperitoneal repair of ventral hernia: a step towards physiological repair. Indian J Surg 2011;73(6):403–8.
[70] Prasad P, Tantia O, Patle NM, et al. Laparoscopic ventral hernia repair: a comparative study of transabdominal preperitoneal versus intraperitoneal onlay mesh repair. J Laparoendosc Adv Surg Tech A 2011;21(6):477–83.
[71] Luque JAB, Luque AB, Menchero JG, et al. Safety and effectiveness of self-adhesive mesh in laparoscopic ventral hernia repair using transabdominal preperitoneal route. Surg Endosc 2017;31(3):1213–8.
[72] Miserez M, Penninckx F. Endoscopic totally preperitoneal ventral hernia repair: surgical technique and short-term results. Surg Endosc 2002;16(8):1207–13.
[73] Costa TN, Abdalla RZ, Santo MA, et al. Transabdominal midline reconstruction by minimally invasive surgery: technique and results. Hernia 2016;20(2):257–65.
[74] Schroeder AD, Debus ES, Schroeder M, et al. Laparoscopic transperitoneal sublay mesh repair: a new technique for the cure of ventral and incisional hernias. Surg Endosc 2013;27(2):648–54.
[75] Belyansky I, Daes J, Radu VG, et al. A novel approach using the enhanced-view totally extraperitoneal (eTEP) technique for laparoscopic retromuscular hernia repair. Surg Endosc 2018;32(3):1525–32.
[76] Belyansky I, Reza Zahiri H, Sanford Z, et al. Early operative outcomes of endoscopic (eTEP access) robotic-assisted retromuscular abdominal wall hernia repair. Hernia 2018;22(5): 837–47.
[77] Ballantyne GH, Hourmont K, Wasielewski A. Telerobotic laparoscopic repair of incisional ventral hernias using intraperitoneal prosthetic mesh. JSLS 2003;7(1):7–14. Available at: http://vb3lk7eb4t.search.serialssolutions.com.libproxy.lib.unc.edu/?sid=Entrez:PubMed&id=pmid:12722992. Accessed October 20, 2018.
[78] Armijo P, Pratap A, Wang Y, et al. Robotic ventral hernia repair is not superior to laparoscopic: a national database review. Surg Endosc 2018;32(4):1834–9.
[79] Altieri MS, Yang J, Xu J, et al. Outcomes after robotic ventral hernia repair: a study of 21,565 patients in the state of New York. Am Surg 2018;84(6):909–15.
[80] Coakley KM, Sims SM, Prasad T, et al. A nationwide evaluation of robotic ventral hernia surgery. Am J Surg 2017;214(6):1158–63.
[81] Liang MK, Clapp ML, Garcia A, et al. Mesh shift following laparoscopic ventral hernia repair. J Surg Res 2012;177(1):e7–13.
[82] Susmallian S, Gewurtz G, Ezri T, et al. Seroma after laparoscopic repair of hernia with PTFE patch: is it really a complication? Hernia 2001;5(3):139–41.

[83] Bittner R, Bingener-Casey J, Dietz U, et al. Guidelines for laparoscopic treatment of ventral and incisional abdominal wall hernias (International Endohernia Society [IEHS])-Part III. Surg Endosc 2014;28(2):380–404.
[84] Franklin ME, Dorman JP, Glass JL, et al. Laparoscopic ventral and incisional hernia repair. Surg Laparosc Endosc 1998;8(4):294–9. Available at: http://www.ncbi.nlm.nih.gov/-pubmed/9703605. Accessed October 25, 2018.
[85] Dunne JR, Malone DL, Tracy JK, et al. Abdominal wall hernias: risk factors for infection and resource utilization. J Surg Res 2003; https://doi.org/10.1016/S0022-4804(03)00000-0.
[86] Razavi SM, Ibrahimpoor M, Kashani AS, et al. Abdominal surgical site infections: incidence and risk factors at an Iranian teaching hospital. BMC Surg 2005; https://doi.org/10.1186/1471-2482-5-2.
[87] Kurz A, Sessler DI, Lenhardt R. Perioperative normothermia to reduce the incidence of surgical-wound infection and shorten hospitalization. N Engl J Med 1996;334(19):1209–16.
[88] Mangram AJ, Horan TC, Pearson ML, et al. Guideline for prevention of surgical site infection. AJIC 1999;27(2):97–134.
[89] Boni L, Benevento A, Rovera F, et al. Infective complications in laparoscopic surgery. Surg Infect (Larchmt) 2006;7(suppl 2); https://doi.org/10.1089/sur.2006.7.s2-109.
[90] Surgery C, Latham R, Lancaster AD, et al. The association of diabetes and glucose control with surgical-site infections among. Infect Control Hosp Epidemiol 2001;22(10):607–12.
[91] Hill GE, Frawley WH, Griffith KE, et al. Allogeneic blood transfusion increases the risk of postoperative bacterial infection: a meta-analysis. J Trauma 2003;54(5):908–14.
[92] Perrone JM, Soper NJ, Eagon JC, et al. Perioperative outcomes and complications of laparoscopic ventral hernia repair. Surgery 2005;138(4):708–16.
[93] Carbonell AM, Cobb WS. Safety of prosthetic mesh hernia repair in contaminated fields. Surg Clin North Am 2013;93(5):1227–39.
[94] Carbonell AM, Criss CN, Cobb WS, et al. Outcomes of synthetic mesh in contaminated ventral hernia repairs. J Am Coll Surg 2013;217(6):991–8.
[95] Bueno-Lledo J, Torregrosa-Gallud A, Sala-Hernandez A, et al. Predictors of mesh infection and explantation after abdominal wall hernia repair. Am J Surg 2017;213(1):50–7.
[96] Liang MK, Berger RL, Li LT, et al. Outcomes of laparoscopic vs open repair of primary ventral hernias. JAMA Surg 2013;148(11):1043–8.
[97] Clapp ML, Hicks SC, Awad SS, et al. Trans-cutaneous Closure of Central Defects (TCCD) in laparoscopic ventral hernia repairs (LVHR). World J Surg 2013;37(1):42–51.
[98] Carter SA, Hicks SC, Brahmbhatt R, et al. Recurrence and pseudorecurrence after laparoscopic ventral hernia repair: predictors and patient-focused outcomes. Am Surg 2014;80(2):138–48.
[99] Liang MK, Clapp M, Li LT, et al. Patient satisfaction, chronic pain, and functional status following laparoscopic ventral hernia repair. World J Surg 2013;37(3):530–7.
[100] Eriksen JR, Poornoroozy P, Jørgensen LN, et al. Pain, quality of life and recovery after laparoscopic ventral hernia repair. Hernia 2009;13(1):13–21.
[101] Carbonell AM, Harold KL, Mahmutovic AJ, et al. Local injection for the treatment of suture site pain after laparoscopic ventral hernia repair. Am Surg 2003;69(8):682–8. Available at: https://www.ncbi.nlm.nih.gov/pubmed/12953827.
[102] Wassenaar E, Schoenmaeckers E, Raymakers J, et al. Mesh-fixation method and pain and quality of life after laparoscopic ventral or incisional hernia repair: a randomized trial of three fixation techniques. Surg Endosc 2010;24(6):1296–302.
[103] Itani KMF, Hur K, Kim LT, et al. Comparison of laparoscopic and open repair with mesh for the treatment of ventral incisional hernia: a randomized trial. Arch Surg 2010;145(4):322–8 [discussion: 328].

[104] Hope WW, Lincourt AE, Newcomb WL, et al. Comparing quality-of-life outcomes in symptomatic patients undergoing laparoscopic or open ventral hernia repair. J Laparoendosc Adv Surg Tech A 2008;18(4):567–71.
[105] Agarwal BB, Sneh AE, Ae A, et al. Laparoscopic ventral hernia repair: innovative anatomical closure, mesh insertion without 10-mm transmyofascial port, and atraumatic mesh fixation: a preliminary experience of a new technique. Surg Endosc 2009; https://doi.org/10.1007/s00464-008-0159-7.
[106] Franklin JE, Gonzalez JJ, Glass JL, et al. Laparoscopic ventral and incisional hernia repair: an 11-year experience. Hernia 2004;8(1):23–7.
[107] Chelala E, Barake H, Estievenart J, et al. Long-term outcomes of 1326 laparoscopic incisional and ventral hernia repair with the routine suturing concept: a single institution experience. Hernia 2016;20(1):101–10.
[108] Orenstein SB, Dumeer JL, Monteagudo J, et al. Outcomes of laparoscopic ventral hernia repair with routine defect closure using "shoelacing" technique. Surg Endosc 2011;25(5):1452–7.
[109] Berger D, Bientzle M, Müller A. Postoperative complications after laparoscopic incisional hernia repair. Surg Endosc 2002;16(12):1720–3.
[110] Rosen M, Brody F, Ponsky J, et al. Recurrence after laparoscopic ventral hernia repair. Surg Endosc 2003;17(1):123–8.

Advances in Surgery 53 (2019) 21–35

ADVANCES IN SURGERY

Ductal Carcinoma In Situ of the Breast

Controversies and Current Management

Andrea V. Barrio, MD*, Kimberly J. Van Zee, MS, MD

Breast Service, Department of Surgery, Memorial Sloan Kettering Cancer Center, 300 East 66th Street, New York, NY 10065, USA

Keywords

• DCIS • Local recurrence • Margin width • Surgery • Radiation • Endocrine therapy

Key points

- Radiation therapy (RT) reduces risk of local recurrence after breast-conserving surgery (BCS) by half, but may be associated with serious side effects.
- Endocrine therapy reduces risk of local recurrence after BCS and RT by 30% in women with estrogen receptor-positive ductal carcinoma in situ (DCIS), but can be associated with side effects that reduce compliance.
- In patients receiving RT, a margin width of 2 mm reduces risk of local recurrence compared with a narrower negative margin.
- In select low-risk subsets of DCIS (ie, low-to-intermediate grade, small tumor size <2.5 cm, and age >50 years), absolute risk of local recurrence following BCS may be sufficiently low that omission of RT may be appropriate.
- Nonoperative management of highly select patients with low-risk DCIS should only be performed in a clinical trial.

INTRODUCTION

Ductal carcinoma in situ (DCIS) is a noninvasive malignancy of the breast, and comprises nearly 20% of all newly diagnosed breast cancers [1]. The standard treatment of DCIS is primarily surgical and includes mastectomy for extensive or multicentric disease, and breast-conserving surgery (BCS) for localized

Disclosure Statement: Dr A.V. Barrio has received speaking honorarium from Roche. Dr K.J. Van Zee has nothing to disclose.

*Corresponding author. *E-mail address:* barrioa@mskcc.org

https://doi.org/10.1016/j.yasu.2019.04.002

lesions. Although the risk of local recurrence (LR) following mastectomy is minimal, long-term LR rates following excision alone in the early randomized trials were 25% to 35%, with half of those recurrences being invasive [2–5].

Four prospective randomized trials begun between 1985 and 1990 have demonstrated a significant reduction in both invasive and DCIS recurrence with the addition of adjuvant radiation therapy (RT) following BCS, with no impact on survival [2–5]. Adjuvant endocrine therapy further reduces LR by approximately 30% in patients with estrogen receptor (ER)-positive DCIS, although the side-effect profile of these medications reduces uptake and compliance [2,4,6–8].

Among select women with low-risk DCIS treated with BCS alone, more recent prospective trials have demonstrated lower rates of LR than seen in the original randomized trials [9–11]. These observed lower rates of LR, coupled with the excellent survival after surgical treatment of DCIS [12], have raised concerns regarding potential overtreatment of patients, particularly with respect to the appropriate use of adjuvant RT and endocrine therapy, and their associated morbidity.

This controversy has led to interest in identifying a subset of "low-risk" patients who could be managed without any surgical excision. Although there is no evidence that omission of surgery is safe in patients with DCIS, trials of observation in very select patients with DCIS are ongoing in the United States and Europe [13–15], leaving many to incorrectly extrapolate that observation is appropriate in certain DCIS subsets outside of a clinical trial.

SIGNIFICANCE

Standard treatment of ductal carcinoma in situ

As a noninvasive cancer, treatment of DCIS is focused on complete surgical removal of disease in the breast with the goal of preventing LR, particularly invasive recurrence. To that end, appropriate treatment options include mastectomy alone or BCS with or without adjuvant RT and/or endocrine therapy. Each of these options results in a low mortality rate, although LR rates vary across treatments [2–5,12,16].

Mastectomy

Mastectomy was once the gold standard for all patients with any type of breast cancer, including DCIS, regardless of disease extent. Following publication of the randomized trials demonstrating equivalent survival between mastectomy and BCS in women with invasive disease [17–22], clinicians surmised that BCS would similarly be acceptable in women with localized DCIS. Currently, mastectomy is considered necessary only for women with more extensive or multicentric DCIS. A meta-analysis of 8 studies that reported outcomes for women with DCIS treated with mastectomy found a 2.6% (95% CI, 0.8%–4.5%) 10-year LR rate [23].

Breast-conserving surgery with or without adjuvant radiation therapy

Even in the absence of randomized data comparing recurrence and overall survival between mastectomy and BCS in women with DCIS, BCS became the preferred approach for patients with localized DCIS, based on inferences from the randomized trials in invasive cancer that showed equivalent long-term survival [17–22].

Data from 4 prospective randomized trials comparing adjuvant RT to no RT following BCS demonstrated an approximately 50% LR reduction with the addition of RT (Table 1) [2–5]. An individual patient-level meta-analysis of the 4 randomized trials performed by the Early Breast Cancer Trialists' Collaborative Group (EBCTCG), which included 3729 women with DCIS, demonstrated an absolute 15.2% 10-year reduction in LR risk with RT use (28.1% without RT, 12.9% with RT, $P<.00001$) [16]. The benefit of RT was observed in all patient subsets regardless of patient age, margin status, focality, grade, or tumor size [16]. Importantly, in the meta-analysis and the individual randomized trials [2–5], RT use also reduced the invasive recurrence risk by approximately half (for example, 15-year invasive LR rates from National Surgical Adjuvant Breast and Bowel Project [NSABP] B-17: 19.4% without RT, 8.9% with RT) [2–5,16].

Despite the LR reduction observed with RT, there was no effect on 10-year breast cancer mortality (3.7% without RT, 4.1% with RT, $P=$ NS) or all-cause mortality (8.2% without RT, 8.4% with RT, $P=$ NS) (Table 2) [16]. Notably, RT is associated with a higher cardiovascular disease rate and rare malignancies such as radiation-associated angiosarcoma [24,25]. Without a benefit in survival observed with RT among patients with DCIS, adjuvant RT use

Table 1
Ipsilateral local recurrence from the randomized trials comparing adjuvant radiotherapy to no radiotherapy following breast-conserving surgery for ductal carcinoma in situ

				Local recurrence		
Study	Study dates	N	Follow-up (y)	No RT (%)	RT (%)	Relative risk reduction (%)
NSABP B-17 [4]	1985–1990	813	15	35	18	50
EORTC 10853 [3]	1986–1996	1010	15	31	18	48
SweDCIS [5]	1987–1999	1046	20	32	20	37.5
UK/ANZ DCIS [2]	1990–1998	475	12.7 median	25	9	69
EBCTCG meta-analysis [16]	1985–1999	3729	10	28.1	12.9	54

Note: The NSABP and EORTC data are 15-year local recurrence rates, the SweDCIS data are 20-year local recurrence rates, and the UK/ANZ data are crude rates for those not receiving tamoxifen, and randomized to no radiotherapy versus radiotherapy. EBCTCG data are 10-year rates from a patient-level meta-analysis of the 4 randomized trials listed above it in the table.

Abbreviations: DCIS, ductal carcinoma in situ; f/u, follow-up; EBCTCG, Early Breast Cancer Trialists' Collaborative Group; EORTC, European Organisation for Research and Treatment of Cancer; NSABP, National Adjuvant Breast and Bowel Project; RT, radiation therapy; SweDCIS, Sweden Ductal Carcinoma In Situ; UK/ANZ; United Kingdom/Australia/New Zealand.

Data from Refs [2–5].

Table 2
Breast cancer mortality from the randomized trials comparing adjuvant radiotherapy to no radiotherapy following breast-conserving surgery for ductal carcinoma in situ

				Breast cancer mortality		Overall mortality	
Study	Study dates	N	Follow-up (y)	No RT (%)	RT (%)	No RT (%)	RT (%)
NSABP B-17 [4]	1985–1990	813	15	3.1	4.7	15.7	17.1
EORTC 10853 [3]	1986–1996	1010	15	5	4	10	12
SweDCIS [5]	1987–1999	1046	20	4.2	4.1	27.0	22.8
UK/ANZ DCIS [2],[a]	1990–1998	811[a]	12.7 median	2.0	1.5	9.6	9.7
EBCTCG meta-analysis [16]	1985–1999	3729	10	3.7	4.1	8.2	8.4

Note: The NSABP and EORTC data are 15-year rates, the SweDCIS data are 20-year rates, and the UK/ANZ data are crude rates for those not receiving tamoxifen. EBCTCG data are 10-year rates from a patient-level meta-analysis of the 4 randomized trials listed above it in the table.

Abbreviations: DCIS, ductal carcinoma in situ; EBCTCG, Early Breast Cancer Trialists' Collaborative Group; EORTC, European Organisation for Research and Treatment of Cancer; NSABP, National Adjuvant Breast and Bowel Project; RT, radiation therapy; SweDCIS, Sweden Ductal Carcinoma In Situ; UK/ANZ; United Kingdom/Australia/New Zealand.

[a]Patients not receiving tamoxifen.

Data from Early Breast Cancer Trialists' Collaborative G, Correa C, McGale P, et al. Overview of the randomized trials of radiotherapy in ductal carcinoma in situ of the breast. J Natl Cancer Inst Monogr 2010;2010(41):162–177.

should be selective, and reserved for those patients at higher risk for LR and thus likely to derive greater benefit from its use.

Adjuvant endocrine therapy following breast-conserving surgery

The use of tamoxifen following BCS in women with DCIS has been demonstrated in 2 large randomized trials to reduce LR with a relative risk reduction of approximately 25% (Table 3). Notably, in the UK/ANZ (United Kingdom/Australia/New Zealand) DCIS trial, the observed reduction in ipsilateral breast events with tamoxifen was limited to those patients *not* receiving RT (hazard ratio [HR] = 0.77), whereas in NSABP B-24, all women received RT, and they experienced a similar reduction in risk (HR = 0.68 for invasive LR; 0.84 for DCIS LR). In both trials, the addition of tamoxifen was also associated with a reduction in contralateral breast cancer (32% in NSABP B-24, 54% in UK/ANZ). As expected, the use of adjuvant tamoxifen was not associated with a reduction in breast cancer or overall mortality in either trial (Table 4) [2,4].

The hormone receptor status of patients enrolled in NSABP B-24 and the UK/ANZ trial was unknown, but retrospective analysis of 732 cases from B-24 confirmed that the benefit of tamoxifen was limited to ER-positive DCIS. In these patients, tamoxifen was associated with a 42% reduction in any breast event ($P = .0015$) and a 32% reduction in any ipsilateral breast cancer ($P = .07$) (see Table 3) [6].

Table 3
Review of the randomized trials comparing ipsilateral local recurrence after breast-conserving surgery with or without adjuvant tamoxifen

				Ipsilateral Local Recurrence		Risk Reduction	
Study	Study Dates	N	Follow-up (y)	No Tam (%)	Tam (%)	HR	*P* value
UK/ANZ DCIS [2],[a]	1990–1998	1576	10	19.6	15.7	0.78	.04
No RT[b]		1053	12.7 median	26.4	20.9	0.77	.04
RT[b]		523	12.7 median	8.8	7.4	0.93	.8
NSABP B-24 [4],[c]	1991–1994	1799	15	18.3	16.0	NR	NR
NSABP B-24 ER+ cases [6],[c]	1991–1994	732	14.5 median	17	14	0.68	.07

Abbreviations: f/u; follow-up; Tam, tamoxifen; HR, hazard ratio; RT, radiation therapy; UK/ANZ; United Kingdom/Australia/New Zealand; NSABP, National Adjuvant Breast and Bowel Project; NR, not reported.

[a]UK/ANZ patients randomized to tamoxifen or placebo include 1053 not receiving RT and 523 receiving RT. Reported percentages are 10-year estimates.

[b]Percentages reflect crude number of events/total number of patients randomized to tamoxifen or no tamoxifen, by receipt of RT, at a median follow-up of 12.7 years.

[c]In NSABP B-24, all patients received RT.

Data from Allred DC, Anderson SJ, Paik S, et al. Adjuvant tamoxifen reduces subsequent breast cancer in women with estrogen receptor-positive ductal carcinoma in situ: a study based on NSABP protocol B-24. J Clin Oncol 2012;30(12):1268–1273.

Anastrozole was compared with tamoxifen in postmenopausal women with hormone receptor-positive DCIS treated with BCS in NSABP B-35 and the International Breast Cancer Intervention Studies (IBIS)-II trials [7,8]. All 3104 women in B-35 and 71% of the 2980 women in IBIS-II received RT. In B-35, the 10-year breast cancer event rate was lower among women randomized to anastrozole compared with tamoxifen (6.9% [anastrozole] vs 10.9% [tamoxifen], HR = 0.73, $P = .02$) [8]. In IBIS-II, at a median follow-up of 7.2 years, anastrozole was demonstrated to be noninferior to tamoxifen with a similar breast cancer event rate in either group (5%) [7].

Notably, although adjuvant endocrine therapy does reduce the incidence of LR in women with DCIS treated with local excision, many patients experience side effects including a higher incidence of thromboembolic events and endometrial cancer with tamoxifen, and arthralgias, osteoporosis, and vaginal dryness with aromatase inhibitors [26]. The lack of survival benefit observed with endocrine therapy in patients with DCIS, combined with their side-effect profile, limits uptake of endocrine therapy, which is reported in only 20% to 48% of DCIS patients [27–29].

Factors associated with local recurrence

Although the randomized trials demonstrated that the risk of LR with excision alone for DCIS was substantial [16], more recent evidence suggests that risk of recurrence is influenced by several clinical and pathologic factors that may be used to estimate risk and make treatment decisions regarding adjuvant therapy.

Table 4
Randomized trials comparing breast cancer and overall mortality after breast-conserving surgery with or without adjuvant tamoxifen

				Breast cancer mortality		Overall mortality	
Study	Receipt of Radiation	N	Follow-up (y)	No Tamoxifen (%) n/N	Tamoxifen (%) n/N	No Tamoxifen (%) n/N	Tamoxifen (%) n/N
UK/ANZ DCIS [2]	No RT	1111	12.7 median	2.0 (11/544)	3.4 (19/567)	9.6 (52/544)	10 (58/567)
UK/ANZ DCIS [2]	RT	583	12.7 median	1.5 (4/267)	1.6 (5/316)	9.7 (26/267)	14 (43/316)
NSABP B-24 [4]	RT	1799	15	2.7[a]	2.3[a]	17.1[b]	14.3[b]

Note: UK/ANZ rates are crude rates. B-24 are 15-year rates.

Abbreviations: NSABP, National Adjuvant Breast and Bowel Project; RT, radiation therapy; UK/ANZ; United Kingdom/Australia/New Zealand.

[a]HR tamoxifen versus no tamoxifen for breast cancer mortality: 0.81 (95% CI, 0.43–1.50).

[b]HR tamoxifen versus no tamoxifen for overall mortality: 0.86 (95% CI, 0.66–1.11).

Data from Cuzick J, Sestak I, Pinder SE, et al. Effect of tamoxifen and radiotherapy in women with locally excised ductal carcinoma in situ: long-term results from the UK/ANZ DCIS trial. Lancet Oncol 2011;12(1):21–29; and Wapnir IL, Dignam JJ, Fisher B, et al. Long-term outcomes of invasive ipsilateral breast tumor recurrences after lumpectomy in NSABP B-17 and B-24 randomized clinical trials for DCIS. J Natl Cancer Inst 2011;103(6):478–488.

Age

Both retrospective [30,31] and randomized trials [2–5] have demonstrated young age to be associated with a higher LR risk among patients with DCIS treated with BCS. Cronin and colleagues [32] examined the relationship between age and LR among nearly 3000 women with DCIS treated with BCS at Memorial Sloan Kettering Cancer Center (MSK); 53% of women received RT. The 10-year rates of any LR were lower among women age ≥80 years (7.5%) compared with women age <40 (27.3%, *P*<.0001), and the effect of age persisted on multivariable analysis, even after adjusting for 8 clinicopathologic and treatment variables. Importantly, women age <40 years were at a significant risk of invasive recurrence, with a 10-year rate of 15.8% compared with 6.5% for those age ≥40. Although young women age <40 years with localized disease are still considered appropriate candidates for BCS, the higher LR risk should be discussed with young patients when considering appropriate surgical and adjuvant treatment options. Alternatively, the lower recurrence risk seen in older women suggests that many of them may be adequately treated with excision alone and may garner only a small absolute benefit to adjuvant therapy.

Volume of ductal carcinoma in situ

The EBCTCG meta-analysis failed to demonstrate a difference in 10-year LR rates between patients with small DCIS tumors (13.1%, 13.1–20 mm) versus larger tumors (13.0%, 20–50 mm) treated with BCS + RT [16]. However, more recent prospective trials [10] of DCIS have demonstrated increasing tumor size to be associated with a higher LR risk following BCS in the absence of adjuvant RT. In the Eastern Cooperative Oncology Group-Radiation Therapy Oncology Group (ECOG-ACRIN) E5194 study, a prospective study of 665 patients with low-risk DCIS treated with excision alone, increasing tumor size was significantly associated with a higher LR risk (5 mm reference group, HR = 1.42 [6–10 mm], HR = 2.11 [>10 mm], $P = .03$) [10]. This lower rate of LR observed among patients with small-volume DCIS raises the question of whether excision alone may be sufficient in these patients. Muhsen and colleagues [33] examined LR risk among 290 patients with minimal volume DCIS, defined as DCIS diagnosed on the core biopsy with no residual disease identified at excision, using the contralateral breast as a control. Overall, 28% of patients received RT and, in this group, the 10-year LR risk was 6.5%, lower than the contralateral breast cancer risk. Contrastingly, among those who did not receive RT, the 10-year LR rate was 14.7% and higher than the contralateral breast cancer risk, highlighting that even patients with small-volume disease are not at negligible risk of local failure when treated with excision alone. Patients with small-volume disease should be considered for adjuvant therapy if other clinical and pathologic factors suggest high-risk disease.

Treatment period

LR rates in women with invasive breast cancer have declined over time, largely because of systemic therapy improvements [34–36]. Similar trends have been noted among women with DCIS treated with BCS, although the reason for this is multifactorial, as most women with DCIS do not receive systemic therapy. Subhedar and colleagues [37] examined temporal trends in recurrence rates among 2996 women treated with BCS at MSK over 3 decades. Between 1978 and 2010, a significant decrease in recurrence rates over time was observed ($P = .001$). Ten-year rates of recurrence significantly decreased from 20% in women treated from 1978 to 1998 to 14% in women treated from 1999 to 2010 ($P < .0001$). Even after controlling for multiple clinicopathologic variables, treatment period remained significant, with a lower recurrence risk in patients treated in the later time period (HR = 0.74, $P = .02$). The association of recurrence with treatment period was limited to those treated without RT (HR = 0.62, $P = .003$), suggesting factors other than improvements in radiation technique, including improved radiologic detection and pathologic assessments, may explain the decline [37].

Margin width

The randomized trials of RT demonstrated that positive margins are associated with a higher rate of LR in women with DCIS treated with BCS [2–5]. In NSABP B-24, a randomized trial of tamoxifen versus placebo in women with DCIS treated with BCS and RT, 25% of the 1799 women enrolled had positive margins and had a more than 2-fold increase in invasive recurrence compared with women with negative margins (HR = 2.61; 95% CI, 1.68–4.05; $P < .001$). In 3 of the 4 randomized trials, a negative margin was defined as no tumor on ink, and, therefore, these studies could not be used to determine the ideal negative margin width to minimize the risk of LR [2–5].

In 2016 the Society of Surgical Oncology, American Society for Radiation Oncology, and the American Society of Clinical Oncology published a consensus statement [38] on margins for women with DCIS treated with BCS and RT based on a study-level meta-analysis of nearly 8000 women for whom margin status was available [39]. A margin width of at least 2 mm was associated with a lower risk of LR compared with a narrower negative margin width (odds ratio [OR] = 0.51; 95% CI, 0.31–0.85, frequentist analysis). In addition, a more widely negative margin (>2 mm) did not further reduce the risk of LR (relative OR = 0.99; 95% CI, 0.61–1.64) [39]. Although a margin width of at least 2 mm is considered optimal, selective re-excision of a narrower margin (<2 mm) may be appropriate in certain cases in which the residual volume of disease in the breast is perceived to be minimal. In addition, if the original disease was associated with calcifications, a postexcision mammogram may be useful to identify the presence of residual calcifications, which would prompt a return trip to the operating room.

Women who underwent BCS without RT were not included in the meta-analysis due to the limited number of studies available. However, Van Zee and colleagues [40] examined 1374 women who were treated with BCS without RT and found that increasing negative margin width was associated with a lower risk of recurrence ($P<.0001$). Among those with a negative margin width of over 10 mm, or who underwent a re-excision with no residual DCIS found, 10-year LR rates were 16% compared with 41% with positive margins, and 27% with close (≤2 mm) margins. After adjusting for several clinicopathologic factors, there was a 69% relative reduction in risk associated with a > 10 mm negative margin width compared with positive margins.

Low-risk subsets of ductal carcinoma in situ: can radiation therapy be avoided?

In addition to evidence from MSK demonstrating a significant decline in LR over time in patients with DCIS treated with BCS [37], more recent prospective studies have similarly demonstrated a lower risk of LR in select modern cohorts of patients treated with BCS without RT compared with the initial randomized trials. These findings have garnered great interest in identifying a low-risk subset of patients in whom RT could be avoided following BCS.

A prospective study by Wong and colleagues [11], the ECOG-ACRIN E5194 study [10], and the Radiation Therapy Oncology Group (RTOG) 9804 study [9] all accrued patients with primarily small (≤2.5 cm), low–intermediate grade DCIS treated with BCS with a minimum of 3 mm margins. Notably, ECOG-ACRIN E5194 also enrolled patients with small-volume (≤1 cm), high-grade DCIS [10], and RTOG 9804 randomized patients to RT versus no RT [9]. Tamoxifen was prohibited in the Wong study, and used by 31% and 62% in the ECOG and RTOG studies, respectively. Overall, at a follow-up of 7 to 12 years, rates of LR among patients with low–intermediate grade DCIS treated with BCS alone ranged from 7% to 16% (Table 5),

Table 5
Outcomes of the modern prospective trials in patients with low-intermediate grade ductal carcinoma in situ treated with breast-conserving surgery alone

Study	Study dates	N	% Women using tamoxifen	Follow-up (y)	Local recurrence (No RT) (%)
Wong et al [11]	1995–2002	143	0	10	15.6
ECOG-ACRIN E5194 cohort 1 [10],[a]	1997–2002	561	31	12	14.4
RTOG 9804 (no-radiation group) [9],[b]	1998–2006	298	62	7	6.7

Abbreviations: BCS, breast-conserving surgery; DCIS, ductal carcinoma in situ; ECOG-ACRIN, Eastern Cooperative Oncology Group-American College of Radiology Imaging Network; RT, radiation therapy; RTOG, Radiation Therapy Oncology Group.

[a]Twelve-year local recurrence rate in the high-grade DCIS cohort was 24.6%.

[b]Seven-year local recurrence rate in the RT group was 0.6%.

Data from Early Breast Cancer Trialists' Collaborative G, Correa C, McGale P, et al. Overview of the randomized trials of radiotherapy in ductal carcinoma in situ of the breast. J Natl Cancer Inst Monogr 2010;2010(41):162–177.

much lower than the 28% 10-year rate of LR reported in the randomized trials for patients treated with BCS alone [16].

Although there is no debate that RT lowers LR risk in all patients with DCIS, the absolute risk of LR in select subsets of patients with non-high-grade DCIS may be sufficiently low that the benefit of RT is outweighed by the potential risks. Understanding LR risk for each individual patient is essential when making decisions regarding the need for adjuvant RT.

Predicting the risk of local recurrence: nomograms and genomic signatures

The prospective trials, along with large retrospective series, have shed light on the risk of LR following BCS for DCIS, which can vary significantly based on a variety of clinical and pathologic factors. Estimation of risk based on the original randomized trials of RT would likely result in overestimation of risk for many, and potential overtreatment. Individualizing risk allows clinicians to counsel patients about risks of recurrence after BCS alone and the additional benefit of adjuvant therapy to tailor therapy.

Rudloff and colleagues [41] developed a DCIS nomogram to better estimate risk of LR following BCS. The nomogram was developed from a cohort of 1681 patients with DCIS treated with BCS from 1991 to 2006, and uses 10 clinical, pathologic, and treatment variables to estimate the risk of LR and invasive recurrence at 5 and 10 years after BCS. Variables in the model include patient age, family history, year of surgery, clinical versus radiologic presentation, nuclear grade, necrosis, margins, and number of re-excisions (as a surrogate for tumor size). Once a patient's individual data are entered, the effect of adjuvant therapy, including RT and endocrine therapy, can be added into the model to estimate benefit with each of these therapies. The model has been internally validated and demonstrates good discrimination (C-index 0.704; bootstrap corrected 0.688); external validation with independent populations has demonstrated similar results (C-index 0.63–0.92) [42–46].

Another method to estimate risk is with molecular profiling of the tumor. The Oncotype DX (Genomic Health, Redwood City, CA) DCIS score is a 12-gene assay that was developed to estimate LR risk in patients with DCIS treated with BCS. The DCIS score was validated using a subset of 327 patients from the ECOG-ACRIN E5194 study in whom tissue was available. In this cohort, the DCIS score was significantly associated with developing any LR (HR = 2.31, $P = .02$) as well as an invasive LR (HR = 3.68, $P = .01$) [47]. However, a "high" score was not associated with a higher LR risk than an intermediate score; in patients with low, intermediate, or high recurrence scores, the 10-year risk of LR was 10.6%, 26.7%, and 25.9%, respectively ($P \leq .0006$). Furthermore, the association with LR risk seemed to be predominantly limited to premenopausal women and those with DCIS size greater than 10 mm.

The Oncotype DCIS score was also assessed in 571 patients from Ontario with DCIS treated with BCS alone [48]. On multivariable analysis, a 50-point increase in the DCIS score was significantly associated with LR (HR = 1.68, $P = .02$). However, multifocality (HR = 1.97, $P = .003$), tumor size greater than 10 mm (HR = 2.07, $P = .01$), age less than 50 years (HR = 1.75, $P = .03$), and DCIS architecture (HR = 2.75, $P = .04$) each had a larger effect on LR risk than the DCIS score, suggesting that, in a heterogeneous DCIS population treated with BCS, clinicopathologic factors are needed to accurately estimate risk of LR.

PRESENT RELEVANCE

Concern for overtreatment

In 2015 Narod and colleagues [12] published a retrospective study using Surveillance, Epidemiology, and End Results data evaluating outcomes among 108,196 women treated for DCIS. The 20-year breast cancer mortality was 3.3%, irrespective of type of surgical treatment or the use of adjuvant therapy. Even though all women in this study received treatment of their DCIS that was appropriate for their clinical situation, many interpreted this study as evidence that DCIS is essentially a "non-lethal" disease that does not require treatment.

Natural progression

Although DCIS may be a nonobligate precursor to invasive carcinoma with a poorly understood natural history, clear evidence supports DCIS to be a precursor to invasive carcinoma versus a marker of increased risk. Studies of "benign" excisional biopsies that were re-reviewed decades later and found to contain DCIS demonstrated development of invasive carcinoma in the same breast as the initial DCIS lesion in 39% to 53% of patients [49–51]. In addition, evidence for progression to invasive carcinoma also comes from prospective studies evaluating LR type after BCS for DCIS. In all of the randomized trials of RT [2–5,9,16], 50% of recurrences were invasive, suggesting that DCIS has the potential to invade. In addition, if DCIS were simply a high-risk lesion, the risk of LR would be unaffected by margin status following BCS, and the incidence of ipsilateral and contralateral cancers would be similar in patients with DCIS. Instead, the risk of LR is doubled in patients with positive versus negative margins [39,40], and ipsilateral invasive recurrences are fourfold higher than contralateral breast cancer incidence in patients with DCIS [16], confirming that DCIS is a true precursor lesion.

Studies of observation

Because of concerns regarding overdiagnosis and overtreatment of DCIS, coupled with the belief that some DCIS may not progress to invasive carcinoma in a woman's lifetime, there has been renewed interest in studying active surveillance in patients with low-risk DCIS as an alternative to surgery. Currently, there are 3 ongoing studies comparing surgery versus observation in women with low-risk DCIS: the surgery versus active monitoring for low-risk DCIS (LORIS) trial [14], the low-risk DCIS (LORD) trial [13], and the Comparison of Operative to Monitoring and Endocrine Therapy (COMET) trial (Table 6) [15].

A major concern regarding the trials of observation is whether these patients are in fact truly low risk for the development of invasive carcinoma. Pilewskie and colleagues [52] reviewed patients with DCIS diagnosed by core needle

Table 6
Eligibility criteria and primary endpoints for the LORIS, LORD, and COMET trials of surgery versus observation in low-risk ductal carcinoma in situ

	LORIS [14]	LORD [13]	COMET [15]
Age, y	≥46	≥45	≥40
Presentation	Screen-detected calcifications	Screen-detected calcifications	Screen-detected calcifications
DCIS grade	Non-high grade	Pure low grade	Non-high grade
Comedo necrosis	No	No	No
Hormone receptors	—	—	ER and/or PR ≥10%
Endocrine therapy	Allowed	Not allowed	Allowed
Primary endpoint	5-y ipsilateral invasive breast cancer-free survival	10-y ipsilateral invasive breast cancer-free survival	2-y ipsilateral invasive breast cancer-free survival

Abbreviations: COMET, Comparison of Operative to Monitoring and Endocrine Therapy; DCIS, ductal carcinoma in situ; ER, estrogen receptor; LORD, low-risk DCIS; LORIS, surgery versus active monitoring for low-risk DCIS; PR, progesterone receptor.

Data from Youngwirth LM, Boughey JC, Hwang ES. Surgery versus monitoring and endocrine therapy for low-risk DCIS: The COMET Trial. Bulletin of the American College of Surgeons 2017;102(1):62–63.

biopsy and subsequently treated at MSK between 2009 and 2012; they identified 296 patients who met LORIS criteria, which represented only 16% of the entire DCIS cohort. At surgical excision, 20% of the LORIS-eligible patients had invasive carcinoma that was not seen on core needle biopsy, suggesting that even low-risk patients with DCIS have a substantial upgrade rate to invasive carcinoma [52]. Furthermore, among women who remained LORIS eligible with pure DCIS even after excision, the 10-year rate of any LR after BCS alone was 12%, with a 6% risk of invasive recurrence [53]. Collectively, these findings reinforce that, outside of a clinical trial, surgical excision is warranted for all patients with biopsy-proven DCIS.

SUMMARY

The treatment of DCIS has evolved significantly over time, from mastectomy to BCS with RT, and now to consideration for BCS alone in select low-risk subsets of DCIS. Complete excision of disease is critical to minimize LR risk and, more importantly, invasive recurrence. With the understanding that LR risk after BCS is variable and influenced by several clinical and pathologic factors, treatment decisions are tailored to the individual patient based on risk estimation. RT reduces LR risk by half in all patients with DCIS following BCS, although the absolute benefit of this adjuvant therapy varies in each patient based on the individual risk. Because RT has no impact on breast cancer mortality, the risks and benefits of RT should be carefully weighed in each patient, particularly given its potentially serious associated side effects. Adjuvant endocrine therapy similarly reduces the risk of LR as well as the incidence of new contralateral cancers; however, the side-effect profile often limits compliance.

When counseling patients with DCIS, it is important to understand the wishes and priorities of the patient. A thorough discussion regarding the advantages and disadvantages of each treatment, as well as the impact of adjuvant therapies on recurrence risk, can help inform decision making so that patients can choose treatments that are best for them.

References

[1] Siegel RL, Miller KD, Jemal A. Cancer statistics, 2018. CA Cancer J Clin 2018;68(1):7–30.

[2] Cuzick J, Sestak I, Pinder SE, et al. Effect of tamoxifen and radiotherapy in women with locally excised ductal carcinoma in situ: long-term results from the UK/ANZ DCIS trial. Lancet Oncol 2011;12(1):21–9.

[3] Donker M, Litiere S, Werutsky G, et al. Breast-conserving treatment with or without radiotherapy in ductal carcinoma in situ: 15-year recurrence rates and outcome after a recurrence, from the EORTC 10853 randomized phase III trial. J Clin Oncol 2013;31(32): 4054–9.

[4] Wapnir IL, Dignam JJ, Fisher B, et al. Long-term outcomes of invasive ipsilateral breast tumor recurrences after lumpectomy in NSABP B-17 and B-24 randomized clinical trials for DCIS. J Natl Cancer Inst 2011;103(6):478–88.

[5] Warnberg F, Garmo H, Emdin S, et al. Effect of radiotherapy after breast-conserving surgery for ductal carcinoma in situ: 20 years follow-up in the randomized SweDCIS Trial. J Clin Oncol 2014;32(32):3613–8.

[6] Allred DC, Anderson SJ, Paik S, et al. Adjuvant tamoxifen reduces subsequent breast cancer in women with estrogen receptor-positive ductal carcinoma in situ: a study based on NSABP protocol B-24. J Clin Oncol 2012;30(12):1268–73.
[7] Forbes JF, Sestak I, Howell A, et al. Anastrozole versus tamoxifen for the prevention of locoregional and contralateral breast cancer in postmenopausal women with locally excised ductal carcinoma in situ (IBIS-II DCIS): a double-blind, randomised controlled trial. Lancet 2016;387(10021):866–73.
[8] Margolese RG, Cecchini RS, Julian TB, et al. Anastrozole versus tamoxifen in postmenopausal women with ductal carcinoma in situ undergoing lumpectomy plus radiotherapy (NSABP B-35): a randomised, double-blind, phase 3 clinical trial. Lancet 2016;387(10021):849–56.
[9] McCormick B, Winter K, Hudis C, et al. RTOG 9804: a prospective randomized trial for good-risk ductal carcinoma in situ comparing radiotherapy with observation. J Clin Oncol 2015;33(7):709–15.
[10] Solin LJ, Gray R, Hughes LL, et al. Surgical excision without radiation for ductal carcinoma in situ of the breast: 12-year results from the ECOG-ACRIN E5194 study. J Clin Oncol 2015;33(33):3938–44.
[11] Wong JS, Chen YH, Gadd MA, et al. Eight-year update of a prospective study of wide excision alone for small low- or intermediate-grade ductal carcinoma in situ (DCIS). Breast Cancer Res Treat 2014;143(2):343–50.
[12] Narod SA, Iqbal J, Giannakeas V, et al. Breast cancer mortality after a diagnosis of ductal carcinoma in situ. JAMA Oncol 2015;1(7):888–96.
[13] Elshof LE, Tryfonidis K, Slaets L, et al. Feasibility of a prospective, randomised, open-label, international multicentre, phase III, non-inferiority trial to assess the safety of active surveillance for low risk ductal carcinoma in situ - the LORD study. Eur J Cancer 2015;51(12): 1497–510.
[14] Francis A, Thomas J, Fallowfield L, et al. Addressing overtreatment of screen detected DCIS; the LORIS trial. Eur J Cancer 2015;51(16):2296–303.
[15] Youngwirth LM, Boughey JC, Hwang ES. Surgery versus monitoring and endocrine therapy for low-risk DCIS: the COMET trial. Bull Am Coll Surg 2017;102(1):62–3.
[16] Early Breast Cancer Trialists' Collaborative Group, Correa C, McGale P, Taylor C, et al. Overview of the randomized trials of radiotherapy in ductal carcinoma in situ of the breast. J Natl Cancer Inst Monogr 2010;2010(41):162–77.
[17] Arriagada R, Le MG, Rochard F, et al. Conservative treatment versus mastectomy in early breast cancer: patterns of failure with 15 years of follow-up data. Institut Gustave-Roussy Breast Cancer Group. J Clin Oncol 1996;14(5):1558–64.
[18] Blichert-Toft M, Rose C, Andersen JA, et al. Danish randomized trial comparing breast conservation therapy with mastectomy: six years of life-table analysis. Danish Breast Cancer Cooperative Group. J Natl Cancer Inst Monogr 1992;(11):19–25.
[19] Fisher B, Anderson S, Bryant J, et al. Twenty-year follow-up of a randomized trial comparing total mastectomy, lumpectomy, and lumpectomy plus irradiation for the treatment of invasive breast cancer. N Engl J Med 2002;347(16):1233–41.
[20] Poggi MM, Danforth DN, Sciuto LC, et al. Eighteen-year results in the treatment of early breast carcinoma with mastectomy versus breast conservation therapy: the National Cancer Institute Randomized Trial. Cancer 2003;98(4):697–702.
[21] van Dongen JA, Voogd AC, Fentiman IS, et al. Long-term results of a randomized trial comparing breast-conserving therapy with mastectomy: European Organization for Research and Treatment of Cancer 10801 trial. J Natl Cancer Inst 2000;92(14):1143–50.
[22] Veronesi U, Cascinelli N, Mariani L, et al. Twenty-year follow-up of a randomized study comparing breast-conserving surgery with radical mastectomy for early breast cancer. N Engl J Med 2002;347(16):1227–32.

[23] Stuart KE, Houssami N, Taylor R, et al. Long-term outcomes of ductal carcinoma in situ of the breast: a systematic review, meta-analysis and meta-regression analysis. BMC Cancer 2015;15:890.
[24] Grantzau T, Mellemkjaer L, Overgaard J. Second primary cancers after adjuvant radiotherapy in early breast cancer patients: a national population based study under the Danish Breast Cancer Cooperative Group (DBCG). Radiother Oncol 2013;106(1):42–9.
[25] Henson KE, McGale P, Taylor C, et al. Radiation-related mortality from heart disease and lung cancer more than 20 years after radiotherapy for breast cancer. Br J Cancer 2013;108(1):179–82.
[26] Ganz PA, Cecchini RS, Julian TB, et al. Patient-reported outcomes with anastrozole versus tamoxifen for postmenopausal patients with ductal carcinoma in situ treated with lumpectomy plus radiotherapy (NSABP B-35): a randomised, double-blind, phase 3 clinical trial. Lancet 2016;387(10021):857–65.
[27] Anderson C, Meyer AM, Wheeler SB, et al. Endocrine therapy initiation and medical oncologist utilization among women diagnosed with ductal carcinoma in situ. Oncologist 2017;22(5):535–41.
[28] Miller ME, Muhsen S, Olcese C, et al. Contralateral breast cancer risk in women with ductal carcinoma in situ: is it high enough to justify bilateral mastectomy? Ann Surg Oncol 2017;24(10):2889–97.
[29] Sagara Y, Freedman RA, Wong SM, et al. Trends in adjuvant therapies after breast-conserving surgery for hormone receptor-positive ductal carcinoma in situ: findings from the National Cancer Database, 2004-2013. Breast Cancer Res Treat 2017;166(2): 583–92.
[30] Van Zee KJ, Liberman L, Samli B, et al. Long term follow-up of women with ductal carcinoma in situ treated with breast-conserving surgery: the effect of age. Cancer 1999;86(9): 1757–67.
[31] Vicini FA, Kestin LL, Goldstein NS, et al. Impact of young age on outcome in patients with ductal carcinoma-in-situ treated with breast-conserving therapy. J Clin Oncol 2000;18(2): 296–306.
[32] Cronin PA, Olcese C, Patil S, et al. Impact of age on risk of recurrence of ductal carcinoma in situ: outcomes of 2996 women treated with breast-conserving surgery over 30 years. Ann Surg Oncol 2016;23(9):2816–24.
[33] Muhsen S, Barrio AV, Miller M, et al. Outcomes for women with minimal-volume ductal carcinoma in situ completely excised at core biopsy. Ann Surg Oncol 2017;24(13):3888–95.
[34] Cabioglu N, Hunt KK, Buchholz TA, et al. Improving local control with breast-conserving therapy: a 27-year single-institution experience. Cancer 2005;104(1):20–9.
[35] Canavan J, Truong PT, Smith SL, et al. Local recurrence in women with stage I breast cancer: declining rates over time in a large, population-based cohort. Int J Radiat Oncol Biol Phys 2014;88(1):80–6.
[36] Mannino M, Yarnold JR. Local relapse rates are falling after breast conserving surgery and systemic therapy for early breast cancer: can radiotherapy ever be safely withheld? Radiother Oncol 2009;90(1):14–22.
[37] Subhedar P, Olcese C, Patil S, et al. Decreasing recurrence rates for ductal carcinoma in situ: analysis of 2996 women treated with breast-conserving surgery over 30 years. Ann Surg Oncol 2015;22(10):3273–81.
[38] Morrow M, Van Zee KJ, Solin LJ, et al. Society of Surgical Oncology-American Society for Radiation Oncology-American Society of Clinical Oncology Consensus Guideline on margins for breast-conserving surgery with whole-breast irradiation in ductal carcinoma in situ. J Clin Oncol 2016;34(33):4040–6.
[39] Marinovich ML, Azizi L, Macaskill P, et al. The association of surgical margins and local recurrence in women with ductal carcinoma in situ treated with breast-conserving therapy: a meta-analysis. Ann Surg Oncol 2016;23(12):3811–21.

[40] Van Zee KJ, Subhedar P, Olcese C, et al. Relationship between margin width and recurrence of ductal carcinoma in situ: analysis of 2996 women treated with breast-conserving surgery for 30 years. Ann Surg 2015;262(4):623–31.
[41] Rudloff U, Jacks LM, Goldberg JI, et al. Nomogram for predicting the risk of local recurrence after breast-conserving surgery for ductal carcinoma in situ. J Clin Oncol 2010;28(23): 3762–9.
[42] Collins LC, Achacoso N, Haque R, et al. Risk prediction for local breast cancer recurrence among women with DCIS treated in a community practice: a nested, case-control study. Ann Surg Oncol 2015;22(Suppl 3):S502–8.
[43] Sedloev T, Vasileva M, Kundurzhiev T, et al. Validation of the Memorial Sloan-Kettering Cancer Center nomogram in the prediction of local recurrence risks after conserving surgery for Bulgarian women with DCIS of the breast. Presented at: 2nd World Congress on Controversies in Breast Cancer (CoBrCa). Barcelona, Spain, September 8–11, 2016. Available at: https://www.researchgate.net/publication/312232507_Validation_of_the_Memorial_Sloan-Kettering_Cancer_Center_nomogram_in_the_prediction_of_local_recurrence_risks_after_conserving_surgery_for_Bulgarian_women_with_DCIS_of_the_breast. Accessed November 7, 2018.
[44] Sweldens C, Peeters S, van Limbergen E, et al. Local relapse after breast-conserving therapy for ductal carcinoma in situ: a European single-center experience and external validation of the Memorial Sloan-Kettering Cancer Center DCIS nomogram. Cancer J 2014;20(1):1–7.
[45] Wang F, Li H, Tan PH, et al. Validation of a nomogram in the prediction of local recurrence risks after conserving surgery for Asian women with ductal carcinoma in situ of the breast. Clin Oncol (R Coll Radiol) 2014;26(11):684–91.
[46] Yi M, Meric-Bernstam F, Kuerer HM, et al. Evaluation of a breast cancer nomogram for predicting risk of ipsilateral breast tumor recurrences in patients with ductal carcinoma in situ after local excision. J Clin Oncol 2012;30(6):600–7.
[47] Solin LJ, Gray R, Baehner FL, et al. A multigene expression assay to predict local recurrence risk for ductal carcinoma in situ of the breast. J Natl Cancer Inst 2013;105(10):701–10.
[48] Rakovitch E, Nofech-Mozes S, Hanna W, et al. A population-based validation study of the DCIS Score predicting recurrence risk in individuals treated by breast-conserving surgery alone. Breast Cancer Res Treat 2015;152(2):389–98.
[49] Betsill WL Jr, Rosen PP, Lieberman PH, et al. Intraductal carcinoma. Long-term follow-up after treatment by biopsy alone. JAMA 1978;239(18):1863–7.
[50] Collins LC, Tamimi RM, Baer HJ, et al. Outcome of patients with ductal carcinoma in situ untreated after diagnostic biopsy: results from the Nurses' Health Study. Cancer 2005;103(9): 1778–84.
[51] Rosen PP. The clinical significance of pre-invasive breast carcinoma. Cancer 1980;46: 919–25.
[52] Pilewskie M, Stempel M, Rosenfeld H, et al. Do LORIS trial eligibility criteria identify a ductal carcinoma in situ patient population at low risk of upgrade to invasive carcinoma? Ann Surg Oncol 2016;23(11):3487–93.
[53] Pilewskie M, Olcese C, Patil S, et al. Women with low-risk DCIS eligible for the LORIS trial after complete surgical excision: how low is their risk after standard therapy? Ann Surg Oncol 2016;23(13):4253–61.

Advances in Surgery 53 (2019) 37–53

ADVANCES IN SURGERY

What Is the Role for Carotid Stenting Versus Endarterectomy?

Kyla M. Bennett, MD[a], John E. Scarborough, MD[b,*]

[a]Department of Surgery, University of Wisconsin-Madison School of Medicine and Publich Health, 600 Highland Avenue, G5/322 Clinical Science Center, Madison, WI 53792, USA; [b]Department of Surgery, University of Wisconsin-Madison School of Medicine and Publich Health, 600 Highland Avenue, G5/340 Clinical Science Center, Madison, WI 53792, USA

Keywords

• Carotid stenosis • Carotid endarterectomy • Carotid stenting
• Carotid atherosclerosis

Key points

- There have been significant advances in medical management of carotid atherosclerosis since early trials comparing endarterectomy to medical therapy were performed.
- Carotid endarterectomy is strongly recommended for patients with symptomatic 70% to 99% carotid stenosis, preferentially within 14 days of symptom onset, but less strongly recommended for symptomatic 50% to 69% stenosis.
- Carotid endarterectomy may be recommended for patients with asymptomatic 60% to 99% stenosis, especially if they have certain imaging characteristics placing them at higher risk of embolic stroke.
- Carotid stenting may be an acceptable alternative to endarterectomy, but should not be performed in symptomatic patients who are greater than 70 years of age or in patients whose revascularization procedure occurs within 14 days of symptom onset.
- Ongoing clinical trials may help to further define the role of endarterectomy and stenting in the management of carotid stenosis.

Disclosure statement: Neither author has any relationship with a commercial company that has a direct financial interest in subject matter or materials discussed in this article.

*Corresponding author. *E-mail address:* scarborough@surgery.wisc.edu

https://doi.org/10.1016/j.yasu.2019.04.003
0065-3411/19/

INTRODUCTION

The optimal management of atherosclerotic carotid arterial disease has been studied extensively over the past 3 decades. From the landmark trials comparing carotid endarterectomy (CEA) to medical therapy in the late 1980s, through the large trials comparing CEA to carotid arterial stenting (CAS) in the 1990s and 2000s, to the present day comparisons of both interventions with modern medical management, carotid stenosis has remained one of the most intensely investigated disease processes in surgery.

Despite the considerable attention allotted to carotid stenosis management in the literature, the recommended therapeutic approach to patients who have this condition has not changed dramatically, especially among those who have sustained symptoms attributable to their carotid disease. In this analysis, the authors will review the major clinical trials that have focused on carotid stenosis management and discuss the increasingly nuanced guidelines for carotid revascularization.

ORIGINAL TRIALS COMPARING ENDARTERECTOMY TO MEDICAL THERAPY

Traditional indications for carotid arterial revascularization originate from several well-known randomized clinical trials performed in the late 1980s and early 1990s. Consistent with the differential risk of subsequent stroke according to the presence or absence of symptoms attributable to carotid stenosis, these trials compared CEA with usual medical therapy in either symptomatic or asymptomatic study populations.

Asymptomatic carotid stenosis: asymptomatic carotid atherosclerosis study and the first asymptomatic carotid surgery trial

Before recent developments in medical management of atherosclerotic disease, the management of asymptomatic patients was largely informed by the results of 2 landmark randomized clinical trials, the Asymptomatic Carotid Atherosclerosis Study (ACAS) and the first Asymptomatic Carotid Surgery Trial (ACST-1).

The ACAS study randomized 1662 patients aged 40 to 79 years with 60% to 99% asymptomatic carotid artery stenosis to either CEA and daily aspirin or BMT (which consisted of daily aspirin and stroke risk factor modification, including lipid-lowering therapy in 13% of patients at trial entry) [1]. The trial excluded patients with comorbid conditions that were deemed likely to produce disability or death within 5 years. The primary outcome for the trial was ipsilateral stroke or any perioperative stroke or death. The estimated 5-year incidence of this outcome was 5.1% for CEA patients compared with 11.0% for BMT patients ($P = .004$), with an aggregate risk reduction of 53% associated with CEA. Subgroup analysis of trial data demonstrated that men aged $\leq$68 years, and those who had prior contralateral CEA or stroke, had the greatest estimated 5-year benefit from CEA.

The ACST-1 study randomized 3120 patients with 70% to 99% asymptomatic stenosis to either immediate CEA or indefinite deferral of any carotid procedure [2]. There were no age exclusions in this trial. The primary outcomes of the trial were 30-day death or stroke, and nonperioperative stroke. The 30-day death or stroke rate for patients undergoing immediate CEA was 3.0%. At 5 years, the risk of stroke was 4.1% in the immediate CEA group compared with 10.0% in the deferred CEA group, and this benefit for immediate CEA persisted at 10 years (stroke risk 10.8% for immediate CEA patients compared with 16.9% for deferred CEA patients). Although medical management of the patients in the ACST-1 trial was left to the discretion of the individual participating clinicians, most of the patients in both arms of the study were on antithrombotic and antihypertensive therapy, and the use of lipid-lowering agents increased significantly over the course of the study period. The investigators in this trial noted that the benefits of immediate CEA were significant for patients who were on lipid-lowering therapy, and for patients of either gender up to 75 years of age.

Symptomatic carotid stenosis: North American symptomatic carotid endarterectomy trial and european carotid surgery trial

The North American Symptomatic Carotid Endarterectomy Trial (NASCET) was performed at 50 centers in the United States and Canada, and included patients less than 80 year old who had sustained symptoms attributable to carotid stenosis within the 120 days preceding enrollment [3]. Patients were randomized to either BMT alone, or BMT and CEA. Patients with high-grade (70%–99%) stenosis were considered separately from those with lower-grade (30%–69%) stenosis. For the high-grade stenosis group, the trial was stopped prematurely at 18 month follow-up because of interim discovery of a clear benefit for CEA, which had an estimated 2-year ipsilateral stroke rate of 9% compared with 26% with BMT alone. The trial was continued for patients with lower-grade stenosis for an average follow-up of 5 years [4]. The NASCET investigators found that the 5-year ipsilateral stroke rate was 15.7% among patients treated with CEA who had 50% to 69% stenosis, compared with 22.2% among patients treated medically ($P = .45$). There were no significant differences between the 2 treatment arms for patients with 30% to 49% stenosis (14.9% for CEA patients vs 18.7% for medical therapy patients, $P = .16$).

Results from the later European Carotid Surgery Trial (ECST) largely confirmed the findings from NASCET [5]. The ECST randomized 3024 patients of any age with carotid stenosis and ipsilateral symptoms within 6 months of enrollment to either CEA or usual medical care. For this trial, patients were stratified by degree of stenosis (0%–19%, 20%–29%, 30%–39%, and so on). Investigators found that the risk of perioperative major stroke or death was 7.0% in patients undergoing CEA, and noted that this adverse perioperative event rate did not vary substantially by the degree of stenosis. Conversely, the investigators found that the major stroke rate for patients who were treated medically did increase with degree of stenosis for approximately 3 years after randomization, especially for patients with ≥80% stenosis. Comparison of the 2 treatment arms in patients with ≥80% stenosis demonstrated an estimated 3-year major stroke or death rate of 14.9% in CEA patients compared with 26.5% in medical therapy patients. For patients with lesser degrees of stenosis, the benefit of CEA was less clear.

Because the methods used to measure degree of stenosis were different in NASCET and ECST, a pooled analysis of these trials and an additional Veterans Administration trial was conducted in which degree of stenosis for ECST patients was recalculated according to NASCET methodology [6]. This study found CEA to increase the 5-year risk of ipsilateral stroke in patients with less than 30% stenosis, have no effect in patients with 50% to 69% stenosis, and have a large benefit (with an absolute risk reduction of 16.0%) in patients with 70% to 99% stenosis.

Summary of original trials

Based on the results of these landmark trials, a standard approach to carotid revascularization developed whereby symptomatic patients with ≥50% stenosis and asymptomatic patients with ≥70% stenosis would be recommended for CEA as long as their anticipated risk of major perioperative stroke or death was sufficiently low (<6% and <3%, respectively, for symptomatic and asymptomatic disease) [7].

CAROTID ARTERIAL STENTING

Although CEA has been considered the mainstay for patients needing carotid revascularization due to atherosclerotic stenosis, the aforementioned trials that established its efficacy over usual medical therapy tended to exclude patients who might be at higher risk for perioperative intervention, either because of significant comorbidity or because of anatomic characteristics that might increase the risk of intraoperative complications during endarterectomy (Table 1). Specific physiologic criteria that have been perceived to place patients at higher risk of perioperative morbidity during CEA include advanced age, class III or

Table 1
Physiologic and anatomic characteristics perceived to place patients at higher risk for complications during carotid endarterectomy

Physiologic high-risk characteristics	Anatomic high-risk characteristics
• Age >80 y	• Contralateral carotid occlusion
• Recent myocardial infarction	• Contralateral laryngeal nerve palsy
• Class III/IV congestive heart failure	• Prior ipsilateral radical neck surgery
• Severe pulmonary disease	• Prior radiation therapy to the neck
• Abnormal stress test	• Prior ipsilateral endarterectomy
• Need for open-heart surgery	

Data from Yadav JS, Wholey MH, Kuntz RE, Fayad P, Katzen BT, Mishkel GJ, et al. Protected carotid-artery stenting versus endarterectomy in high-risk patients. N Engl J Med 2004;351:1493–1501.

IV congestive heart failure, unstable angina or significant multivessel coronary artery disease, recent myocardial infarction, or severe chronic pulmonary or renal disease [8]. Specific anatomic criteria, meanwhile, include stenotic lesions located at or above the second cervical verterbral level, a prior history of ipsilateral radical neck surgery or radiation, occlusion of the contralateral carotid artery, previous ipsilateral CEA, contralateral laryngeal nerve palsy, or tracheostoma [8]. Although CAS was initially proposed as an alternative treatment option for patients who possessed 1 or more of these high-risk characteristics, the early clinical trials that compared this intervention to CEA were applied to the broader population of carotid stenosis patients who met traditional criteria for endarterectomy.

Early trials comparing carotid arterial stenting to carotid endarterectomy

The Carotid and Vertebral Artery Transluminal Angioplasty Study, published in 2001, was the first major randomized trial to compare the 2 interventions [9]. The trial was conducted at 22 centers in Europe, Australia, and Canada, and included patients with any degree of carotid stenosis, with or without symptoms, who were considered to be eligible for both procedures. Stenting after carotid angioplasty was not required. A total of 504 patients were assigned to either CEA (n = 253) or endovascular treatment (n = 251), and the mean degree of stenosis in these patients was 85.1% and 86.4%, respectively. The 30-day rate of disabling stroke or death did not differ between the 2 groups (9.9% after CEA vs 10.0% after endovascular treatment). At 1-year follow-up, patients undergoing endovascular treatment had a significantly greater incidence of severe (70%–99%) ipsilateral carotid stenosis (14% after endovascular therapy vs 4% after CEA; $P<.001$), but the estimated 3-year rate of ipsilateral stroke did not differ between the 2 groups. Importantly, only 26% of patients in the endovascular arm of this trial received a stent.

The Endarterectomy versus Angioplasty in Patients with Symptomatic Severe Carotid Stenosis (EVA-3S) trial, published in 2006, was performed across 30 centers starting in November 2000, but was stopped prematurely for safety reasons in 2005 after enrolling 527 patients [10]. Patients were eligible for this trial if they had 60% to 99% carotid stenosis and ipsilateral symptoms within 120 days before enrollment. All patients in the endovascular arm of this trial received stents, and 91.9% of the endovascular procedures used a distal embolic protection device. The primary outcome of the trial was 30-day postoperative death or any stroke, a composite endpoint which occurred in 9.6% of CAS patients and 3.9% of CEA patients (relative risk with CAS 2.5; 95% CI, 0.5–4.2). Notably, investigators in this trial reported that the rate of periprocedural stroke or death was significantly higher in the small group of CAS patients whose procedure was performed without a distal embolic protection device (25% without vs 7.9% with embolic protection; $P = .03$), a finding that emphasizes the importance of such devices for perioperative stroke prevention during stenting procedures. Longer-term follow-up demonstrated that the cumulative probability of any procedural stroke or death or any ipsilateral stroke after randomization remained statistically higher at 5 years (11.0% after CAS vs 6.3%; $P = .04$), but not at 10 years (11.5% vs 7.6%; $P = .07$) [11].

The Stent-Protected Angioplasty versus Carotid Endarterectomy (SPACE) trial randomized patients with symptomatic severe (≥70%) stenosis to CEA or CAS, and was designed as a noninferiority study [12]. The use of embolic protection devices during this trial were left to the discretion of the proceduralist. A total of 1183 patients were included in the analysis. The 30-day rate of death or ipsilateral stroke was 6.84% in CAS patients and 6.34% in CEA patients, which resulted in a 1-sided P value for noninferiority of .09. Despite failing to demonstrate noninferiority at 30 days, the SPACE investigators did find the estimated 2-year incidence of death or stroke to be no different in the 2 treatment groups, although they found recurrent severe (≥70%) restenosis at 2 years to be significantly higher after stenting (10.7% after CAS vs 4.6% after CEA; $P = .0009$) [13].

The International Carotid Stenting Study (ICSS) enrolled 1713 patients worldwide who had ≥50% symptomatic stenosis and who were deemed to be well-suited for either revascularization intervention [14]. Use of embolic protection devices was recommended but not mandated in this trial, with 72% of stenting procedures ultimately using such devices. At 120 days after randomization, the ICSS investigators found a significantly higher incidence of stroke, death, or myocardial infarction in the CAS group (8.5% after CAS vs 5.2% after CEA; $P = .006$), although the rate of disabling stroke or death did not differ between the 2 groups. Longer-term follow-up demonstrated no difference between the 2 groups in terms of cumulative 5-year risk of fatal or disabling stroke, but a significantly higher risk of any stroke in the CAS group [15]. Importantly, the functional outcomes of patients who sustained strokes did not differ between the 2 groups, as determined by distribution of modified Rankin scores, suggesting that the higher stroke rate observed among CAS patients did not translate into increased disability.

The Stenting and Angioplasty with Protection in Patients at High Risk for Endarterectomy trial was unique among carotid revascularization trials in that it has been the only one to date to confine its study population to those patients with one of the previously described physiologic and/or anatomic characteristics that presumably place them at higher risk for endarterectomy [16]. Symptomatic patients with ≥50% stenosis and asymptomatic patients with ≥80% stenosis were eligible for enrollment if they were deemed to be suitable candidates for either revascularization technique. All stenting procedures used distal embolic protection. The median total stenting experience of the proceduralists in this trial was 64 (range 20–700) procedures. The primary endpoint for the study was the composite incidence of death, stroke, or myocardial infarction within 30 days after the intervention, or death by ipsilateral stroke between 31 days and 1 year. This endpoint occurred in 12.2% of CAS patients and 20.1% of CEA patients ($P = .004$ for noninferiority, and $P = .053$ for superiority). When extended to 3 years, the incidence of the primary endpoint did not differ significantly between the 2 groups [17].

Although the previously described trials included either only symptomatic patients, or a combination of symptomatic and asymptomatic patients, the Asymptomatic Carotid Trial-1 has been the only large randomized trial to compare revascularization techniques in an exclusively asymptomatic population of carotid stenosis patients [18]. This trial randomized 1453 patients aged less than 80 years with asymptomatic 70% to 99% carotid stenosis to either CAS or CEA. All CAS procedures were performed using distal embolic protection. The primary endpoint for the trial, composite death, stroke, or myocardial infarction during the first 30 postprocedure days or ipsilateral stroke within the first postprocedure year, occurred in 3.8% of CAS patients and 3.4% of CEA patients, indicating noninferiority for stenting. The rate of ipsilateral stroke in the 2 groups was also statistically similar from 30 days to 5 years postprocedure.

The carotid revascularization endarterectomy versus stenting trial

Perhaps unavoidably, the aforementioned trials have faced critique since their publications. The major criticisms of this group of trials involve issues of heterogeneity in patient-eligibility criteria, experience levels of the interventionalists in the CAS arms, and technical aspects of the stenting procedures performed.

Because of its size, ample funding, and meticulous design, the Carotid Revascularization Endarterectomy versus Stenting Trial (CREST) is widely considered the preeminent study for comparison of revascularization techniques for carotid stenosis [19]. Importantly, the protocol for this trial seemed to overcome many of the notable weaknesses of earlier comparisons of revascularization techniques. The trial was conducted at 108 centers in the United States and 9 in Canada. Surgeons who participated in the trial required a minimum annual volume of CEA of 13 procedures pear year and documented perioperative death and complication rates of less than 3% in asymptomatic patients and less than 5% in symptomatic patients. Interventionists, meanwhile, were required to certification based on evaluation of previous endovascular experience, review of prior carotid stenting outcomes, pretrial hands-on training, and performance of stenting procedures during a lead-in phase before being able to participate in the trial. The same type of stent was used for all CAS procedures, and distal embolic protection use was protocolized when technically feasible.

Patients were considered eligible if they were symptomatic within 180 days before randomization and had a minimum threshold degree of stenosis based on imaging technique (≥50% by angiography, ≥70% by ultrasonography, or ≥70% on computed tomographic angiography [CTA] or magnetic resonance angiography [MRA] if the stenosis was 50%–69% on ultrasound). Although not included in the original study protocol, asymptomatic patients became eligible in 2005 if they had ≥60% stenosis on angiography, ≥70% on ultrasonography, or ≥70% on CTA or MRA if stenosis on ultrasound was 50% to 69%. Patients also had to be suitable for management by either technique to be eligible for participation in this trial, whereas patients with a recent history of atrial fibrillation, myocardial infarction, or unstable angina were excluded from participation. A total of 2522 patients were randomized (1271 to CAS and 1251 to CEA).

The primary outcome of the CREST was the composite of any stroke, myocardial infarction, or death within 30 days of procedure or ipsilateral stroke within 4 years after randomization. The incidence of the primary outcome was 7.2% in CAS patients and 6.8% in CEA patients (hazard ratio with stenting 1.11; 95% CI, 0.81–1.51; $P = .51$). Analysis of the individual components of the periprocedural outcomes demonstrated that CAS patients had a higher risk of stroke (4.1% after CAS vs 2.3% after CEA; $P = .01$), but a lower risk of myocardial infarction (1.1% after CAS vs 2.3% after CEA; $P = .03$). The incidence of stroke after the periprocedural period was similar for both groups. Subgroup analyses of the primary endpoint in this trial revealed no differences between treatment groups based on preoperative symptom status or patient gender, although women in the CAS group did seem to have a higher risk of perioprocedural adverse events compared with women in the CEA group [20,21]. Investigators also found that the primary endpoint increased with patient age in CAS patients but not CEA patients, primarily due to age-related increase in stroke [22]. Perhaps in testament to the rigorous training and credentialing requirements contained within the CREST protocol, investigators failed to find an association between periprocedural event rates and the enrollment volume of the different centers that participated in this trial [23].

After 10-year follow-up, there was not a significant difference in the rate of the trial's composite endpoint between groups (11.8% for CAS patients and 9.9% for CEA patients [hazard ratio with CAS 1.10; 95% CI, 0.83–1.44]), either as a whole or once stratified by preoperative symptom status [24]. There was also no difference in the primary long-term endpoint of postprocedural ipsilateral stroke over the 10-year follow-up (6.9% after CAS and 5.6% after CEA). A prominent criticism of CREST was its inclusion of myocardial infarction (MI) as a component of the primary endpoint, which contributed to the ultimate trial conclusion that there was no difference in overall outcome between the 2 procedures [25,26]. Concern was raised because the criteria used to define MI in the trial allowed for the possibility that some asymptomatic infarcts would be captured, and that such events could therefore be weighted equally with stroke and death in terms of clinical import. However, CREST investigators showed that even those patients with biomarker elevation only (without electrocardiographic changes or chest pain) had increased mortality at 4 years, and that the 4-year risk of death after CREST-defined MI (hazard ratio = 3.4; 95% CI, 1.7–6.9) was similar to that observed for patients who sustained CREST-defined perioperative stroke of 2.78 (95% CI, 1.63–4.76) [27,28]. At the same time, the investigators also found that periprocedural stroke had a greater and more prolonged impact on health-related quality of life than MI at 1-year postprocedure [29].

BEYOND THE TRIALS

Improvements in medical therapy

There have been dramatic improvements in the medical management of carotid stenosis since the landmark trials of the 1980s and 1990s comparing CEA with usual medical therapy. Typical specified medical therapy in those trials consisted only of daily aspirin. In the interim, however, numerous studies have demonstrated the important impact that lipid-lowering agents and control of hypertension have on stroke prevention in patients with atherosclerotic disease.

In the Justification for the Use of Statins in Prevention: an Intervention Trial Evaluating Rosuvastatin trial, 17,802 healthy patients with low-density lipoprotein (LDL) cholesterol levels of less than 130 mg/dL and high C-reactive protein levels were randomized to receive either 20 mg rosuvastatin or placebo daily [30]. After this trial was stopped at a median follow-up of 1.9 years, patients in the treatment arm had a reduction in LDL cholesterol levels of 50%, and had a significantly lower incidence of stroke compared with patients in the placebo arm (0.18 stroke events per 100 person-years of follow-up in the rosuvastatin group versus 0.34 in the placebo group [hazard ratio = 0.52; 95% CI, 0.34–0.79; $P = .002$]). In a meta-analysis of 18 randomized controlled trials comparing statins versus placebo or usual care, and which had ≤10% of participants with a history of cerebrovascular disease, Taylor and colleagues [31] found that the use of statins was associated with a relative risk of combined fatal and nonfatal stroke of 0.78 (95% CI, 0.68–0.89; vs placebo or usual care). Additional evidence exists for a strong benefit for blood pressure-lowering medications in terms of stroke prevention. As a result, present day BMT for patients with asymptomatic carotid disease consists of statin therapy, antihypertensive medication to maintain long-term blood pressure less than 140/90 mm Hg, and aspirin therapy (or clopidogrel in patients who cannot tolerate aspirin) [32].

This important advance in BMT for carotid stenosis has essentially made trials such as ACAS and NASCET, which relied primarily on antiplatelet therapy for stroke prevention in their nonsurgical arms, obsolete. On the other hand, general awareness of the importance of statin therapy for patients with atherosclerotic carotid disease increased over the longer study period of the ACST-1, as demonstrated by the fact that the percentage of patients in that trial who were taking lipid-lowering therapy increased from less than 10% at the beginning of the trial to 80% by the end of the follow-up period [2]. As improved BMT has reduced the annual stroke risk for patients with asymptomatic carotid stenosis who forego revascularization, it is now necessary to conduct new trials that compare revascularization (using endarterectomy or stenting) with modern BMT [32,33].

Identification of high-risk characteristics of asymptomatic stenosis

Advances in medical therapy for atherosclerosis, and the resulting reduction in stroke risk with modern medical management of carotid stenosis, have led some to reconsider whether carotid revascularization need be performed in patients with asymptomatic disease. Nevertheless, from prospective multicenter studies, several imaging characteristics (which are summarized in Box 1) have been associated with increased stroke risk among patients with asymptomatic carotid disease.

In a prospective, multicenter cohort study of patients undergoing medical therapy for asymptomatic 50% to 99% carotid stenosis, investigators from the Asymptomatic Carotid Stenosis and Risk of Stroke (ACSRS) Study Group found contralateral ischemic symptoms, large plaque area, large juxta-luminal hypoechoic area on ultrasonography to be independent predictors of ipsilateral cerebrovascular or retinal ischemic events [34,35]. This same group performed a multicenter natural history study of 821 patients with asymptomatic stenosis who were monitored with head computed tomography scans every 6 months for a maximum of 8 years, finding that the presence of silent embolic infarcts in the setting of 60% to 99% stenosis placed patients at higher risk of subsequent stroke [36]. Later analysis of a larger cohort from this study also demonstrated that 19.8% of patients with 50% to 99% asymptomatic stenosis sustained progression of their stenosis at a mean follow-up of 4 years, and that the stroke rate in the presence of progression was 21% compared with 12% in the absence of progression [37]. A separate retrospective of data from medically treated patients from ACST confirmed the prognostic import of fast progression of carotid stenosis, but the ACSRS investigators stopped short of recommending screening for progression in the absence of cost-effectiveness data [37,38].

The Asymptomatic Carotid Emboli Study (ACES) performed transcranial Doppler ultrasounds and then followed 106 patients with $\geq$70% asymptomatic stenosis, and found a nonsignificant trend toward increased stroke risk in patients with severely impaired cerebrovascular reactivity [39]. Given that their study was underpowered, they then completed a meta-analysis of the

Box 1: Imaging characteristics that increase the risk of stroke in patients with asymptomatic carotid stenosis

- Silent infarction on computed tomography of head
- Progression of stenosis on serial ultrasonography
- Large plaque area on computerized plaque analysis
- Large juxta-luminal hypoechoic area on ultrasonography
- Intraplaque hemorrhage on magnetic resonance imaging
- Impaired cerebrovascular reactivity on transcranial Doppler ultrasonography
- Plaque lucency on Duplex ultrasonography
- Spontaneous embolization on transcranial Doppler ultrasonography
- Contralateral transient ischemic attack or stroke

Data from Naylor AR, Ricco JB, de Borst GJ, Debus S, de Haro J, Halliday A, et al. Editor's choice - Management of atherosclerotic and verterbral disease: 2017 Clinical Practice Guidelines of the European Society for Vascular Surgery (ESVS). Eur J Vasc Endovasc Surg 2018;55:3–81.

ACES data with previous analysis, and found a significant association between reactivity and subsequent stroke risk. Similar analyses by the same group also demonstrated increased stroke risk for patients with spontaneous embolization during transcranial Doppler ultrasound [40]. Other investigators have demonstrated an increased risk of stroke for asymptomatic patients who demonstrate intraplaque hemorrhage on magnetic resonance imaging or plaque lucency on ultrasound to be associated with increased stroke risk [41,42].

Although the import of the above characteristics in terms of stroke risk prediction, and the subsequent usefulness of carotid revascularization in reducing that risk, has not been validated in randomized, multicenter trials, the presence of one or more of these characteristics is presently considered as potential justification for considering carotid revascularization for patients with asymptomatic carotid disease.

Age-associated increase in risk of periprocedural stroke with carotid arterial stenting

The Carotid Stenting Trialists' Collaboration (CSTC) conducted a meta-analysis of symptomatic patients from 4 of the stenting versus endarterectomy trials (EVA-3S, SPACE, ICSS, and CREST) to determine whether patient age was associated with treatment differences between the 2 revascularization techniques [43]. The CSTC investigators found no evidence of increased periprocedural risk of ipsilateral stroke or death by age in patients undergoing CEA, but did note that the risk of periprocedural stroke increased in patients undergoing CAS beyond the age of 70 years. The investigators concluded that CEA was superior to CAS in patients aged 70 years or older.

Several carotid anatomic and plaque characteristics have been shown to increase the risk of periprocedural stroke during CAS (Table 2), which may be more likely to be present in older patients with carotid disease and thus may help to explain the increased risk of periprocedural embolic stroke in aged patients who undergo CAS [25].

Timing of revascularization in symptomatic patients

The CSTC also performed a meta-analysis of 3 trials (EVA-3S, SPACE, and ICSS) to determine the association of time between symptom onset and risk periprocedural stroke or death in patients undergoing carotid revascularization [44]. The investigators found that the lowest periprocedural stroke or death rates occurred in patients who underwent CEA within 7 days of symptoms, although they found that patients undergoing endarterectomy between 8 and 14 days also had a lower risk of periprocedural events than patients undergoing the operation more than 14 days after symptom onset. Conversely, the investigators found that the risk of periprocedural stroke for patients undergoing CAS was highest in the first 7 days (9.4% risk), and decreased as the interval between symptom onset and stenting increased (8.1% if CAS performed between 8–14 days, 7.3% if performed after 14 days).

Table 2
Carotid plaque and vessel characteristics found to place patients at higher risk for periprocedural stroke during carotid arterial stenting

Plaque characteristics	Anatomic high-risk characteristics
• Soft, lipid-rich plaque • Extensive plaque (>1.5 cm) • Intraplaque hemorrhage • Thin fibrous cap • Heavily calcified plaque • Preocclusive lesion • Bifurcation stenosis • Lesion located at a curve	• Aortoiliac tortuosity • Type III or IV arch anatomy • Bovine anatomy • Arch disease • Proximal or distal internal carotid toruosity

Data from Noiphithak R, Liengudom A. Recent update on carotid endarterectomy versus carotid artery stenting. Cerebrovasc Dis 2017;43:68–75.

CURRENT RECOMMENDATIONS AND FUTURE DIRECTIONS

Numerous guidelines have been published regarding the appropriateness of carotid revascularization (be it CEA or CAS) for patients with carotid stenosis. Not surprisingly, given the ever-increasing volume of data generated from randomized clinical trials and clinical registries, there is some discordance among guidelines in terms of when and which type of revascularization is recommended [45]. The following review of current recommendations for carotid stenosis management are based primarily on the 2017 Clinical Practice Guidelines of the European Society for Vascular Surgery (ESVS), which are the most recent to be published [32].

Asymptomatic stenosis

The only recommendations achieving class I status (Table 3) and backed by level I evidence in the ESVS guidelines are for daily low-dose aspirin, statin therapy, and maintenance of long-term blood pressure less than 140/90 mm Hg [32]. Notably, there are no class 1 recommendations promoting carotid revascularization, be it by endarterectomy or stenting, for asymptomatic disease. The only ESVS recommendation for revascularization that achieved class IIa status (based on level B evidence) was for patients with 60% to 99% carotid stenosis to be considered for CEA if (1) the procedure is performed by a surgeon with documented perioperative stroke/death rates of less than 3%, (2) the patient's life expectance exceeds 5 years, and (3) the patients has one or more characteristics on imaging that place them at higher risk for embolic stroke (see Box 1). Carotid stenting, meanwhile, received IIb classification as a potential alternative to CEA if the aforementioned criteria were met, irrespective of the presence or absence of anatomic/physiologic characteristics that would potentially place patients at high risk during endarterectomy.

Table 3
Classes of recommendation and levels of evidence described

Class of recommendation	Class I	Evidence and/or general agreement that given treatment or procedure is beneficial, useful, and effective
	Class II	Conflicting evidence and/or divergence of opinion about the usefulness/efficacy of given treatment or procedure
	Class IIa	Weight of evidence/opinion in favor of usefulness/efficacy
	Class IIb	Usefulness/efficacy less well established by evidence/opinion
	Class III	Evidence of general agreement that treatment or procedure is not useful/effective, and in some cases may be harmful
Level of evidence	Level A	Data derived from multiple randomized clinical trials or meta-analyses
	Level B	Data derived from a single randomized clinical trial or large nonrandomized studies
	Level C	Consensus of opinion of experts and/or small studies, retrospective studies, registries

Symptomatic stenosis

Regarding patients with symptomatic carotid stenosis, the ESVS makes a class 1 recommendation (based on level A evidence) for CEA in patients who report carotid territory symptoms within the past 6 months, and who have 70% to 99% stenosis, as long as the documented procedural death/stroke rate of the surgeon is less than 6% [32]. The ESVS also recommended CEA in patients with 50% to 69% symptomatic stenosis, but only as a class IIa recommendation (albeit based on level A evidence). Importantly, an additional class I recommendation from these most recent guidelines that concerned revascularization in symptomatic patients was that patients aged more than 70 years who had 50% to 99% stenosis should preferentially undergo CEA and not CAS. For younger patients, CAS was recommended with class IIb status as an alternative to CEA. Finally, the ESVS recommended (with class I status) that any symptomatic patient with 50% to 99% stenosis in whom revascularization is deemed appropriate should be performed within 14 days of symptom onset, and by endarterectomy (not stenting) when done within that timeframe.

Ongoing trials

Several clinical trials may serve to further clarify if revascularization has a role in the management of carotid disease in the modern era. CREST-2, which began enrolling patients in December of 2014, is being conducted as 2 parallel multicenter, randomized, observer-blinded endpoint clinical trials: one comparing CAS with BMT and the other comparing CEA to BMT [46]. BMT for this trial includes aggressive antihypertensive and antilipid treatment as well as patient enrollment in a lifestyle management program for promotion of weight loss, smoking cessation, glucose control, and exercise. Adult patients with ≥70% stenosis, no ipsilateral stroke, or transient ischemic attack within 180 days of randomization, and no other serious medical problems will be eligible for enrollment. The primary endpoints of the trial with be combined stroke or death within 44 days of randomization or ipsilateral stroke within the first 4 years from randomization. MI is not a component of the primary endpoint in this trial. The ACST-2 trial, meanwhile, will compare CAS and CEA in asymptomatic patients with 70% to 99% stenosis [47]. Early results suggest near-universal compliance with BMT in trial participants, and suggest a 1-month risk of 30-day disabling stroke, fatal MI, or death of 1.0% in those patients undergoing revascularization.

SUMMARY

Indications for revascularization for carotid artery stenosis have become more nuanced since the results of NASCET and ACAS were first released. Revascularization for patients with asymptomatic disease has been approached more wearily, because the risk of stroke in patients who are treated medically is now lower. However, certain imaging characteristics confer a higher risk of stroke in patients with asymptomatic stenosis, and revascularization in patients with these symptoms is generally viewed as acceptable. Symptomatic patients with 70% to 99% stenosis are clearly recommended for revascularization, and patients with 50% to 69% less strongly so. Revascularization within 14 days of onset is increasingly preferred, although when it is possible to intervene within this timeframe, CEA is clearly preferred to CAS. At this time, there is no population in whom CAS is clearly preferred to CEA. The balance of evidence from randomized clinical trials tends to favor endarterectomy over stenting, although ongoing trials may serve to better define patient subgroups in whom CAS is an equal alternative to CEA. As a practical consideration, Medicare only reimburses for CAS procedures that are performed in symptomatic patients with ≥70% stenosis and a physiologic and/or anatomic condition that places them at high risk during endarterectomy (see Table 1) [48]. Symptomatic patients with 50% to 69% stenosis and asymptomatic patients with ≥80% stenosis may be also be covered if they are at high risk for CEA and if their stenting procedure is performed within the context of a clinical trial. Medicare will only cover procedures if certain approved stenting systems are used, and if the procedure includes an embolic protection device.

References

[1] Executive Committee for the Asymptomatic Carotid Athersosclerosis Study. Endarterectomy for asymptomatic carotid artery stenosis. JAMA 1995;273:1421–8.

[2] Halliday A, Harrison M, Hayter E, et al. 10-year stroke prevention after successful carotid endarterectomy for asymptomatic stenosis (ACST-1): a multicentre randomized trial. Lancet 2010;376:1074–84.

[3] North American Symptomatic Carotid Endarterectomy Trial Collaborators, Barnett HJM, Taylor DW, Haynes RB, et al. Beneficial effect of carotid endarterectomy in symptomatic patients with high-grade carotid stenosis. N Engl J Med 1991;325:445–53.

[4] Barnett HJ, Taylor DW, Eliasziw M, et al. Benefit of carotid endarterectomy in patients with symptomatic moderate or severe stenosis. North American Symptomatic Carotid Endarterectomy Trial Collaborators. N Engl J Med 1998;339:1415–25.
[5] Randomised trial of endarterectomy for recently symptomatic carotid stenosis: final results of the MRC European Carotid Surgery Trial (ECST). Lancet 1998;351:1379–87.
[6] Rothwell PM, Eliasziw M, Gutnikov SA, et al. Analysis of pooled data from the randomized controlled trials of endarterectomy for symptomatic carotid stenosis. Lancet 2003;361:107–16.
[7] Brott TG, Halperin JL, Abbara S, et al. 2011 ASA/ACCF/AHA/AANN/AANS/ACR/ASNR/CNS/SAIP/SCAI/SIR/SNIS/SVM/SVS guideline on the management of patients with extracranial carotid and vertebral artery disease: executive summary. Catheter Cardiovasc Interv 2013;81:E76–123.
[8] Bates ER, Babb JD, Casey DE, et al. A report of the American College of Cardiology Foundation Task Force on Clinical Expert Consensus Documents ACCF/SCAI/SVMB/SIR/ASITN Clinical Expert Consensus Document Committee on Carotid Stenting. J Am Coll Cardiol 2007;49:126–70.
[9] Endovascular versus surgical treatment in patients with carotid stenosis in the Carotid and Verterbral Artery Transluminal Angioplasty Study (CAVITAS): a randomized trial. Lancet 2001;357:1729–37.
[10] Mas JL, Chatellier G, Beyssen B, et al. Endarterectomy versus stenting in patients with symptomatic severe carotid stenosis. N Engl J Med 2006;355:1660–71.
[11] Mas JL, Arquizan C, Calvert D, et al. Long-term follow-up study of endarterectomy versus angioplasty in patients with symptomatic severe carotid stenosis trial. Stroke 2014;45:2750–6.
[12] Ringleb PA, Allenberg J, Bruckman H, et al. 30 day results from the SPACE trial of stent-protected angioplasty versus carotid endarterectomy in symptomatic patients: a randomized non-inferiority trial. Lancet 2006;368:1239–47.
[13] Eckstein HH, Ringleb P, Allenberg JR, et al. Results of the stent-protected angioplasty versus carotid endarterectomy (SPACE) study to treat symptomatic stenosis at 2 years: a multinational, prospective, randomized trial. Lancet Neurol 2008;7:893–902.
[14] Ederle J, Dobson J, Featherstone RL, et al. Carotid artery stenting compared with endarterectomy in patients with symptomatic carotid stenosis (International Carotid Stenting Study): an interim analysis of a randomized controlled trial. Lancet 2010;375:985–7.
[15] Bonati LH, Dobson J, Featherstone RL, et al. Long-term outcomes after stenting versus endarterectomy for treatment of symptomatic carotid stenosis: the International Carotid Stenting Study (ICSS) randomized trial. Lancet 2015;385:529–38.
[16] Yadav JS, Wholey MH, Kuntz RE, et al. Protected carotid-artery stenting versus endarterectomy in high-risk patients. N Engl J Med 2004;351:1493–501.
[17] Gurm HS, Yadav JS, Fayad P, et al. for the SAPHHIRE Investigators. Long-term results of carotid stenting versus endarterectomy in high-risk patients. N Engl J Med 2008;358:1572–9.
[18] Rosenfield K, Matsumura JS, Chatuverdi S, et al. for the ACT-1 Investigators. Randomized trial of stent versus surgery for asymptomatic carotid stenosis. N Engl J Med 2016;374:1011–20.
[19] Brott TG, Hobson RW, Roubin GS, et al, for the CREST Investigators. Stenting versus endarterectomy for treatment of carotid-artery stenosis. N Engl J Med 2010;363:11–23.
[20] Silver FL, Mackey A, Clark WM, et al. Safety of stenting and endarterectomy by symptomatic status in the Carotid Revascularization Endarterectomy versus Stenting Trial (CREST). Stroke 2011;42:675–80.
[21] Howard VJ, Lutsep HL, Mackey A, et al. Influence of sex on outcomes of stenting versus endarterectomy: a subgroup analysis of the Carotid Revascularization Endarterectomy versus Stenting Trial (CREST). Lancet Neurol 2011;10:530–7.

[22] Voeks JH, Howard G, Roubin GS, et al. Age and outcomes after carotid stenting and endarterectomy: the carotid revascularization endarterectomy versus stenting trial. Stroke 2011;42:3484–90.
[23] Gonzales NR, Demaerschalk BM, Voeks JH, et al. Complication rates and center enrollment volume in the carotid revascularization endarterectomy versus stenting trial. Stroke 2014;45:3320–4.
[24] Brott TG, Howard G, Roubin GS, et al, for the CREST Investigators. Long-term results of stenting versus endarterectomy for carotid artery stenosis. N Engl J Med 2016;374:1021–31.
[25] Noiphithak R, Liengudom A. Recent update on carotid endarterectomy versus carotid artery stenting. Cerebrovasc Dis 2017;43:68–75.
[26] Jones DW, Brott TG, Schermerhorn ML. Trials and frontiers in carotid endarterectomy and stenting. Stroke 2018;49:1776–83.
[27] Blackshear JL, Cutlip DE, Roubin GS, et al. CREST Investigators. Myocardial infarction after carotid stenting and endarterectomy: results from the carotid revascularization endarterectomy versus stenting trial. Circulation 2011;123:2571–8.
[28] Hill MD, Brooks W, Mackey A, et al, CREST Investigators. Stroke after carotid stenting and endarterectomy in the Carotid Revascularization Endarterectomy versus Stenting Trial (CREST). Circulation 2012;126:3054–61.
[29] Cohen DJ, Stolker JM, Wang K, et al, CREST Investigators. Health-related quality of life after carotid stenting versus carotid endarterectomy: results from CREST (Carotid Revascularization Endarterectomy versus Stenting Trial). J Am Coll Cardiol 2011;58:1557–65.
[30] Ridker PM, Danielson E, Fonseca FA, et al, for the JUPITER Study Group. Rosuvastatin to prevent vascular events in men and women with elevated C-reactive protein. N Engl J Med 2008;459:2195–207.
[31] Taylor F, Huffman MD, Macedo AF, et al. Statins for the primary prevention of cardiovascular disease. Cochrane Database Syst Rev 2013;(1):CD004816.
[32] Naylor AR, Ricco JB, de Borst GJ, et al. Editor's choice - management of atherosclerotic and verterbral disease: 2017 clinical Practice guidelines of the European Society for Vascular Surgery (ESVS). Eur J Vasc Endovasc Surg 2018;55:3–81.
[33] den Hartog AG, Achterberg S, Moll FL, et al, SMART Study Group. Asymptomatic carotid artery stenosis and the risk of ischemic stroke secondary to subtype in patients with clinical manifest arterial disease. Stroke 2013;44:1002–7.
[34] Nicolaides A, Kakkos SK, Kyriacou E, et al. Asymptomatic internal carotid artery stenosis and cerebrovascular risk stratification. J Vasc Surg 2010;52:1486–96.
[35] Kakkos SK, Griffin MB, Nicolaides AN, et al. The size of the juxta-luminal hypoechoic area in ultrasound images of asymptomatic carotid plaques predicts the occurrence of stroke. J Vasc Surg 2013;57:609–18.
[36] Kakkos SK, Sabetai M, Tegos T, et al. Silent embolic infarcts on computed tomography brain scans and risk of ipsilateral hemispheric events in patients with asymptomatic internal carotid artery stenosis. J Vasc Surg 2009;49:902–9.
[37] Kakkos SK, Nicolaides AN, Charambous I, et al. Predictors and clinical significance of progression or regression of asymptomatic carotid stenosis. J Vasc Surg 2014;49:956–67.
[38] Hirt LS. Progression rate and ipsilateral neurologic events in asymptomatic carotid stenosis. Stroke 2014;45:702–6.
[39] King A, Serena J, Bornstein NM, et al, on behalf of the ACES Investigators. Does impaired cerebrovascular reactivity predict stroke risk in asymptomatic carotid stenosis: a prospective substudy of the asymptomatic carotid emboli study. Stroke 2011;42:1550–5.
[40] Topakian R, King A, Kwon U, et al. Ultrasonic plaque echolucency and emboli signals predict stroke in asymptomatic carotid stenosis. Neurology 2011;77:751–8.
[41] Gupta A, Baradaran H, Schweitzer AD, et al. Carotid plaque MRI and stroke risk: a systematic review and meta-analysis. Stroke 2013;44:3071–7.
[42] Gupta A, Kesavabhotta K, Baradaran H, et al. Plaque echolucency and stroke risk in asymptomatic carotid stenosis: a systematic review and meta-analysis. Stroke 2015;46:91–7.

[43] Howard G, Roubin GS, Jansen O, et al, Carotid Stenting Trialists' Collaboration. Association between age and risk of stroke or death from carotid endarterectomy and carotid stenting: a meta-analysis of pooled patient data from four randomized trials. Lancet 2016;387: 1305–11.
[44] Rantner B, Goebel G, Bonati LH, et al, Carotid Stenting Trialists' Collaboration. The risk of carotid artery stenting compared with carotid endarterectomy is greatest in patients treated within 7 days of symptoms. J Vasc Surg 2013;57:619–26.
[45] Abbott AL, Paraskevas KI, Kakkos SK, et al. Systematic review of guidelines for the management of asymptomatic and symptomatic carotid stenosis. Stroke 2015;46:3288–301.
[46] Mott M, Koroshetz W, Wright CB. CREST-2: identifying the best method of stroke prevention for carotid artery stenosis: National Institute of Neurologic Disorders and Stroke Organizational Update. Stroke 2017;48:e130–1.
[47] ACST-2 Collaborative Group, Halliday A, Bulbulia R, Gray W, et al. Status update and interim results from the Asymptomatic Carotid Surgery Trial-2 (ACST-2). Eur J Vasc Endovasc Surg 2013;46:510–8.
[48] Decision memo for carotid artery stenting (CAG-00085R). Centers for Medicare and Medicaid Services. Available at: https://www.cms.gov/medicare-coverage-database/details/nca-decision-memo.aspx?NCAId=157&ver=29&NcaName=Carotid+Artery+Stenting+(1st+Recon)&bc=BEAAAAAAEAAA&&fromdb=true. Accessed November 10, 2018.

Advances in Surgery 53 (2019) 55–68

ADVANCES IN SURGERY

ELSEVIER
MOSBY

Managing Complications of Bariatric Surgery

Richard M. Peterson, MD, MPH[a,*], John D. Scott, MD[b]

[a]7703 Floyd Curl Drive, Mail Code 7842, San Antonio, TX 78229-3900, USA; [b]905 Verdae Boulevard, Suite 202, Greenville, SC 29607, USA

Keywords

• Emergency • Bariatric surgery • General surgeon • Gastric bypass • Sleeve gastrectomy • Laparoscopic adjustable gastric band • Nutrition emergencies

Key points

- The general surgeon will most likely be faced with bariatric surgical emergencies at some time in their career.
- Having a plan for the most common emergencies (surgical and nutritional) that one will encounter can save time for the surgeon and the patient.
- Applying good surgical principles with some of the specialized considerations covered in this article can have a dramatically positive effect for the patient.

INTRODUCTION

Since 2011, more than 1.4 million bariatric surgeries have been performed in the United States [1]. There has been a slow but steady increase of about 6.5%, on average, in the number of surgeries performed each year over the last 5 years. The last 2 years have seen the number increase to more than 200,000 cases annually. These numbers are based on estimates from the American Society for Metabolic and Bariatric Surgery (ASMBS) and the American College of Surgeons combined national database known as the Metabolic and Bariatric Surgery Accreditation and Quality Improvement Program. Additional information can be gleaned from the National Inpatient Sample Data. What is not included in these estimates are the number of patients who are seeking surgical care abroad, with the highest volume of procedures being

Disclosure Statement: The authors have nothing to disclose.

*Corresponding author. *E-mail address:* petersonr3@uthscsa.edu

https://doi.org/10.1016/j.yasu.2019.04.004
0065-3411/19/

done in Mexico. The primary factor leading patients to centers outside of the United States is a lower cost of surgery due to the lack of universal national insurance coverage for bariatric surgical procedures. With the increase in volume from accredited centers or international surgical tourism, the general surgeon will undoubtedly face a growing number of bariatric surgical emergencies, regardless of where patients have their index procedure performed. This article addresses the most common surgical emergencies following the 3 most common bariatric surgeries currently performed in the United States and its international neighbors.

GASTRIC SLEEVE COMPLICATIONS

Although laparoscopic sleeve gastrectomy (LSG) has been championed as a safer, less-invasive, alternative bariatric procedure compared with the Roux-en-Y gastric bypass [2], complications of this procedure can still have severe consequences for patients. Thankfully, the rate of such devastating complications is relatively low compared with other abdominal operations [3]. The 4 most common sleeve-specific perioperative complications of the procedure include staple line leaks, bleeding, stenosis, and portal vein thrombosis (PVT).

Leaks

One of the more feared complications after LSG is a leak along a disrupted staple line. The incidence of leaks after sleeve gastrectomy is 2.1%, with most leaks occurring after discharge from the hospital [4]. The causes of leaks can include poor surgical technique, staple line failure, and, most commonly, a distal gastric obstruction (such as a midbody stricture) that causes increased intragastric pressure with disruption of the staple line near the gastroesophgeal junction [5]. Patients can present with tachycardia, fevers and chills, and worsening abdominal pain; and surgeons need to maintain a high index of suspicion when postoperative patients present with these symptoms [6]. Computed tomography (CT) with oral contrast is the diagnostic test of choice, with a greater sensitivity (84%) than swallow studies with gastrograffin (50%) [7]. Even though the definitive management of leaks after sleeve gastrectomy has evolved as the prevalence of the technique has increased, the treatment algorithm remains dependent on the hemodynamic stability of the patient, regardless of the number of postoperative days since surgery. Patients that are unstable should be explored either open or laparoscopically, controlling the area of leakage with drains and assessing the gastric tissue for debridement or repair. Unfortunately, most simple repairs tend to fail, but prompt treatment and control of sepsis often buys time for a more definitive solution. Patients who are stable and can be drained using interventional radiologic techniques should be maintained with broad-spectrum antibiotics and withheld oral feeds for at least 2 weeks, when they can then be reassessed radiographically for fistula healing. Patients who have chronic nonhealing leaks should be transferred to a tertiary bariatric center, where treatment options include endoscopic stent placement [8], intragastric drainage [9], or a Roux-en-Y fistulojejunostomy [10].

Bleeding

The prevalence of bleeding requiring blood transfusion after LSG is estimated to be 1.0% [11]. Bleeding can be intraluminal from the staple line itself or extraluminal from the greater curve and perisplenic vasculature, both of which require dissection during the procedure. Intraluminal bleeding often presents with hematemesis or melena, whereas extraluminal bleeding can present quickly with signs and symptoms of hemodynamic compromise. There has been vigorous debate among bariatric surgeons on a preventative strategy to minimize staple line bleeding, including the use of reinforcement materials and other adjuncts [12]. Regardless of the source of bleeding, the first step in management of bleeding is resuscitation of the patient with intravenous fluids and the possible transfusion of packed red blood cells. For unstable patients, a prompt evaluation with an endoscope in the operating room can quickly differentiate between intraluminal and extraluminal bleeding. Some cases of mild intraluminal bleeding can be controlled with the application of endoscopically placed clips, but should that intervention fail, a fallback measure would be the oversewing of the gastric staple line. For unstable extraluminal bleeding, control of the source should be done quickly, either laparoscopically or in an open surgical fashion. For stable patients, most bleeding episodes will resolve spontaneously; however, vigilance is required for close monitoring, stopping anticoagulation, and replacement of blood products, if necessary. A worsening clinical appearance (dropping hematocrit or multiple transfusions) necessitates surgical exploration.

Stenosis

Gastric sleeve stenosis occurs with a prevalence of 3.9% [13]. Most patients present with:

- Food intolerance (especially solids)
- Nausea and vomiting
- Severe reflux

The most common location for narrowing is the midgastric body near the incisura. This may be due to technical factors during sleeve creation or corkscrewing of the sleeve. The diagnosis is easily confirmed with an upper gastrointestinal contrast study. Pneumatic balloon dilation has been shown to be modestly effective in almost 80% of cases [14]. For refractory cases, endoscopic treatment with covered stents is justified; however, a more permanent solution to a chronic stenosis is conversion to a laparoscopic Roux-en-Y gastric bypass.

Portal vein thrombosis

The incidence of PVT after bariatric surgery is reported at 1% to 3% of cases and it is estimated that there is an unexplained higher incidence after LSG [15–17]. Presentation of this complication usually occurs from 1 to 6 weeks after surgery. The symptoms of PVT are usually nonspecific, highlighted by malaise, abdominal pain, and nausea. A diagnosis can usually be made with contrasted CT scanning, demonstrating partial or complete venous occlusion, as well as bowel compromise if present. Duplex ultrasonography can demonstrate the presence of portal venous flow but has limited information on potential bowel ischemia. The mainstay of treatment of nonocclusive clots is heparinization to prevent propagation. An algorithm [12] has been proposed for more difficult cases. For example, high-grade nonocclusive clots may be best treated with systemic or catheter-directed tissue plasminogen activator followed by heparinization; and occlusive disease (associated with potential bowel compromise and a high mortality rate) may be amenable to operative thrombectomy. The goal of all therapies should be achieving portal vein patency.

GASTRIC BYPASS

The open gastric bypass has been described in various forms since the 1970s, but the development of the laparoscopic Roux-en-Y gastric bypass (LRYGB), first described by Wittgrove in the 1990s, led to an expansion in the performance of bariatric operations. This was mainly due to the overall decrease in complications associated with fewer open incisions, development of laparoscopic endostaplers, and refinement of the technique. Although safer than its open surgical predecessor, the LRYGB is not immune to potential complications.

To quickly assess and treat postoperative LRYGB patients in distress, one can begin by classifying a complication as being part of an obstructive process or one associated with peritonitis. First and foremost, the stability of the patient must be addressed. As with all patients, good surgical principles should be applied. Unstable patients will likely require earlier and more invasive measures as guided by the surgeon's experience.

Looking at the 2 categories of obstruction and peritonitis, they can be further characterized by:

- Peritonitis
  - Early
    - Gastrojejunostomy leak
    - Jejunostomy leak
  - Late
    - Perforated marginal ulcer
- Obstruction
  - Early
    - Gastrojejunostomy stricture (6–8 weeks)
  - Early or late
    - Internal hernia
      - Jejunojejunostomy (JJ) mesentery
      - Retro-roux limb (Petersen's hernia)
      - Mesocolic
      - Adhesive disease
    - Intussusception

Early peritonitis

Gastrojejunostomy leak

As peritonitis from a gastrojejunostomy (GJ) leak typically occurs on average at 10 days following surgery (range 5–15 days), it should be considered one of the early sources of peritonitis after LRYGB [18]. Leak rates in the most recent literature suggest that the rate ranges from 1% to 3% [19].

The typical patient who presents to an emergency room will have been discharged home on a standard postoperative diet, which in the early phase is typically a sugar-free liquid diet or purees. The presentation of a leak is often heralded by tachycardia, fever, and increasing abdominal pain. Other less-specific signs can include nausea, vomiting, tachypnea, shortness of breath, and altered mental status. Patients who present with these less-specific symptoms after bariatric surgery may be indicators of 1 of the 2 most concerning postsurgical complications: leak and pulmonary embolism. These presentations may be similar, with the most common sign being tachycardia. Imaging is critical in this setting, and CT scan remains a more sensitive test to detect a GJ leak.

Source control is of paramount importance [20,21]. Lavage and drainage should be the main focus of the initial approach. One may find a primary repair possible, but in the setting of significant contamination and/or a robust inflammatory response, primary closure may not be possible. In this setting, using the remnant stomach for placement of a gastrostomy tube provides both access for decompressing the gastrointestinal (GI) tract from an impending ileus as well as enteral feeding remote from the site of leak as the ileus improves. Use of broad-spectrum antibiotics is necessary here.

Endoscopic approaches have also been used in the setting of a GJ leak. This is typically initiated after primary source control is obtained. In a study by Puli and colleagues [22], the use of self-expanding covered stents allowed patients to begin a clear liquid or high-protein liquid diet within 24 to 48 hours after stent placement. The reported success rate in their series of stenting after GJ leaks was noted at 87% [22].

Although interventional radiology may have some role in the approach to these patients as possible early source control, they lack the ability to thoroughly lavage the abdomen.

Jejunojejunostomy leak

A less-often considered postoperative source of leak is that at the JJ. Although much less frequent than a GJ leak, because of the difficulty of recognizing the diagnosis, it carries a 40% higher mortality rate [23]. The delay in detection relates to it not being considered in cases, and that the modalities to detect suspected leaks are often focused on the GJ anastomosis. Many surgeons use an upper gastrointestinal study to evaluate the GJ, but continuing the evaluation to the JJ is not routinely carried out. With the more frequent use of CT scans, more subtle fluid collections in the area of the JJ should raise the suspicion of this being the potential source. If all imaging modalities have not produced an adequate source, visualization in the operating room is merited. Good surgical principles of sepsis control with lavage and drainage are the foundation of care. Broad-spectrum antibiotics should also be initiated.

Late peritonitis

Perforated marginal ulcer

Perforated marginal ulcer (MU) can be considered in the setting of late peritonitis given that the typical time of presentation after gastric bypass is approximately 18 months. Although less frequent than the other complications seen after gastric bypass, MU still seems to have a rate of about 0.5% to 1% [24,25]. The risk factors in the development of MU are listed here:

- Smoking[a]
- NSAIDs[a]
- Steroids[a]
- Nonabsorbable suture material
- Gastric acid hypersecretion
- *H. pylori* infection
- Recent surgery
- Alcohol use
- Stress

[a]More frequently associated with perforation.

A study by Felix found that the perforation rate was highest in patients who were smoking, taking nonsteroidal anti-inflammatory drugs (NSAIDs), or on steroids [26]. Their retrospective analysis of 3430 patients found that 35 (1%) had MU perforation. The factors most associated with perforation in their series were notable with 51% of patients actively smoking, 29% were taking NSAIDs, and 6% were taking steroids. The classic signs of perforated MU are tachycardia, fever and severe abdominal pain with abdominal rigidity and peritoneal signs. Imaging with plain films or CT scan will typically exhibit free air.

The operative approach can be laparoscopically or open and should be dictated by the surgeon's comfort level. Primary repair of the ulcer with omental patch or Graham patch is successful in the vast majority of patients [27,28]. Most authors advocate that the outcomes are improved when performed within the first 24 to 48 hours after the perforation. In addition to repair of the perforation, the abdomen should be washed out, as there will be contamination within the peritoneal cavity. Placement of a gastrostomy tube in the remnant stomach as a means for enteral access and as a decompressive tube in the setting of an expected ileus is similar to the treatment of an early GJ leak. Once the repair is complete, it is imperative to counsel the patient and identify the cause to prevent continued marginal ulceration. In addition to the use of antibiotics, one should also consider use of an antifungal given the flora in the contaminant.

Obstructive

Much like the categorization of peritoneal complications of gastric bypass, obstructive symptoms can be broken down into early and late complications.

Early obstruction

Gastrojejunostomy stricture

GJ strictures most commonly present in the sixth to eighth week after surgery and may occur in 3% to 27% of these cases [29,30]. The symptoms are progressive in nature, and based on timing most patients will have already advanced to a more regular postsurgical diet and then will relate classic symptoms of progressive inability to tolerate solids and then liquids. Dehydration is a primary concern in these patients, and they will require fluid resuscitation. Diagnosis can be made with an upper GI radiology examination. An upper endoscopy will be both diagnostic and therapeutic because dilation is the basis of treatment. Strictures can occur after any of the techniques for fashioning the GJ anastomosis. These include hand sewn, linear stapler, and circular staplers. In each of these instances the anastomosis size to achieve is approximately 15 mm. Pneumatic dilation is the recommended treatment of choice, with dilations achieving 15 mm [31]. The success of the dilation is higher if the stricture is treated earlier. Early dilations have a 98% success rate versus late interventions (61%) [32].

Late obstruction

Internal hernia

Obstruction following gastric bypass must be handled expeditiously. The reformed anatomy of the gastric bypass limits conventional conservative "bowel obstruction" techniques and requires urgent exploration in the operating room. General surgical postoperative obstructions can often be managed conservatively in more than 40% to 78% of patients [33,34]. However, in the setting of LRYGB, with a small gastric pouch and small gastrojejunal anastomosis, these patients cannot be treated with nasogastric tube decompression and bowel rest.

Symptoms for obstruction from an internal hernia mirror those of any postoperative bowel obstruction, with the classic symptoms of nausea, emesis, and abdominal pain. Because the overwhelming majority of gastric bypasses are done laparoscopically, one should always consider an internal hernia in the differential for abdominal pain. It is much more common to have an internal hernia after a laparoscopic gastric bypass compared with an open gastric bypass, in which adhesion formation is more common and tends to prevent internal hernias [35]. For example, the rate of internal hernia after open gastric bypass is 0% to 0.7% [36]. whereas the overall rate of internal hernia after LRYGB is about 2.5%, with study results ranging from as low as 0.2% to as high as 8%

[37,38]. Internal hernias most commonly present after the first year of surgery [39,40].

There are 2 defects of concern in the antecolic gastric bypass: the mesomesenteric or JJ mesenteric defect and Petersen's hernia (also known as the retro-roux limb hernia). Internal herniation most commonly occurs at the JJ mesenteric defect, occurring in 50% to 62% of all internal hernia cases. Petersen's hernia occurs in approximately 12% to 15% of internal hernia cases. In the retrocolic gastric bypass a third site of internal hernia is found at the transverse mesocolon [41,42].

Computed tomographic imaging of patients presenting with abdominal pain after gastric bypass can have some classic findings to suggest an internal hernia in the acute setting. The most sensitive and specific of these is a swirl sign of the mesentery [43]. Other signs suggestive of internal hernia are gastric remnant distention with or without air and the JJ on the patient's right side. Laboratory examination may reveal increased amylase and lipase in the setting of obstruction after gastric bypass. Spector found that when the biliopancreatic limb was obstructed there was an increase in the amylase and lipase levels, with 48% of all patients with a small bowel obstruction noted to have elevated levels [44]. When it was the biliopancreatic limb that was obstructed, 94% of patients had elevated amylase and lipase levels.

The surgeon should proceed directly to the operating room. Dependent on the surgeon's comfort level, either a laparoscopic or open approach can be performed, with the goal of reducing the internal hernia in a timely fashion before bowel ischemia is irreversible. Most surgeons advocate for directing their attention to the cecum and run the bowel proximally. By approaching the bowel from this direction, the hernia is reduced and the appropriate anatomy restored. There will be 3 limbs to identify. The common channel will have been identified as it is the distal bowel, now reduced. At this point the 2 proximal limbs will be the roux limb and the biliopancreatic limb. In the case of antecolic, this will be the roux limb that is encountered as it passes anterior to the colon. In the retrocolic bypass the most lateral small bowel at the mesentery should be the roux limb. The biliopancreatic limb will be medial and the ligament of Treitz can be identified.

All defects of the mesentery should be closed with permanent suture. The antecolic bypass can have 2 defects. The first defect, the retro-roux limb defect, should be closed from the colon to the root of the mesentery. The JJ mesenteric defect is the second area to be inspected and is the most common area for internal hernia. Any gap or opening here should also be closed. With the retrocolic gastric bypass there will be 3 defects that should be evaluated. Two of these defects are smaller and occur at the mesocolic window created by the retrocolic dissection and the retro-roux limb defect. The third potential defect is at the JJ mesentery as in the antecolic gastric bypass.

Intussusception

An uncommon presentation of obstruction after gastric bypass is intussusception, and it should be considered in the differential diagnosis of a patient presenting with obstructive symptoms. If a CT scan is performed during the patient's active episode, then imaging will likely reveal a "target sign." This is pathognomonic for intussusception. This most commonly occurs at the JJ. Although not completely understood, hypothetical mechanisms include a patulous JJ, disruption of intestinal pacemakers, and orientation of the JJ (isoperistaltic vs antiperistaltic) [45]. These patients will require a surgical intervention to reduce the bowel and will most likely need a revision or resection of the JJ.

GASTRIC BAND COMPLICATIONS

Before the rise of popularity of the LSG, the laparoscopic adjustable gastric band (LAGB) was seen by many bariatric surgeons as a reasonable, lower-risk yet lower-reward alternative to the LRYGB. Although once one of the most commonly performed bariatric operations in the United States, the LAGB has fallen out of favor as a primary bariatric operation and has been supplanted by the LSG. Nevertheless, a significant number of gastric bands remain implanted and, unfortunately, many patients have been lost to follow-up from their original bariatric surgeon. The gastric band has been associated with unique, device-related complications that can have devastating consequences if not managed appropriately or if care providers do not have an awareness of their impact.

Erosion

Erosion of the gastric band, either partially or completely, into the gastric lumen has an incidence between 0.2% and 4% [46]. Patients can present with weight regain, a loss of restriction, or infection of the access port or tubing. Imaging studies such as a swallow study or a CT scan can demonstrate orally ingested contrast material leaking around the gastric balloon portion. Occasionally, CT scanning will demonstrate fluid around the access port or tubing itself. Upper endoscopy can be used to confirm the diagnosis, although often band erosions are detected serendipitously during band removals for other diagnoses, such as prolapse or weight regain. Eroded bands can be removed laparoscopically or endoscopically, depending on the intragastric or extragastric location of the "buckle" of the balloon [47].

Slippage

Although the device is often anchored in place by a plication of gastric tissue, the LAGB balloon can be displaced cephalad or caudally, in a manner akin to a napkin sliding through a napkin ring. Patients can present with a nonemergent, chronic band slippage that often manifests as nausea, regurgitation, and loss of satiety. Emergent slippages can present with acute epigastric abdominal pain, obstruction, and sepsis from gastric ischemia. Acute band slippages can be diagnosed with a plain film radiograph that demonstrates a change in the angle of the band to an upright or flat position [48]. For patients with obstructive symptoms, an upper GI series will demonstrate the pooling of oral contrast above the band without passage of contrast through the balloon. Emergency measures include the removal of all fluid from the device, and if oral contrast passes through the band and no signs of gastric ischemia are present, the band can be removed in a less urgent setting. In all situations in which gastric ischemia is suspected or obstructions are not relived by the removal of fluid, the device should be removed urgently through a laparoscopic or open approach.

Esophageal dilation

A long-term consequence of the LAGB is development of esophageal dilation, with an estimated incidence as high as 50% [49]. With the progression of the dilation, esophageal motility can be affected, leading to reflux, dysphagia, regurgitation, loss of satiety, and eating-behavior modification [50]. It is speculated that overinflation of the balloon can lead to a chronic subclinical gastric obstruction. Often patients will have been lost to follow-up for some time, possibly unaware that their symptoms of reflux, nausea, or regurgitation are related to their LAGB. Esophageal dilation is diagnosed during a gastrograffin swallow. The standard initial treatment for this condition is removal of all fluid from the band circuit, as there is evidence that this "pseudoachalasia" is potentially reversible and salvageable [51]. It is unknown what the long-term implications are for chronic dilation of the esophagus related to LAGB, therefore, many bariatric surgeons elect to remove the band and perform a revisional, secondary salvage procedure such as a gastric bypass or sleeve [52].

NUTRITIONAL EMERGENCIES

Although there are various nutritional deficiencies that patients can exhibit after bariatric surgery, there are 2 that are considered emergent and should be on the forefront of the surgeon's mind.

Thiamine

Unrecognized thiamine (B1) deficiency can have permanent and disastrous consequences. It only takes 2 weeks to deplete the body's B1 stores. Several studies have found preoperative deficiency of B1 in patients ranging from 12% to 29% [53,54]. The primary location for B1 absorption occurs in the first part of the small intestine, and as such the altered anatomy of the gastric bypass or duodenal switch can exacerbate this deficiency. Limited oral intake and emesis can exacerbate this deficiency.

Nutritional guidelines as published by the ASMBS classifies B1 deficiency in 2 categories [55] (Table 1).

When this deficiency is suspected, rapid treatment is imperative. The guidelines for treatment include avoiding glucose in initial intravenous (IV) fluids, as this can worsen the symptoms and increase risk of permanent neurologic impairment. Lactated ringers or normal saline with an ampule of multivitamin

Table 1
Thiamine (B1) deficiency symptoms

Early:	Advanced:
• *Dry beriberi (without edema)*: characterized by brisk tendon reflexes, peripheral neuropathy and/or polyneuritis, muscle weakness and/or pain of the upper and lower extremities • *Wet beriberi*: heart failure with high cardiac output, edema in lower extremities, tachycardia or bradycardia, lactic acidosis, dyspnea, heart hypertrophy and dilation, respiratory distress, systemic venous hypertension, bounding arterial pulsations • *Other/gastroenterologic*: slow gastric emptying, nausea, vomiting, jejunal dilation or megacolon, constipation	• *Wernicke's encephalopathy*: polyneuropathy and ataxia, ocular changes (ophthalmoplegia and nystagmus), confabulation, short-term memory loss

can be initiated in the emergency room. In the advanced or severe form, the deficiency is treated with B1 500 mg IV q8 hours for up to 5 days followed by 250 mg IV daily until symptoms resolve. When switching to oral therapy, the dose is 100 mg 2 to 3 times per day.

Cobalamin (B12)

Preoperative B12 deficiency occurs in up to 18% of patients with obesity [56,57]. As with B1, there are also early and advanced manifestations of B12 deficiency. B12 stores are much greater than B1 stores, but it is still critical to recognize the signs and symptoms of this deficiency, as the consequences can be dire when left untreated (Table 2).

Treatment should consist of 1000 μg intramuscular or IV dose. For severe deficiencies treatment includes B12 1000 μg daily for 1 week and then weekly injections of 1000 μg for 1 month [58].

Table 2
Cobalamin (B12) deficiency symptoms

Early:	Advanced:
• Pernicious anemia, fatigue, anorexia, diarrhea • Numbness and paresthesia in extremities, ataxia • Lightheadedness or vertigo • Tinnitus • Palpitations	• Angina or congestive heart failure • Altered mental status

SUMMARY

The general surgeon will most likely be faced with bariatric surgical emergencies at some time in their career. Having a plan for the most common emergencies (surgical and nutritional) that one will encounter can save time for the surgeon and the patient. Applying good surgical principles with some of the specialized considerations covered in this article can have a dramatically positive effect for the patient.

References

[1] American Society for Metabolic and Bariatric Surgery. Estimate of bariatric surgery numbers, 2011-2017. Available at: https://asmbs.org/resources/estimate-of-bariatric-surgery-numbers. Accessed October 20, 2018.

[2] Sippey M, Kasten KR, Chapman WH, et al. 30-day readmissions after sleeve gastrectomy versus Roux-en-Y gastric bypass. Surg Obes Relat Dis 2016;12(5):991–6.

[3] Osland E, Yunus RM, Khan S, et al. Postoperative early major and minor complications in laparoscopic vertical sleeve gastrectomy (LVSG) versus laparoscopic Roux-en-Y gastric bypass (LRYGB) procedures: a meta-analysis and systematic review. Obes Surg 2016;26(10):2273–84.

[4] Gagner M, Buchwald JN. Comparison of laparoscopic sleeve gastrectomy leak rates in four staple-line reinforcement options: a systematic review. Surg Obes Relat Dis 2014;10(4): 713–23.

[5] Aurora AR, Khaitan L, Saber AA. Sleeve gastrectomy and the risk of leak: a systematic analysis of 4,888 patients. Surg Endo 2011;26:1509–15.

[6] Gonzalez R, Sarr MG, Smith CS, et al. Diagnosis and contemporary management of anastomotic leaks after gastric bypass for obesity. J Am Coll Surg 2007;204:47–55.

[7] Sakran N, Goiten D, Raziel A, et al. Gastric leaks after sleeve gasteectomy: a multicenter experience with 2834 patients. Surg Endosc 2012;27:240–5.

[8] Nguyen NT, Nguyen X-MT, Dholakia C. The use of endoscopic stent in management of leaks after sleeve gastrectomy. Obes Surg 2010;20:1289–92.

[9] Campos JM, Ferreira FC, Teixeira AF, et al. Sptotomy and balloon dilation to treat chronic leak after sleeve gastrectomy: technical principals. Obes Surg 2016;26(8):1992–3.

[10] Thomopoulos T, Thoma M, Navez B. Roux-En-Y fistulojejunostomy: a new therapeutic option for complicated post-sleeve gastric fistulas, video report. Obes Surg 2017;27(6):1638–9.

[11] Guerrier JB, Dietch ZC, Schirmer BD, et al. Laparoscopic sleeve gastrectomy is associated with lower 30-day morbidity versus laparoscopic gastric bypass: an analysis of the American College of Surgeons NSQIP. Obes Surg 2018;28(11):3567–72.

[12] Wang Z, Dai X, Xie H, et al. The efficacy of staple line reinforcement during laparoscopic sleeve gastrectomy: a meta-analysis of randomized controlled trials. Int J Surg 2016;25: 145–52.

[13] Deslauriers V, Beauchamp A, Garofalo F, et al. Endoscopic management of post-laparoscopy sleeve gastrectomy stenosis. Surg Endosc 2018;32(2):601–9.

[14] Rebibo L, Hakim S, Dhahri A, et al. Gastric stenosis after laparoscopic sleeve gastrectomy: diagnosis and management. Obes Surg 2016;26(5):995–1001.

[15] Alsina E, Ruiz-Tovar J, Alpera MR, et al. Incidence of deep vein thrombosis and thrombosis of the portal-mesenteric axis after laparoscopic sleeve gastrectomy. J Laparoendosc Adv Surg Tech A 2014;24:601–5.

[16] Belnap L, Rodgers GM, Cottam D, et al. Portal vein thrombosis after laparoscopic sleeve gastrectomy: presentation and management. Surg Obes Relat Dis 2016;12:1787–94.

[17] Tan SBM, Greenslade J, Martin D, et al. Portomesteric vein thrombosis in sleeve gastrectomy: a 10-year review. Surg Obes Relat Dis 2018;14:271–5.

[18] Spaniolas K, Kasten KR, Sippey ME, et al. Pulmonary embolism and gastrointestinal leak following bariatric surgery: when do major complications occur? Surg Obes Relat Dis 2016;12:379–83.
[19] Varban OA, Cassidy RB, Sheetz KH, et al. Technique or technology? Evaluating leaks after gastric bypass. Surg Obes Relat Dis 2016;12:264–72.
[20] Kim J, Azagury D, Eisenberg D, et al. ASMBS position statement on prevention, detection, and treatment of gastrointestinal leak after gastric bypass and sleeve gastrectomy, including the roles of imaging, surgical exploration, and nonoperative management. Surg Obes Relat Dis 2015;11:739–48.
[21] Augustin T, Aminian A, Romero-Talamás H, et al. Reoperative surgery for management of early complications after gastric bypass. Obes Surg 2015;26:345–9.
[22] Puli SR, Spofford IS, Thompson CC. Use of self-expandable stents in the treatment of bariatric surgery leaks: a systematic review and meta-analysis. Gastrointest Endosc 2012;75: 287–93.
[23] Lee S, Carmody B, Wolfe L, et al. Effect of location and speed of diagnosis on anastomotic leak outcomes in 3828 gastric bypass cases. J Gastrointest Surg 2007;11:708–13.
[24] Fringeli Y, Worreth M, Langer I. Gastrojejunal anastomosis complications and their management after laparoscopic Roux-en-Y gastric bypass. J Obes 2015;2015:698425.
[25] Lublin M, Mccoy M, Waldrep DJ. Perforating marginal ulcers after laparoscopic gastric bypass. Surg Endosc 2005;20:51–4.
[26] Felix EL, Kettelle J, Mobley E, et al. Perforated marginal ulcers after laparoscopic gastric bypass. Surg Endosc 2008;22:2128–32.
[27] Wheeler AA, de la Torre RA, Fearing NM. Laparoscopic repair of perforated marginal ulcer following Roux-en-Y gastric bypass: a case series. J Laparoendosc Adv Surg Tech A 2011;21:57–60.
[28] Wendling MR, Linn JG, Keplinger KM, et al. Omental patch repair effectively treats perforated marginal ulcer following Roux-en-Y gastric bypass. Surg Endosc 2012;27:384–9.
[29] Cusati D, Sarr M, Kendrick M, et al. Refractory strictures after Roux-en-Y gastric bypass: operative management. Surg Obes Relat Dis 2011;7:165–9.
[30] Qureshi A, Podolsky D, Cumella L, et al. Comparison of stricture rates using three different gastrojejunostomy anastomotic techniques in laparoscopic Roux-en-Y gastric bypass. Surg Endosc 2014;29:1737–40.
[31] Ukleja A, Afonso BB, Pimentel R, et al. Outcome of endoscopic balloon dilation of strictures after laparoscopic gastric bypass. Surg Endosc 2008;22:1746–50.
[32] Yimcharoen P, Heneghan H, Chand B, et al. Successful management of gastrojejunal strictures after gastric bypass: is timing important? Surg Obes Relat Dis 2012;8:151–7.
[33] Williams SB, Greenspon J, Young HA, et al. Small bowel obstruction: conservative vs. surgical management. Dis Colon Rectum 2005;48:1140–6.
[34] Aquina CT, Becerra AZ, Probst CP, et al. Patients with adhesive small bowel obstruction should be primarily managed by a surgical team. Ann Surg 2016;264:437–47.
[35] Monkhouse S, Morgan J, Norton S. Complications of bariatric surgery: presentation and emergency management – a review. Ann R Coll Surg Engl 2009;91:280–6.
[36] Capella R, Iannace V, Capella J. Bowel obstruction after open and laparoscopic gastric bypass surgery for morbid obesity. J Am Coll Surg 2006;203:328–35.
[37] Elms L, Moon RC, Varnadore S, et al. Causes of small bowel obstruction after Roux-en-Y gastric bypass: a review of 2,395 cases at a single institution. Surg Endosc 2014;28: 1624–8.
[38] Obeid A, Mcneal S, Breland M, et al. Internal hernia after laparoscopic Roux-en-Y gastric bypass. J Gastrointest Surg 2013;18:250–6.
[39] Ahmed AR, Rickards G, Husain S, et al. Trends in internal hernia incidence after laparoscopic Roux-en-Y gastric bypass. Obes Surg 2007;17:1563–6.
[40] Rogula T, Yenumula PR, Schauer PR. A complication of Roux-en-Y gastric bypass: intestinal obstruction. Surg Endosc 2007;21:1914–8.

[41] Harakeh ABA, Kallies KJ, Borgert AJ, et al. Bowel obstruction rates in antecolic/antegastric versus retrocolic/retrogastric Roux limb gastric bypass: a meta-analysis. Surg Obes Relat Dis 2016;12:194–8.
[42] Paroz A, Calmes J, Giusti V, et al. Internal hernia after laparoscopic Roux-en-Y gastric bypass for morbid obesity: a continuous challenge in bariatric surgery. Obes Surg 2006;16:1482–7.
[43] Karila-Cohen P, Cuccioli F, Tammaro P, et al. Contribution of computed tomographic imaging to the management of acute abdominal pain after gastric bypass: correlation between radiological and surgical findings. Obes Surg 2017; https://doi.org/10.1007/s11695-017-2601-1.
[44] Spector D, Perry Z, Shah S, et al. Roux-en-Y gastric bypass: hyperamylasemia is associated with small bowel obstruction. Surg Obes Relat Dis 2015;11:38–43.
[45] Stephenson D, Moon RC, Teixeira AF, et al. Intussusception after Roux-en-Y gastric bypass. Surg Obes Relat Dis 2014;10:666–70.
[46] Brown WA, Egberts KJ, Franke-Richard D, et al. Erosions after laparoscopic adjustable gastric banding. Ann Surg 2013;257:1047–52.
[47] Spann MD, Aher CV, English WJ, et al. Endoscopic management of erosion after banded bariatric procedures. Surg Obes Relat Dis 2017;13(11):1875–9.
[48] Keane T, Margulis AR, Dakin GF, et al. Imaging of patients after the Lap-Band System application. Abdom Imaging 2012;37:690–6.
[49] De Jong JR, Tiehof C, van Ramshorst B, et al. Esophageal dilation after laparoscopic adjustable gastric banding: a more systematic approach is needed. Surg Endosc 2009;23(12):2802–8.
[50] La Page PA, Kwon S, Lord SJ, et al. Esophageal dysmotility after laparoscopic gastric band surgery. Obes Surg 2014;24(4):625–30.
[51] Khan A, Ren-Fielding C, Traube M. Potenially reversible pseduoachalasia after laparoscopic adjustable banding. J Clin Gastroenterol 2011;45(9):775–9.
[52] Zhou R, Poirier J, Torquati A, et al. Short-term outcomes of conversion of failed gastric banding to laparoscopic sleeve gastrectomy or Roux-en-Y gastric bypass: a meta-analysis. Obes Surg 2018; https://doi.org/10.1007/s11695-018-3538-8.
[53] Carrodeguas L, Kaidar-Person O, Szomstein S, et al. Preoperative thiamine deficiency in obese population undergoing laparoscopic bariatric surgery. Surg Obes Relat Dis 2005;1:517–22.
[54] Flancbaum L, Belsley S, Drake V, et al. Preoperative nutritional status of patients undergoing Roux-en-Y gastric bypass for morbid obesity. J Gastrointest Surg 2006;10:1033–7.
[55] Parrott J, Frank L, Rabena R, et al. American Society for metabolic and bariatric surgery integrated health nutritional guidelines for the surgical weight loss patient 2016 update: micronutrients. Surg Obes Relat Dis 2017; https://doi.org/10.1016/j.soard.2016.12.018.
[56] Aasheim ET, Johnson LK, Hofsø D, et al. Vitamin status after gastric bypass and lifestyle intervention: a comparative prospective study. Surg Obes Relat Dis 2012;8:169–75.
[57] Majumder S, Soriano J, Cruz AL, et al. Vitamin B12 deficiency in patients undergoing bariatric surgery: preventive strategies and key recommendations. Surg Obes Relat Dis 2013;9:1013–9.
[58] Szomstein S, Nguyen DM. Nutritional complications and emergencies. In: Herron DM, editor. Bariatric surgery complications and emergencies. Cham (Switzerland): Springer; 2016. p. 269–82.

Advances in Surgery 53 (2019) 69–81

ADVANCES IN SURGERY

Trends in Palliative Surgical Care

Allison R. Wilcox, MD[a],
Sandra L. Wong, MD, MS[a,b,*]

[a]Department of Surgery, Dartmouth-Hitchcock Medical Center, 1 Medical Center Drive, Lebanon, NH 03756, USA; [b]Dartmouth Geisel School of Medicine, Hanover, NH 03755-1404, USA

Keywords

• Palliative surgery • Decision making • Palliative care • Metastasis

Key points

- Surgical palliative care addresses goals of care for a patient with a surgical problem including preservation of quality of life, reduction of suffering, and even prolongation of survival.
- In the setting of advances in systemic treatment, the indications for surgical intervention are rapidly shifting and now encompass considerations beyond hopeful preemption or end-of-the-line treatment.
- Expansion of palliative surgery now encompasses "adjuvant surgery" and a surgeon's role in determining the appropriateness of nonoperative management.
- Decision making in surgical palliative care involves data, but must also incorporate the presentation of treatment options in the context of a patient's preferences and treatment goals.

INTRODUCTION

A 1990 report from the World Health Organization offers one of the first and most widely referenced definitions of palliative care: "Palliative care is the active total care of patients whose disease is not responsive to curative treatment. Control of pain, of other symptoms, and of psychological, social and spiritual problems is paramount. The goal of palliative care is achievement of the best possible quality of life for patients and their families. Many aspects of palliative care are also applicable earlier in the course of the illness, in conjunction with anticancer treatment" [1].

Disclosure Statement: None.

*Corresponding author. Department of Surgery, Dartmouth-Hitchcock Medical Center, 1 Medical Center Drive, Lebanon, NH 03756. *E-mail address:* Sandra.L.Wong@hitchcock.org

https://doi.org/10.1016/j.yasu.2019.04.016
0065-3411/19/

The subspecialty of hospice and palliative medicine was not recognized with a certificate by the American Board of Medical Specialties until 2006 [2,3], but there has been a steady momentum of rapid growth and increasing recognition of palliative care benefits for patients and their families, as well as to hospitals and health care systems [4–9]. Palliative care specific to the surgical setting has benefitted from the recent growth of the field more broadly. Surgeons' academic interest in palliative care continues to evolve but use of more formalized palliative care services in surgery continues to lag behind that of medical specialties, and specific roles for palliative interventions are often less clear.

This article summarizes recent trends in palliative surgical care. We briefly provide an overview of the history of palliative care in the surgical setting and then review some of the most recent research findings in palliative surgical procedures for common diseases. To close, we look into the future of this discipline by considering the changing nature of how advanced surgical disease is managed.

EVOLUTION OF PALLIATIVE SURGICAL CARE

Surgical intervention is predominantly undertaken as a curative endeavor. Fix the broken arm. Remove the ureteral stone. Cut out the cancer. In the not-so-distant past, surgical palliative care primarily consisted of operative interventions designed to treat symptoms and/or preempt sequelae of the natural history of advanced and possibly incurable disease.

There are several overarching paradigms to consider in the palliative care of the surgical patient (Table 1) [2]. First, there is the generalized notion of palliative care, broadly encompassing an interdisciplinary team that addresses physical, psychological, spiritual, and practical burdens of illness. Surgical palliative care, or what might classically be thought of as palliative care for the surgical patient, addresses goals of care for a patient with a surgical problem including preservation of quality of life, reduction of suffering, and even prolongation of survival (eg, obstructing metastatic colon cancer relieved with diverting colostomy and treated with systemic chemotherapy). In turn, palliative surgery, although often a part of surgical palliative care, is a specific surgical intervention designed to treat the patient but not necessarily to cure the disease. There is clearly overlap of these concepts and strategies. It is also important to understand the opportunity to incorporate both concepts as part of a patient's overall care plan, including efforts aimed at treatment and cure.

There has been directed leadership from the American College of Surgeons (ACS) to advance research and education in surgical palliative care. In 1998 the ACS produced the Statement on Principles Guiding Care at the End of Life [10], and from there created the Surgical Palliative Care Workgroup, which first met in 2000 [11,12]. The ACS has promoted educational offerings in palliative care, with forums at national surgical meetings and the development of didactic curricula [13,14]. However, despite this increased attention, researchers recently found that there has been no meaningful improvement in surgeons' education in palliative care over the past decade, as measured by a regional survey of surgeons, medical oncologists, intensivists, and palliative

Table 1
Palliative care definitions

Palliative care	Medical care provided by an interdisciplinary team, including the professions of medicine, nursing, social work, chaplaincy, counseling, nursing assistant, and other health care professions, focused on the relief of suffering and support for the best possible quality of life for patients facing serious life-threatening illness and their families. It aims to identify and address the physical, psychological, spiritual, and practical burdens of illness.
Palliative medicine	Palliative medicine is the study and management of patients with active, progressive, and far-advanced disease, for which the prognosis is limited and the focus of care is the quality of life.
Surgical palliative care	Surgical palliative care is the treatment of suffering and the promotion of quality of life for patients who are seriously or terminally ill under surgical care [1].
Palliative surgery	A surgical procedure used with the primary intention of improving quality of life or relieving symptoms caused by advanced disease. Its effectiveness is judged by the presence and durability of patient-acknowledged symptom resolution.
Hospice	Hospice is variably used to describe (1) a philosophy of care; (2) a place of care; or (3) an insurance benefit, such as the Medicare Hospice Benefit. Hospice describes supportive care for patients and their families during the patients' final phase of life-limiting illness. The traditional goal of hospice care is to enable patients to be comfortable and free of pain, so that they live each day as contentedly as possible.

From Dunn GP. Surgical palliative care: recent trends and developments. Anesthesiol Clin 2012;30(1):13–28; with permission.

care physicians [15]. Deficiencies in palliative care training were associated with more aggressive treatment recommendations in advanced cancer case scenarios. Other research corroborates these findings, including one study that identified that few fellows in surgical oncology and hepatobiliary surgery programs report exposure to palliative care education during their training, although the impact on practice patterns was not evaluated [16].

Given the evidence demonstrating persistently low levels of exposure to palliative care education and training for surgeons, it follows that use of palliative care services for surgical patients may lag behind that for medical patients. A study published in 2018 by Olmsted and colleagues [17] evaluated the frequency of interventions in the last year of life for nearly 200,000 patients within the Veteran's Health Administration. The retrospective study found that surgical patients were significantly less likely than medical patients to receive palliative or hospice services in the last year of life and that more than 20% of patients had at least one surgical procedure in the last year of life.

Indeed, surgeons themselves identify barriers to offering palliative care for their patients, including inadequate education and training in palliative care and difficulty communicating around these difficult topics. Difficulty with prognostication and uncertainty were also reported as barriers to offering palliative care to their patients [18]. This reluctance to fully embrace palliative care may be in part because of its historic association with hospice care, which promotes an antiquated construct that palliative care is synonymous with end-of-life care or hopelessness. Although palliation is a goal unto itself, it should also be used as a means of complementing disease-targeted therapy and not viewed as either an aggressive or nihilistic approach per se.

Research reports in palliative surgical care have arguably been of variable quality, largely because they represent retrospective reviews, often of small cohorts of patients. Because these are often patients with advanced disease states, reported end points do not always convey meaningful outcomes and the retrospective nature of these studies is fraught with patient selection bias and they do not reflect the complex decision-making processes inherent in decisions to undergo (or defer) a palliative procedure. In 2016, Lilley and colleagues [19] published a systematic review of interventions aimed at improving quality and delivery of palliative care for surgical patients. The report found that palliative care interventions for surgical patients are beneficial, improving communication and reducing overall health care resources. However, the authors stated they were unable to perform a meta-analysis or draw many meaningful conclusions in light of dissimilar study methods across the studies they identified. In short, their review demonstrated that research into the paradigm of palliative care for the surgical patient is limited.

It is also worth noting that palliative care has largely been a service available to those in well-resourced settings. This has led to disparities in access to interdisciplinary palliative care services [20,21]. However, even in the absence of a palliative care team, all surgeons must be ready to incorporate palliative care principles into their scope of practice.

THERAPEUTIC TRENDS

Disease-specific guidelines in surgical palliative care remain scarce. Many have associated surgical intervention in patients with advanced conditions with significant morbidity and mortality [22,23]. Careful patient selection was the cornerstone of improved results, and there were, at best, modest gains in the ability to effectively prevent or treat symptoms related to incurable or advanced disease. On the other end of the spectrum, many took the nihilistic perspective that surgical palliation could have no benefit.

In the setting of advances in systemic treatment of some disease types, however, the indications for surgical intervention are rapidly shifting and now encompass considerations beyond hopeful preemption or end-of-the-line treatment. With this evolution is the expansion of the broader field of "palliative surgery" to include "adjuvant surgery" and a surgeon's role in determining the appropriateness of nonoperative management.

SURGICAL ONCOLOGY

Surgical oncologists have been the traditional prototype of surgeons who deal with palliative issues. Palliative surgery considerations were classically used to treat symptoms associated with advanced cancers at the end of life. Palliative surgery served to alleviate obstructive symptoms, as is the case with proximal colonic diversion in the setting of obstruction or placement of pleural drainage catheters to manage symptomatic malignant effusions. Indications broadened with preemptive procedures when unresectable cancers were encountered. For instance, surgical palliation in the setting of unresectable pancreatic cancer has long been a part of clinical practice and used to preempt downstream sequelae of tumor growth and subsequent gastric outlet obstruction and obstruction of the biliary tract [24]. Even in this classic example, the open gastrojejunostomy with biliary-enteric bypass option has evolved to include minimally invasive approaches, such as laparoscopic gastrojejunostomy (with or without jejunostomy) and consideration of an endoscopically placed biliary stent, noting the trade-offs between operative morbidity and durable palliation with patient performance status and overall life expectancy.

With the discovery of more effective systemic treatment regimens, surgical interventions that were previously purely palliative in intent began to form the foundation of multimodality, cancer-focused treatment. For example, there is well-accepted evidence over the past several years supporting improved survival (and survival that continues to improve) following palliative resection of asymptomatic primary tumors in stage IV colon cancer [25–27]. A meta-analysis published in 2018 found that overall and cancer-specific survival improved following tumor resection after years of evolving practice patterns [26]. "Successful" two-staged resections for stage IV colorectal cancer in the early 2000s have evolved, along with increasingly effective systemic options into more nuanced curative-intent management strategies for those with metastatic disease.

Similar findings were recently published in metastatic cervical cancer, demonstrating another solid organ tumor with improved survival associated with definitive local therapy in the setting of advanced disease [28]. All of these are retrospective studies, but their findings support resection of the primary tumor even in the setting of metastatic disease, largely a testament to the increasing effectiveness of systemic treatments.

In contrast, the results of the Carmena study [29], a randomized-controlled trial, were published in 2018 and challenged the role of primary surgical management in metastatic renal-cell carcinoma (RCC). The standard of care for the past two decades in metastatic RCC has been cytoreductive nephrectomy, and this was in fact one of the seminal examples of such a cytoreductive strategy followed by interleukin-2-immunomodulation. Yet in the past decade, more highly effective targeted therapies have emerged in the treatment of RCC. In this trial, patients with synchronous metastatic RCC were randomized to receive sunitinib (a receptor protein-tyrosine kinase inhibitor) or to undergo nephrectomy followed by sunitinib. Survival was not worse with sunitinib alone compared with sunitinib after surgery (18.4 vs 13.9 months, respectively, in a noninferiority trial). In the so-called Surgery Time (SURTIME) trial [30], investigators sought to investigate the approach of deferred cytoreductive nephrectomy, comparing sunitinib followed by nephrectomy (and subsequent sunitinib) with nephrectomy followed by use of sunitinib. The findings of the study were underpowered, but suggested noninferiority of deferred nephrectomy. Both studies challenge the long-held belief that primary nephrectomy plays an essential role in the management of metastatic RCC and herald a changing paradigm. New, highly effective targeted molecular therapy and immunotherapy regimens for a host of metastatic tumors are now accompanied by evolving indications for surgical intervention in the setting of advanced cancer; considerations for "palliative" resection of metastatic disease has morphed to that of "adjuvant surgery."

EMERGENCY SURGERY AND MALIGNANT BOWEL OBSTRUCTION

Comprehensive palliative care is often considered in patients with chronic terminal illnesses, and there is an increasing role for the same services in acute illnesses. Indeed, just as there is often an urgent or emergent need for surgical intervention in the acute setting, there is an increasing appreciation for the role of palliative care concomitant to these emergent evaluations. Moreover, acute changes in chronic conditions can challenge previously established goals of care and quality-of-life concerns.

Compared with elective surgical care, emergency surgery, particularly in older populations and those with chronic illness, is associated with greater morbidity and mortality for patients, and increased cost to hospitals and health systems [31–34]. Reports vary, but in patients with disseminated malignancy undergoing emergency surgery, 30-day morbidity and mortality rates have been found to be 50% and 27.9%, respectively [22]. A recent study specifically evaluated the outcomes of emergency major abdominal surgery in adults older than 65 years of age. The authors characterized study subjects by illness burden before undergoing emergency major abdominal surgery and found, unsurprisingly, that higher preoperative illness burden was associated with a higher risk of poor outcomes, such as in-hospital death and death within the first year after surgery [35]. These findings confirm inherent patient selection bias and, importantly, challenge us to more carefully consider all treatment alternatives. Surgical decision making for older adults is often complex, and only so much more so in the setting of an acute illness.

Better risk assessment and prognostication are ways to better inform decision-making processes. A 2017 study found reduced postoperative mortality for patients who underwent preoperative frailty screening [36]. Note that this study was conducted in the preoperative setting for patients undergoing elective, rather than emergency, surgery. Postoperative mortality decreased for all patients in the study, but most considerably for frail patients. Another study by the same group studied the impact of frailty screening on palliative care in the preoperative setting, demonstrating that preoperative palliative care consultation was associated with decreased postoperative mortality [37]. Although not explicitly able to be captured in either study, it may be inferred that in some instances operative decision making changed as a result of the frailty assessment and/or the palliative care consultation, including the decision not to operate.

Indeed, not operating is an important and emerging concept in surgical palliative care. Researchers have shown that even in patients who achieve initial symptom relief following palliative surgical intervention, more than half will have recurrent or new symptoms within months [23]. Several studies have been recently published raising questions about the role of operative intervention in a common surgical problem encountered in patients with advanced cancer: malignant bowel obstruction (MBO). MBO is most frequently associated with colorectal and ovarian cancers, but can also be seen in the setting of many malignancies ranging from melanoma to gastric cancer [38]. Obstruction can be secondary to new discrete masses or more diffuse processes, such as carcinomatosis. The presence or absence of these features often guides management strategies, but diagnosis of the latter can be elusive in the preoperative setting. The guiding principle of treatment, regardless of the cause, is symptom relief. However, the widely variable outcomes after operative intervention have made palliative surgery in these settings often frustrating and increasingly controversial.

An updated MBO systematic review [39,40] found that the operative intervention itself varied widely and reported outcomes were not routinely stratified by operation. In addition, patients experienced clinical resolution between 26.7% to more than 68% of the time, whereas return to oral intake ranged from 30% to 100%. The durability of symptom relief is incompletely reported and just one of many important end points for these patients. Quality of life is infrequently measured in an explicit fashion and the authors are often unable to draw reliable conclusions about the merits of operative intervention for MBO. A clinical trial comparing surgical and nonsurgical management strategies for MBO is underway (ClinicalTrials.gov identifier NCT02270450) [41]. Primary outcome measures include number of days alive and outside hospital; secondary end points include a focus on gastrointestinal function, such as ability to eat, days with nasogastric tube, days of intravenous hydration, and days of solid food. There is also specific measurement of quality of life outcomes.

BURNS AND SURGICAL CRITICAL CARE

Traditionally, the academic and clinical focus of palliative care has been on patients with malignant disease. There is also increasing integration of palliative care in surgical intensive care units (ICUs), where patients across the spectrum of surgical disease require interdisciplinary care to address their complex and varied needs.

For example, care for burn patients has been credited as one of the first areas of surgical palliative care [2,11]. Burn care involves intensive pain management while managing complex physiology and severe injuries. Because of historically low survival rates, burn care became a discipline well suited for integration of palliative care services [42]. However, a recent nationwide study published in 2018 evaluated the use of palliative care services in burn care and found that palliative care services may be underused in this population. The study found that elderly, comorbid, and more extensively burned patients were more likely to receive palliative care consultation. Encouragingly, there was also a linear increase in palliative care use over the course of the 10 years studied. Yet even at its peak, less than 6% of burn patients received formal palliative care consultation as part of their multimodality management [43].

In addition to the care of burn patients, critical care more broadly is a discipline ripe with opportunity for the engagement of palliative care. The extent of need is so great that some centers have even included an automatic palliative care consultation for all patients on admission to the ICU. Providers in surgical ICUs benefit from working with dedicated palliative care teams to assist in the care of critically ill patients [44]. The ACS Trauma Quality Improvement Program *Palliative Care Best Practice Guidelines*, published in 2017, supports the essential role for interdisciplinary palliative care in surgical ICUs while recommending that trauma care providers themselves should have a basic knowledge and skillset in palliative care. The *Guidelines* also reinforce the important theme that palliative care for trauma patients must proceed alongside, rather than instead of, life-saving care [14].

OVERARCHING WORK IN SURGICAL PALLIATIVE CARE

Given degrees of uncertainty, a research and action agenda becomes increasingly clear and there are ongoing efforts to help surgeons and their patients in their clinical decision making with regard to palliative intervention. Physicians crave prognostic certainty in quantifying outcomes, especially if risks of the procedure and the underlying condition may outweigh benefits hoped to be gained with an intervention. The use of the frailty index is helpful in guiding patient discussions, as are other risk calculators. Many prediction tools are being developed to better assess probability of specific outcomes given a set of measurable variables. Resultant estimates are incorporated into discussions about prognosis and likelihood of favorable outcomes or adverse events. A nomogram recently developed by researchers at the University of California at Davis Medical Center uses ACS National Surgical Quality Improvement Program data to estimate risk of 30-day morbidity and mortality following surgical intervention in patients with disseminated malignancy [22]. Efforts like these are designed to help providers better understand the risks of palliative interventions, so that they may be better informed when guiding patients in decision making.

Important work in the process of shared decision making is ongoing. Although risk assessment may take expected or anticipated best or worst-case outcomes into account and help present complex data in a more simplified manner, important information support for decision-making processes is still evolving. Decision making involves data, but must also incorporate the presentation of treatment options in the context of a patient's preferences, and treatment goals. Truly shared decision making requires dialogue in addition to information so that patient preferences are elicited and gains are matched with trade-offs that are assumed in exchange for the desired outcome. Education around the balance between medical recommendations and patient autonomy must inform surgeons' use of data and prognostic tools [45]. Efforts to develop conversation frameworks are a starting point for more patient-centered decisions and improved care in difficult acute and/or end-of-life settings, and there is an evolving concept that merely providing patients with evidence and inviting them to choose a treatment option is inadequate for true patient empowerment.

The relative weighting of "more is more" and "less is more" becomes less important. Conversation as "instrument of care" leverages evidence and an opportunity to uncover the best decision given a patient's circumstances and values [46], possibly avoiding futile surgical procedures or, conversely, possibly understanding trade-offs for a best case scenario and hoped-for outcome (Fig. 1). Work by the Schwarze group [45,46] has led to the development of a novel communication tool called "Best Case/Worst Case" to promote goal-concordant care following discussions about risk-risk acute surgical issues.

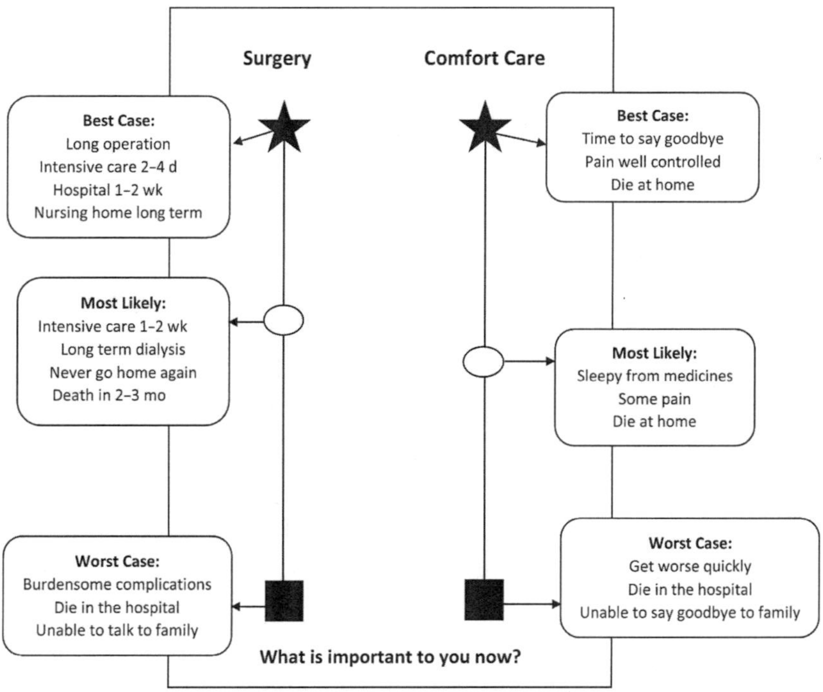

Fig. 1. Representative graphic aid example of "Best Case/Worst Case" communication tool. (*From* Taylor LJ, Adkins S, Hoel AW, et al. Using implementation science to adapt a training program to assist surgeons with high-stakes communication. J Surg Educ 2019;76:166; with permission.)

There remain appropriate scenarios for palliative surgery, and the importance of considering each case individually remains paramount. However, equally important to knowing when to operate is knowing when not to, and efforts continue to help guide surgeons and their patients through these complex decisions.

EVOLUTION OF PALLIATION AND FUTURE DIRECTIONS

Among the central challenges of palliative care, and certainly of palliative surgery, is that what is considered curable or treatable disease is a constantly moving target. Arguably, in light of the definitions of palliative care provided throughout this article and elsewhere, improved survival should be viewed as an important secondary benefit, rather than a primary aim, of palliative care. Patients with incurable diseases are living much longer than before because of advances in multimodal treatments including, among others:

- Surgery
- Chemotherapy
- Radiation
- Immunotherapy

However, among the more recently lauded benefits of palliative care is improved survival [9]. There is a dyad of optimal care for patients with incurable diseases; one suggests that operative intervention is beneficial, and the other suggests that operative intervention is, perhaps, unnecessary. A recent white paper defining research priorities for surgical palliative care included: measuring outcomes that matter to patients, communication and decision making, and a focus on how to deliver palliative care to surgical patients [47].

What is clear from these recent trends is that uncertainty is unavoidable. Better treatments and better predictive models are important advances, but engaging in patient discussions for shared decision-making trumps incremental improvements in surgical outcomes. Strategies for managing uncertainty and discussing uncertainty with patients can and should be taught so that decisions are made using data and patient preferences collectively, prioritizing patients' goals of care.

SUMMARY

Surgical palliative care, including considerations for palliative surgery, must be approached with the intention to relieve suffering and pursue therapeutic benefit where possible and desired. There are ongoing opportunities to provide palliative care to many who stand to benefit from it. Truly integrated and interprofessional palliative care services benefit the patient and their families; timely and comprehensive care improve quality and quantity of life. Although the medical and surgical nuances of palliation continue to evolve with practice-changing discoveries and continued innovations at the bench and in the operating room, "precision medicine" for surgical palliative care may come in the form of enhanced communication skills around decision making in the palliative setting.

References

[1] World Health Organization. Cancer pain relief and palliative care. Technical report series 804. Geneva (Switzerland): World Health Organization; 1990.

[2] Dunn GP. Surgical palliative care: recent trends and developments. Anesthesiol Clin 2012;30(1):13–28.

[3] ABMS subspecialty certification in hospice and palliative medicine. American Academy of Hospice and Palliative Medicine. Available at: http://aahpm.org/certification/subspecialty-certification. Accessed May 9, 2019.

[4] Moore S, Corner J, Haviland J, et al. Nurse led follow up and conventional medical follow up in management of patients with lung cancer: randomised trial. BMJ 2002;325(7373):1145.

[5] Morrison RS, Penrod JD, Cassel JB, et al. Cost savings associated with US hospital palliative care consultation programs. Arch Intern Med 2008;168(16):1783.

[6] Morrison RS, Meier DE. Palliative care. N Engl J Med 2004;350(25):2582–90.

[7] Zimmermann C, Riechelmann R, Krzyzanowska M, et al. Effectiveness of specialized palliative care. JAMA 2008;299(14):1698.

[8] Gade G, Venohr I, Conner D, et al. Impact of an inpatient palliative care team: a randomized controlled trial. J Palliat Med 2008;11(2):180–90.

[9] Temel JS, Greer JA, Muzikansky A, et al. Early palliative care for patients with metastatic non–small-cell lung cancer. N Engl J Med 2010;363(8):733–42.

[10] Statement on principles guiding care at the end of life. 1998. Available at: https://www.journalacs.org/article/S1072-7515(01)01019-5/pdf. Accessed October 8, 2018.

[11] Dunn GP, Milch RA. Introduction and historical background of palliative care: where does the surgeon fit in? J Am Coll Surg 2001;193(3):325–8. Available at: http://www.ncbi.nlm.nih.gov/pubmed/11548803. Accessed October 29, 2018.

[12] Dunn PG. Surgery, palliative care, and the American College of Surgeons. Ann Palliat Med 2015;4(1):5–9. Available at: http://apm.amegroups.com/article/view/5640/6427. Accessed October 8, 2018.

[13] Dunn GP. Surgical palliative care: a resident's guide. Available at: https://www.facs.org/~/media/files/education/palliativecare/surgicalpalliativecareresidents.ashx. Accessed October 28, 2018.

[14] ACS Committee on Trauma. ACS TQIP palliative care best practice guidelines 2017. Available at: https://docs.wixstatic.com/ugd/e37642_4cbc5155f36d42d492def2bd10d04455.pdf. Accessed September 18, 2018.

[15] Bateni SB, Canter RJ, Meyers FJ, et al. Palliative care training and decision-making for patients with advanced cancer: a comparison of surgeons and medical physicians. Surgery 2018;164(1):77–85.

[16] Amini A, Miura JT, Larrieux G, et al. Palliative care training in surgical oncology and hepatobiliary fellowships: a national survey of the fellows. Ann Surg Oncol 2015;22(6):1761–7.

[17] Olmsted CL, Johnson AM, Kaboli P, et al. Use of palliative care and hospice among surgical and medical specialties in the veterans health administration. JAMA Surg 2014;149(11):1169.

[18] Suwanabol PA, Reichstein AC, Suzer-Gurtekin ZT, et al. Surgeons' perceived barriers to palliative and end-of-life care: a mixed methods study of a surgical society. J Palliat Med 2018;21(6):780–8.

[19] Lilley EJ, Khan KT, Johnston FM, et al. Palliative care interventions for surgical patients. JAMA Surg 2016;151(2):172.

[20] Colibaseanu DT, Osagiede O, Spaulding AC, et al. The determinants of palliative care use in patients with colorectal cancer: a national study. Am J Hosp Palliat Care 2018;35(10):1295–303.

[21] Rauenzahn SL, Schmidt S, Aduba I, et al. Disparities in access to palliative care services among cancer patients in south Texas. J Clin Oncol 2016;34(26_suppl):130.

[22] Tseng WH, Yang X, Wang H, et al. Nomogram to predict risk of 30-day morbidity and mortality for patients with disseminated malignancy undergoing surgical intervention. Ann Surg 2011;254(2):333–8.
[23] Miner TJ, Brennan MF, Jaques DP. A prospective, symptom related, outcomes analysis of 1022 palliative procedures for advanced cancer. Ann Surg 2004;240(4):719–26 [discussion: 726–7].
[24] Sarr MG, Cameron JL. Surgical palliation of unresectable carcinoma of the pancreas. World J Surg 1984;8(6):906–18.
[25] Tarantino I, Warschkow R, Worni M, et al. Prognostic relevance of palliative primary tumor removal in 37,793 metastatic colorectal cancer patients: a population-based, propensity score-adjusted trend analysis. Ann Surg 2015;262(1):112–20.
[26] Ha GW, Kim JH, Lee MR. Meta-analysis of oncologic effect of primary tumor resection in patients with unresectable stage IV colorectal cancer in the era of modern systemic chemotherapy. Ann Surg Treat Res 2018;95(2):64–72.
[27] Lau JWL, Chang HSY, Lee KY, et al. Survival outcomes following primary tumour resection for patients with incurable metastatic colorectal carcinoma. experience from a single institution. J Dig Dis 2018;19(9):550–60.
[28] Venigalla S, Guttmann DM, Horne ZD, et al. Definitive local therapy is associated with improved overall survival in metastatic cervical cancer. Pract Radiat Oncol 2018;8(6): e377–85.
[29] Méjean A, Ravaud A, Thezenas S, et al. Sunitinib alone or after nephrectomy in metastatic renal-cell carcinoma. N Engl J Med 2018;379(5):417–27.
[30] Bex A, Mulders P, Jewett MAS, et al. LBA35 – Immediate versus deferred cytoreductive nephrectomy (CN) in patients with synchronous metastatic renal cell carcinoma (mRCC) receiving sunitinib (EORTC 30073 SURTIME). Presented at ESMO 2017, the Annual Congress of the European Society for Medical Oncology in Madrid, Spain, September 8–12, 2017.
[31] Scott JW, Olufajo OA, Brat GA, et al. Use of national burden to define operative emergency general surgery. JAMA Surg 2016;151(6):e160480.
[32] Cooper Z, Mitchell SL, Gorges RJ, et al. Predictors of mortality up to 1 year after emergency major abdominal surgery in older adults. J Am Geriatr Soc 2015;63(12):2572–9.
[33] Ingraham AM, Cohen ME, Raval MV, et al. Comparison of hospital performance in emergency versus elective general surgery operations at 198 hospitals. J Am Coll Surg 2011;212(1):20–8.e1.
[34] Ingraham AM, Cohen ME, Bilimoria KY, et al. Comparison of hospital performance in nonemergency versus emergency colorectal operations at 142 hospitals. J Am Coll Surg 2010;210(2):155–65.
[35] Cooper Z, Lilley EJ, Bollens-Lund E, et al. High burden of palliative care needs of older adults during emergency major abdominal surgery. J Am Geriatr Soc 2018;66(11):2072–8.
[36] Hall DE, Arya S, Schmid KK, et al. Association of a frailty screening initiative with postoperative survival at 30, 180, and 365 days. JAMA Surg 2017;152(3):233.
[37] Ernst KF, Hall DE, Schmid KK, et al. Surgical palliative care consultations over time in relationship to systemwide frailty screening. JAMA Surg 2014;149(11):1121.
[38] Roses RE, Folkert IW, Krouse RS. Malignant bowel obstruction: reappraising the value of surgery. Surg Oncol Clin N Am 2018;27(4):705–15.
[39] Feuer DD, Broadley KE, Shepherd JH, et al. Surgery for the resolution of symptoms in malignant bowel obstruction in advanced gynaecological and gastrointestinal cancer. Cochrane Database Syst Rev 2000;(4):CD002764. In: Feuer DD, editor. Chichester (United Kingdom): John Wiley & Sons, Ltd.
[40] Cousins SE, Tempest E, Feuer DJ. Surgery for the resolution of symptoms in malignant bowel obstruction in advanced gynaecological and gastrointestinal cancer. Cochrane Database Syst Rev 2016;(1):CD002764.

[41] Surgery or non-surgical management in treating patients with intra-abdominal cancer and bowel obstruction. Available at: https://clinicaltrials.gov/ct2/show/NCT02270450. Accessed May 9, 2019.
[42] Jeschke MG, Pinto R, Kraft R, et al. Morbidity and survival probability in burn patients in modern burn care. Crit Care Med 2015;43(4):808–15.
[43] Sheckter CC, Hung K, Rochlin D, et al. Trends and inpatient outcomes for palliative care services in major burn patients: a 10-year analysis of the nationwide inpatient sample. Burns 2018;44(8):1903–9.
[44] Tilden LB, Williams BR, Tucker RO, et al. Surgeons' attitudes and practices in the utilization of palliative and supportive care services for patients with a sudden advanced illness. J Palliat Med 2009;12(11):1037–42.
[45] Kopecky KE, Urbach D, Schwarze ML. Risk calculators and decision aids are not enough for shared decision making. JAMA Surg 2019;154(1):3–4.
[46] Taylor LJ, Adkins S, Hoel AW, et al. Using implementation science to adapt a training program to assist surgeons with high-stakes communication. J Surg Educ 2019;76:165–73.
[47] Lilley EJ, Cooper Z, Schwarze ML, et al. Palliative care in surgery: defining the research priorities. Ann Surg 2018;267:66–72.

Advances in Surgery 53 (2019) 83–101

ADVANCES IN SURGERY

Management of Difficult Dialysis Access Issues for Dialysis Patients

Matthew J. Dougherty, MD[a,*], Douglas A. Troutman, DO[a], Krystal C. Maloni, MD[b]

[a]Section of Vascular Surgery, Pennsylvania Hospital, University of Pennsylvania, 700 Spruce Street, Suite 101, Philadelphia, PA 19106, USA; [b]Pennsylvania Hospital, University of Pennsylvania, 700 Spruce Street, Suite 101, Philadelphia, PA 19106, USA

Keywords

• Arteriovenous fistula • Arteriovenous graft • Tunneled dialysis catheter • Stenosis • Thrombosis • Steal syndrome • Erosions • Aneurysm

Key points

- The demand for hemodialysis access is increasing and many challenges remain.
- Improvements in prevalence of autogenous access has not reduced the need for improvements in maintenance and treatment of complications of hemoaccess.
- The usefulness of endovascular technologies has increased, but surgical therapies will remain important for the foreseeable future.

HEMODIALYSIS ACCESS

Tunneled dialysis catheters

Tunneled dialysis catheters (TCD) are an essential component of the dialysis access armamentarium, despite many shortcomings [1]. These devices serve as a nidus for infection, stenosis, and thrombosis, and are associated with more complications than any other mode of dialysis access. TCD use often comes down to necessity, allowing for immediate use. They are often used as a bridge until more durable hemoaccess is achieved. Eighty percent of US patients initiate hemodialysis with TCDs, and mean time of TCD dialysis exceeds 3 months [2].

Disclosure Statement: The authors have nothing to disclose.

*Corresponding author. *E-mail address:* mdougherty@pavascular.com

https://doi.org/10.1016/j.yasu.2019.04.005

The preferred site for TCD placement is the right internal jugular vein, because of better patency, likely reflecting a straighter path to the superior vena cava (SVC) than the left jugular vein [3]. Subclavian veins should rarely be used, as approximately 50% will develop stenosis that will complicate upper extremity access [3]. For patients who have exhausted conventional sites for access, transhepatic and translumbar catheters can be considered [4,5].

Arteriovenous fistula

Since its first description in 1966, the creation of an accessible primary arteriovenous fistula (AVF) has been considered the first option for hemoaccess [6]. Duplex vein mapping is essential to hemoaccess planning. Larger vein size correlates with increased maturation success as well as long-term patency [7]. A vein diameter greater than 3 mm is generally sufficient, provided adequate arterial inflow is obtained. When planning for hemoaccess, dialysis dependence should be a consideration. Patients on dialysis with a TCD may require months of catheter use awaiting AVF maturation. Upper extremity access is much preferred to lower extremity options, as the latter entail more complications and morbidity.

The radiocephalic fistula is the best first choice, as it does not compromise more proximal future options. A brachial-cephalic fistula is the most common conformation in today's dialysis population. The brachial-basilic transposition fistula has increased in prevalence in the last 2 decades. There remains controversy as to whether staging the transposition procedure is beneficial [8].

Obesity poses a challenge in AVF creation [9]. Increased subcutaneous tissue and depth of veins increases the technical challenge of the surgery and decreases the likelihood of optimal cannulation. These patients may require a secondary superficialization procedure such as lipectomy, liposuction, and/or surgical elevation; prolonging maturation time [9].

Lower extremity access is often pursued after upper extremity options have been exhausted, generally in the setting of central venous occlusion. The saphenous vein is a poor autogenous option, but femoral vein transposition is a durable, albeit morbid, option [10].

Although surgical AVF construction generally involves minimal incisional morbidity, percutaneous techniques of establishing autogenous access have been developed and are of increasing interest, with early results that seem promising [11].

Arteriovenous grafts

For patients who do not have adequate vein for fistula creation in the upper extremity, an arteriovenous graft (AVG) can be constructed. AVGs can be configured in either looped or straight conformation, and tunneled in a fashion to allow for convenient cannulation and hemostasis. The brachial artery is most commonly used for inflow.

More exotic options for AVG placement include brachial artery to jugular vein, axillary artery to contralateral/ipsilateral jugular or axillary vein. Patency has been reported to be equivalent to upper extremity grafts, with fewer complications than lower extremity AVGs [12]. Lower extremity AVGs are generally constructed in the thigh, and carry higher risks of infectious and ischemic complications than upper extremity grafts [13,14]. Avoidance of a groin incision with lower extremity AVGs construction may reduce infection risk.

The "Fistula First" effort spearheaded in the United States by the National Kidney Foundation in 2003 aimed to reduce TCD and AVG use, and the complications associated with these. The effort successfully increased autogenous access prevalence in the United States from 22% to 58% [15]. However, this approach has resulted in a significant primary failure rate for autogenous access, which has prolonged catheter use time. Patients with borderline vein quality and limited life expectancy may be better served by graft construction, especially in the octogenarian population [2].

Conduit options for arteriovenous graft

Considerations for graft material include size match, mechanical strength, thrombogenicity, tissue incorporation, ease of handling, resilience to repeated punctures, infection, myointimal hyperplasia, resistance, and cost. Biologic (primarily bovine xenograft) and prosthetic conduits (dacron and expanded polytetrafluoroethylene [PTFE]) have been used for nearly 5 decades. Multiple modifications have been attempted at improving primary patency rates, which remain poor, averaging 6 months or less [16].

PTFE has been by far the most common prosthetic material used; however there are several alternatives and modifications available. These include carbon coating, heparin binding, and multilayer design for early cannulation. Biologic grafts commercially available include bovine mesenteric vein (ProCol, LeMaitre); bovine ureter (SynerGraft, CryoLife); and bovine carotid artery (Artegraft). Human cryopreserved allografts have also been used in limited applications (CryoLife).

For xenografts, the bovine carotid graft has been received most recent attention. A small but provocative randomized trial demonstrated a large patency advantage compared with PTFE [17]. Several larger series in the last few years have also suggested, but not proven, possible patency and infection advantages over PTFE [18,19]. Early cannulation, often within 24 hours, has been used in 1 report (UCLA data), which may avoid the need for catheter access [20].

Tissue-engineered grafts

An area of ongoing interest is the development of a bioengineered vascular conduit. No such conduits are currently commercially available, but phase 2 and 3 trials are underway. These consist of tissue-cultured conduit scaffolds that have been implanted with some success [21]. This may prove a promising alternative to currently available prosthetic materials, with their manifest limitations of poor patency.

Arteriovenous fistula versus arteriovenous graft

AVFs experience higher patency and lower reintervention rates than AVGs, in the range of a 2- to 4-fold advantage. However, high primary maturation failures for AVF skews these data, and individual considerations should influence access choice [22]. Advanced age has been identified as a risk factor for failure of maturation of fistula and decreased patency [23]. In 1 series, patients over 65 had a 1.7 relative risk of maturation failure compared with younger patients [24], and radial-cephalic AVF do poorly in patients over 75 [25]. Longevity and frailty are important considerations [26,27]: 2-year mortality exceeds 50% in patients initiating dialysis over the age of 75 years (Fig. 1) [27,28].

COMPLICATIONS

Thrombosis/stenosis

Of complications and problems associated with hemoaccess, none is more prevalent than the development of stenosis and occlusion of these circuits. The biology is different than observed with arterial bypass grafts, and patency results are far inferior. Although surveillance to identify stenosis before occlusion is an attractive concept, no patency advantage has been demonstrated with routine duplex surveillance protocols for hemoaccess [29].

Clinical monitoring for efficacy of dialysis, excessive pulsatility, puncture site bleeding, recirculation, or other evidence of declining access function, is the usual approach to identify hemoaccess that warrants imaging. In the last 2 decades, endovascular treatment has supplanted surgical revision as first-line therapy for most patients. In the setting of hemoaccess occlusion, despite previous trials suggesting superior results with surgical treatment, catheter-based intervention is first choice for secondary patency, primarily due to decreased morbidity and easier access to intervention facilities than the operating room [30–32].

There are a variety of mechanical thrombectomy catheters used to restore hemoaccess patency. These include the AngioJet catheter (Boston Scientific, Watertown, MA), Arrow-Treratola Device (Teleflex, Inc, Morrisville, NC),

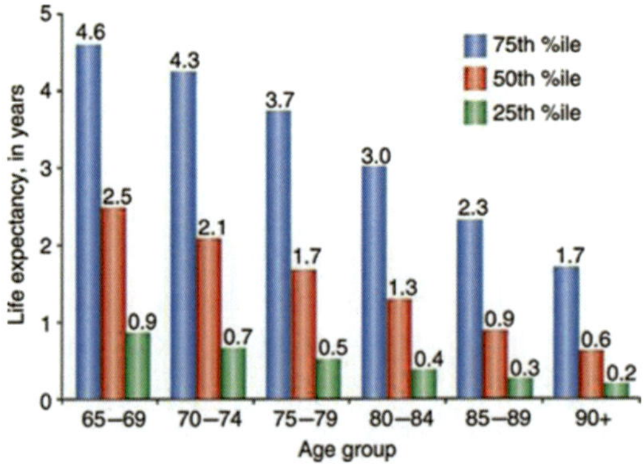

Fig. 1. Life expectancy in years after initiating dialysis. (*From* Tamura MK, Tan JC, O'Hare AM. Optimizing renal replacement therapy in older adults: a framework for making individualized decisions. Kidney Int. 2012;82:262; with permission.)

and Penumbra catherer (Penumbra, Inc, Almeda, CA). Thrombolytic agents, combined with catheter aspiration have also proved effective for declotting hemoaccess. Most thromboses are associated with an underlying stenotic lesion, which is then treated with balloon angioplasty. As lesions tend to be fibrous in nature, elastic recoil is common. High-pressure and cutting balloons may offer advantages, but stenting is sometimes needed to achieve technical success [33].

In the early 1990s, comparative studies of primary bare metal stenting demonstrated no long-term benefit compared with angioplasty alone; however, several recent randomized trials have documented the superiority of covered stents to angioplasty alone when treating lesions in patients with dialysis grafts [34–36]. A recent randomized trial looking specifically at treatment of in-stent stenosis in AVFs likewise showed superiority of stent graft treatment compared with angioplasty alone (Fig. 2) [36,37].

There are no randomized controlled trials comparing stent grafts to bare metal stents, which is unfortunate given the marked cost difference (covered stents are approximately double the cost of bare metal stents). Recurrent myointimal hyperplasia is the primary cause of hemoaccess failure, whether treated with angioplasty alone or stented. Therefore, drug-eluting stents and drug-coated balloons offer promise in this regard, although data are still limited (Fig. 3) [38,39].

Central venous stenosis and occlusion can be difficult to treat. The 2 most common factors causing central stenosis or occlusion are the presence of pacemaker leads and the prolonged use of TCDs. These lesions at the central level are less likely than peripheral lesions to precipitate hemoaccess thrombosis. More typically they cause increased venous pressure, prolonged access site bleeding, recirculation, upper extremity edema, as well as cervicocephalic edema (sometimes SVC syndrome).

Percutaneous intervention is the preferred approach for central venous stenosis/occlusions, but recurrent stenosis is common and often leads to multiple interventions. A venous area particularly prone to development of stenosis is within the subclavian vein at the thoracic inlet. Because of extrinsic compression, these are often recalcitrant lesions. Stents should be avoided as they are prone to fracture due to extrinsic forces. Surgical decompression with first rib excision can be used, but is often also avoided in these patients because of considerable comorbidity [40].

Central venous occlusions have been a recent focus of attention. Recanalization (laser, radiofrequency, and sharp needle) have been combined with stent graft or HeRO device deployment to allow for continued upper extremity dialysis access [41]. The "inside out" approach has been described, accessing the SVC via the femoral vein. A long sheath and dilator are advanced with a stiff wire into the cervical soft tissue. The wire is retrieved and a sheath advanced from above, through which a TCD or HeRO device can be advanced into the SVC [42].

Infection

Infection is the second leading cause of mortality in dialysis patients, accounting for 15% to 20% of deaths, with about 20% of these infections due to

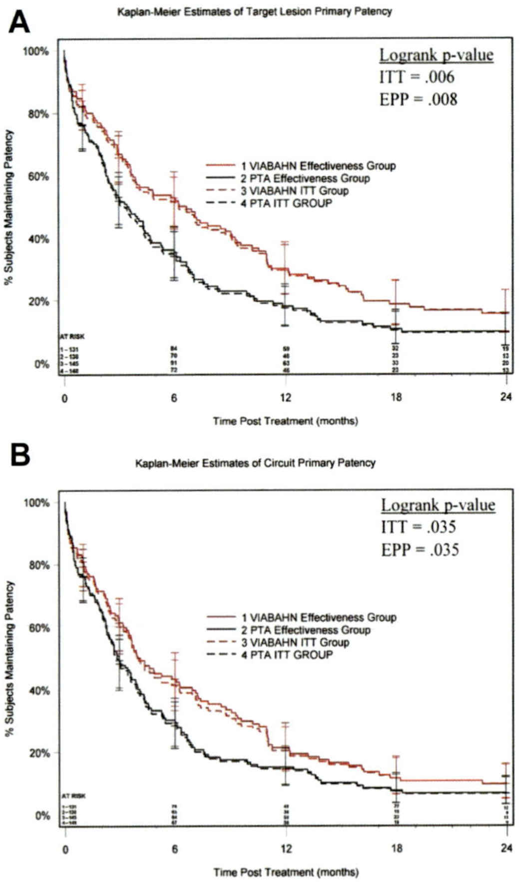

Fig. 2. Stent grafts improve primary patency of target lesion and access circuit compared with balloon angioplasty. (*A*) Kaplan-Meier estimates of primary patency of the target lesion and (*B*) access circuit. In all cases, stent grafts demonstrated statistical superiority in patency compared with balloon angioplasty. (*P* values shown in each panel were calculated using the log-rank test.) EPP, effectiveness-per-protocol; ITT, intention to treat; PTA, percutaneous transluminal angioplasty. (*From* Vesely T, Davanzo W, Behrend T, Dwyer A, Aruny J. Balloon angioplasty versus Viabahn stent graft for treatment of failing or thrombosed prosthetic hemodialysis grafts. Journal of Vascular Surgery. 2016;64(5): 1408; with permission.)

hemoaccess [43]. TCD infections are very common, and when associated with bacteremia, are best treated with removal of the infected catheter and antibiotic therapy. It is important to remove infected TCDs in a timely matter to help prevent bacterial seeding of other prosthetic implants. Catheter salvage rates are poor (25%–32%) with antibiotic treatment alone [15,44].

AVFs have the lowest infection risk, whereas infection rates of 4% to 17% have been reported for AVGs [15,18]. Biological grafts may confer a lower infection risk than prosthetic grafts [18]. Location of AVG implantation also

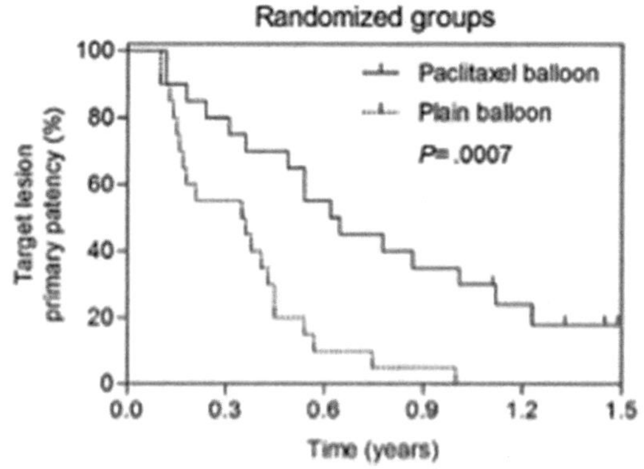

Fig. 3. Kaplan-Meier survival analysis of target lesion primary patency of all cases (those with AVF as well as grafts) randomized between drug-eluting balloon and brachio-axillary angioplasty treatment. (*From* Kitrou PM, Katsanos K, Spiliopoulos S, Karnabatidis D, Siablis D. Drug-eluting versus plain balloon angioplasty for the treatment of failing dialysis access: Final results and cost-effectiveness analysis from a prospective randomized controlled trial (NCT01174472). European Journal of Radiology. 2015;84(3):420; with permission.)

influences the rate of infection, with lower extremity AVG rates reported up to 41% [45,46].

An infected AVG requires a more complicated algorithm for treatment. *Staphylococcus aureus* (methicillin-susceptible and -resistant) is responsible for 70% of all access infections, whereas Gram-negative bacteria cause about 25% of infections [47]. In the presence of systemic sepsis or hemorrhage, urgent excision of the access is required. If a more indolent or localized infection is present, then complete or partial salvage of the access can be attempted. Usually a "jump graft" is performed around the infected portion of the graft. Once incisions are isolated, the infected remnant of the graft is excised. This technique is acceptable with the presence of less-virulent Gram-positive organisms [47]. More virulent infections (eg, methicillin-resistant *S aureus* and Gram-negative bacteria) are best treated with total or subtotal graft excision. Reconstruction of a brachial artery in the setting of gross infection can be technically difficult. Ligation of the brachial artery below the level of the profunda brachii is tolerated in most individuals and can be used when arterial reconstruction is either difficult or not feasible.

Dialysis-associated steal syndrome

Creation of an arteriovenous shunt causes an alteration of flow dynamics both systemically and locally. Although compensatory increases in inflow occur rapidly, sometimes as much as 20-fold, the perfusion bed distal to the arterial anastomosis has more limited adaptation [48]. The physiologic drop in pulse volume and pressure measurements in the extremity become pathologic in a proportion of patients, producing ischemic symptoms. The most common presentation involves:

- Numbness
- Coldness
- Paresthesias
- Pain in the digits and hand (for upper extremity access)

Acral ulceration and gangrene can occur in more advanced cases. The incidence of such complications ranges from 4% to 20%, and is more common in patients with diabetes mellitus and peripheral vascular disease [49,50]. Female gender and tobacco use may also increase dialysis-associated steal syndrome (DASS) risk [51]. Diminished digital plethysmography on preoperative studies can predict elevated risk of DASS, but no threshold value has been validated [52]. Distal brachial artery inflow seems to carry the highest risk of producing a steal syndrome. In most patients having prosthetic access, symptoms develop soon after the surgery. In patients with AVFs, symptoms may develop slowly and progress as the venous resistance diminishes with venous dilatation [53].

Diagnosis

DASS is a clinical diagnosis because it is a dynamic pathology and there is a significant variability of symptoms and examination findings depending on systemic hemodynamics. Low blood pressure states exacerbate steal symptoms, and use of the access for hemodialysis will typically worsen symptoms. Indeed, many patients *only* have steal symptoms while on the dialysis circuit.

It is important to discriminate ischemic symptoms from neuropathic symptoms. Hemodialysis patients, many of whom have preexisting neuropathies, are particularly prone to such symptoms. Most, but not all, patients with clinically significant steal will have absent radial and ulnar pulses to palpation. In many, compression of the access restores the pulse, and, when this causes immediate symptom relief, it is highly predictive of reversibility.

Diagnostic imaging

Arterial physiologic studies can be very helpful in the diagnosis and assessing of severity of steal syndrome [54]. A positive study will show markedly diminished digital pressures and pulse volume recordings at baseline, with significant normalization with access compression (Fig. 4). Some authors have suggested that flow reversal in the donor artery distal to the AVF is indicative of steal [55]. However flow reversal at this location is quite common in asymptomatic patients, and therefore very nonspecific in diagnosing DASS. Duplex calculated volume flow parameters can be helpful in identifying high flow fistulae, which may be more prone to producing steal symptoms. This parameter may also inform treatment options.

Arteriography is not particularly useful as a diagnostic modality but may be crucial to planning treatments. Inflow lesions of the subclavian and axillary artery may be identified in a small percentage of steal patients. Angiography is performed with a catheter placed proximal to the arterial anastomosis. In patients who experience ischemic steal, there will generally be no visualization of the distal vessels unless one performs digital compression of the access. In

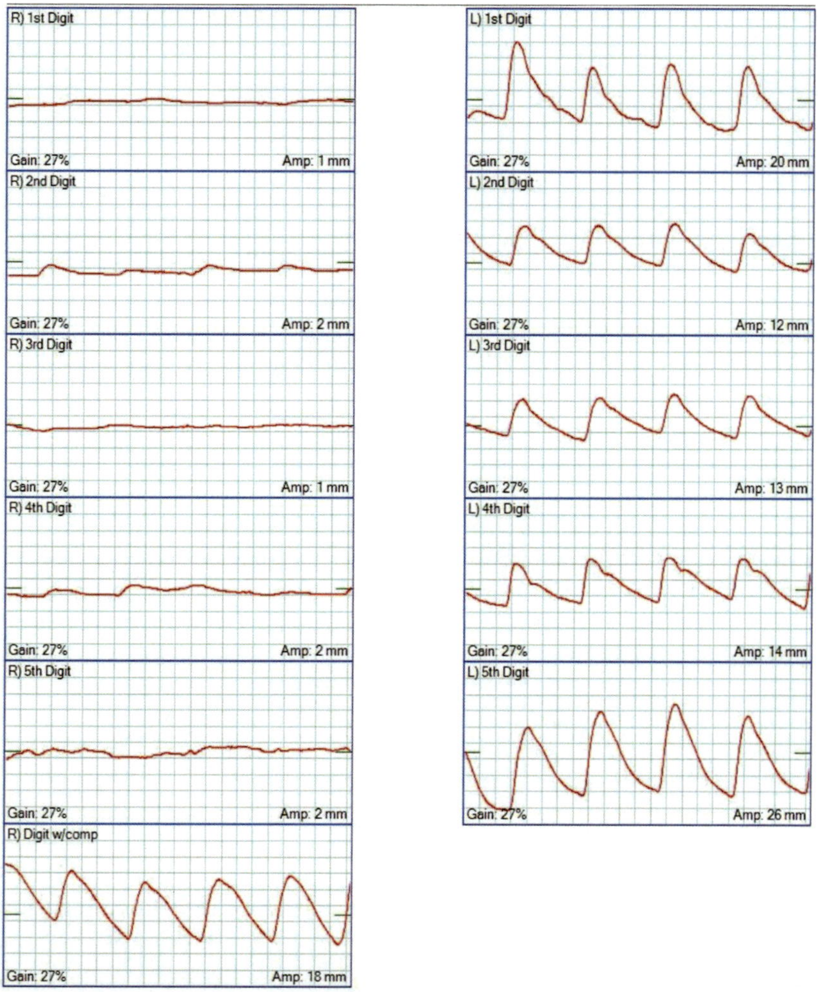

Fig. 4. This is an example of a steal study. The right digital waveforms are flat consistent with ischemia. This is compared with the left digits, which have normal waveforms. As seen in the last waveform on the right, the flow to the right digit augments with compression of the fistula/graft, indicative of steal.

our experience the most common arteriographic finding in patients with symptomatic steal is that of diffuse outflow disease affecting the radial, ulnar, and interosseous arteries in the forearm and hand. This anatomy is important to consider when surgical or endovascular intervention is recommended.

Interventions for steal

Ligation. Closing the access that caused ischemic steal syndrome is the simplest and most immediately effective mechanism to restore distal perfusion to baseline. In patients who develop *severe* steal symptoms *immediately* after access creation, immediate ligation is appropriate to minimize postischemic neuropathy that can occur in this setting. Simple surgical ligation is the most common approach, but coil embolization can also be used. This has been reported for interruption of flow reversal in the radial artery, and is an attractive option in patients with normal arterial outflow and a complete palmar arch [56]. For AVGs, occlusion can sometimes be accomplished with prolonged digital or tourniquet compression.

Unfortunately, complete ligation leaves the patient without durable hemoaccess, and many have limited alternatives. If a patient has developed steal in one extremity, the likelihood of similar symptoms with contralateral access is high. However history of DASS on the ipsilateral side does not preclude more proximal graft placement [57].

Banding. Restricting rather than eliminating access flow is a logical option. Unfortunately the variability and complexity of the hemodynamic responses make the results of this approach somewhat unpredictable. Thrombosis is a common event in AVGs, and lowering flow in a prosthetic graft will likely increase this risk. High flow and autogenous accesses are better suited for banding.

Banding has been performed surgically with a variety of techniques to interpose a higher-resistance segment in the shunt circuit, usually at that arterial end to avoid recirculation and elevated pressure at puncture sites. A midaccess banding may be appropriate in patients with low-flow fistulae to allow an arterial cannula below the band to improve dialysis circuit flow. Endovascular banding has been described, but data are limited and we do not believe this provides a reliable and adjustable flow restriction [58]. Our technique for banding uses surgical clips to produce a smooth tapered narrowing of varying length and diameter.

We use either palmar arch Doppler flow signals or digital plethysmography cuffs to assess the hemodynamic effect of various degrees of plication. Restoration of biphasic Doppler flow with good pulsatile waveforms, while maintaining an adequate fistula flow as assessed by thrill palpation, is the goal. Once this has been accomplished, several mattress sutures are placed at the base of the clips, as it is not uncommon for clips to migrate off the fistula or graft over time (Fig. 5).

Distal revascularization with interval ligation. First reported by Schanzer in 1988, the DRIL procedure (distal revascularization with interval ligation) has come to be considered the most effective access-preserving procedure for dialysis-related steal syndrome. The technique involves placing a bypass originating at least 5 cm (ideally 10 cm) proximal to the arterial anastomosis, and ligating the artery just below the anastomosis (Fig. 6). The bypass is then performed distal to the ligation, ideally with saphenous vein conduit. Although reported results suggest a greater than 90% efficacy (compared with banding success in 70%–80%) the procedure involves significant morbidity and may not be suitable for many patients [59,60]. Ligation of the native artery in patients with

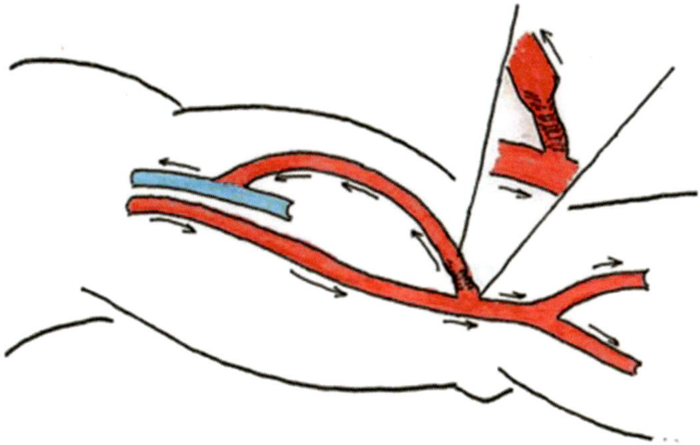

Fig. 5. Demonstrating banding of an arteriovenous fistula with surgical clips placed just distal to the anastomosis as well as mattress sutures to reinforce clips.

hand ischemia is unappealing to many, and some have suggested this can be omitted [59].

Revascularization using distal inflow. Distal brachial inflow for hemoaccess seems to carry the highest risk of producing steal symptoms, and an alternative to proximalization is to use a more distal inflow source, usually the radial artery (Fig. 7). First reported by Minion in 2005, there are only a few published reports involving a few dozen patients [61]. Results seemed comparable with DRIL in 1 comparative study [62]. Like banding, this is a flow restrictive approach, suggesting that results should not significantly differ [61,62].

Proximalization of arterial inflow. First reported by Zanow in 2006, this technique involves effectively re-siting the proximal anastomosis by constructing

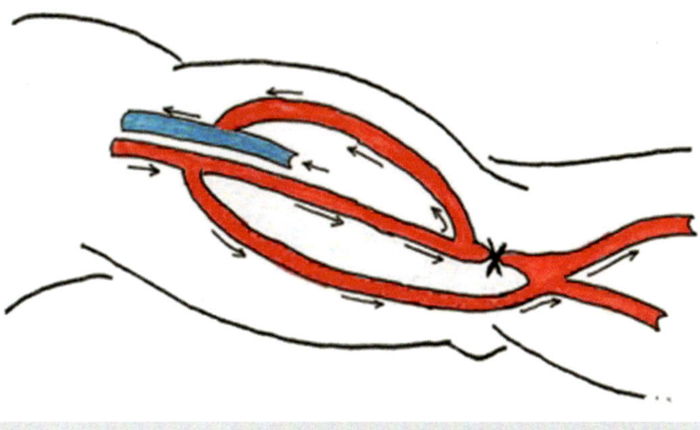

Fig. 6. DRIL procedure with ligation of the artery just distal to the anastomosis. Bypass is created 5 to 10 cm proximal to the anastomosis to beyond the ligated artery.

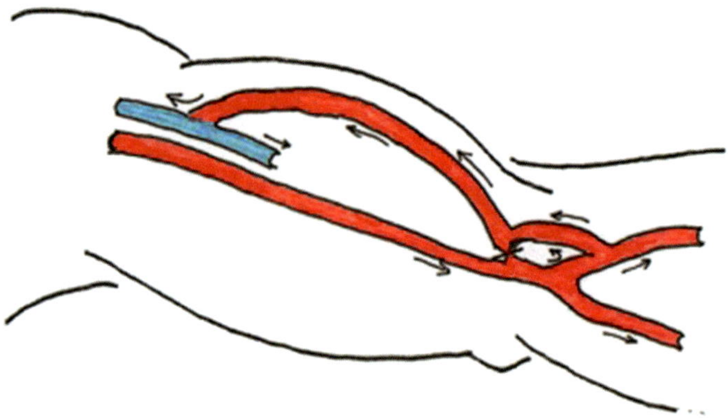

Fig. 7. Revascularization using distal inflow procedure showing ligation of the anastomosis and revascularization by using more distal inflow, generally the radial artery.

an interposition graft from the axillary artery to the arterial aspect of the fistula, ligating the fistula anastomosis rather than the artery (Fig. 8) [63]. There are only a few reports published, but results seem to be similar to those achieved with DRIL. This may be a more appealing option in patients with low-flow prosthetic grafts.

Dialysis-associated steal syndrome treatment algorithm. Our approach has been to use banding as the initial approach in patients with high flow accesses and those with prosthetic grafts, unless there is profound hand ischemia or tissue loss. Banding is a simple and minimally morbid procedure, and in the one-third of patients in whom it is ineffective, more aggressive options can be pursued. For patients with tissue loss, DRIL would be preferred in those with autogenous access and suitable saphenous conduit. We prefer proximalization in patients with prosthetic grafts and in low-flow situations, and consider

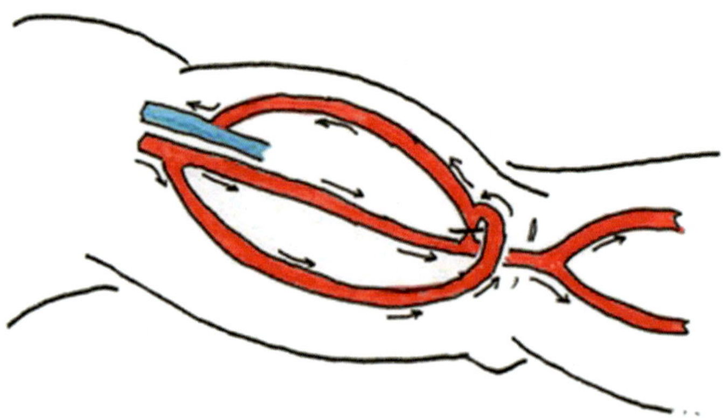

Fig. 8. Proximalization of arterial inflow, with ligation of the anastomosis and creating a bypass from the axillary artery to the most distal aspect of the fistula.

revascularization using distal inflow an alternative method of banding [49]. Fig. 9 depicts a systematic approach to the diagnosis and management of DASS. Whatever intervention is elected should be undertaken with the appreciation that patients with DASS have significantly all-cause mortality risk compared with other dialysis patients, 28% and 79% at 1 and 5 years, respectively in 1 review [60].

Pseudoaneurysm and aneurysm

Aneurysm and pseudoaneurysm (PA) formation in hemodialysis access is common, requiring intervention in 2% to 10% of patients [64]. PAs are false aneurysms that do not contain all the layers of the vessel wall and typically arise from AVGs. In contrast, aneurysms typically arising from AVFs, are more often true aneurysms that contain all the layers of the vessel wall. Although PAs and aneurysms can be unsightly, there are few absolute indications for treatment: bleeding or impending rupture. Soft indications for aneurysm repair are pain, compressive neuropathies, cosmetic, or cannulation difficulty.

PAs and aneurysms arising from hemoaccess can be treated by open or endovascular approach [64,65]. Open techniques include aneurysmorrhaphy, patch angioplasty, and interposition grafting [65,66]. For AVFs we try to keep the access autogenous. For multiple aneurysms, staged revision may be used to preserve accessibility and avoid TCD. Open revision involves an

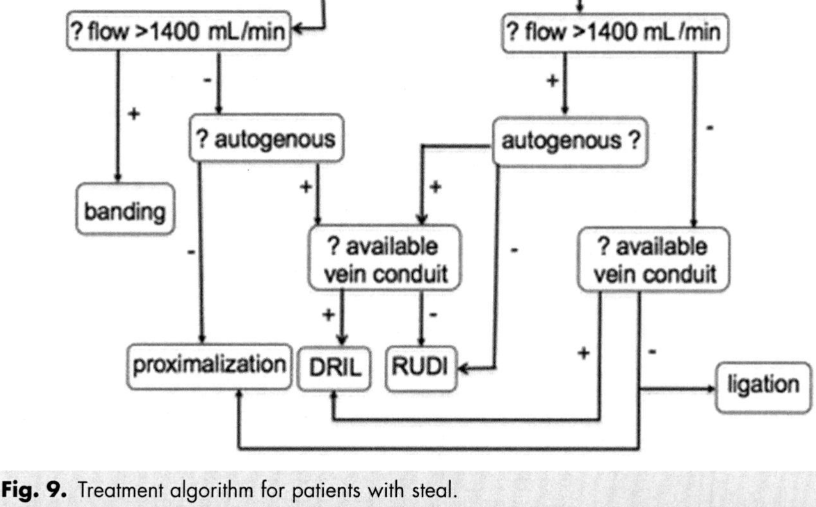

Fig. 9. Treatment algorithm for patients with steal.

elliptical incision over the aneurysm to remove the compromised portion of skin (Fig. 10). Mural thrombus is removed if present, and redundant tissue is excised. The aneurysmorrhaphy is performed by plicating healthy vessel wall over an 18F catheter as a mandrill. Tortuousity is common with AVF aneurysms, often allowing excision and end-to-end anastomosis. The revised portion can be accessed after 4 weeks.

Endovascular treatment with stent grafting is appropriate if the aneurysm is localized and access diameter normal adjacent to it [64,67]. We have used this technique more often with PAs arising from AVGs. Stent grafts can be technically difficult to cannulate, especially through a thrombosed PA/aneurysm sac, so it is avoided when cannulation length is limited.

Erosion/bleeding

Persistent bleeding after access cannulation suggests venous hypertension, usually secondary to a venous outflow stenosis. The hemoaccess is best evaluated with either duplex ultrasonography or fistulogram followed by treatment with balloon angioplasty and/or stent [68]. Erosions can result from repetitive puncture, thinned skin cover, inflammation, and infection [69]. Use of a "ladder technique" to cannulate the access may help prevent these lesions. Once established, treatment of infection, local excision of compromised skin and eschar, or stent graft exclusion, are all acceptable measures for treatment. Fatal hemorrhage can occur when an erosion bleeds, and it is important to treat these lesions in a timely fashion when they present [70]. Scabbing is very common with access cannulation, but if a scab larger than 5 mm persists, and the surrounding skin is not mobile over the fistula, urgent repair is indicated (Fig. 11).

Diabetic neuropathy and uremic neuropathy are both systemic conditions that affect a significant percentage of hemodialysis patients. Diabetic neuropathy is caused from large fiber demyelination leading to clinical manifestations of numbness, paresthesia, and pain. This most commonly occurs in the lower extremities, but can also occur in the upper extremities [71]. Uremic neuropathy is secondary to axonal degeneration with secondary segmental demyelination. It affects 50% to 70% of patients on hemodialysis and is more prevalent in men than women. Clinical symptoms include loss of sensation/vibration and loss of

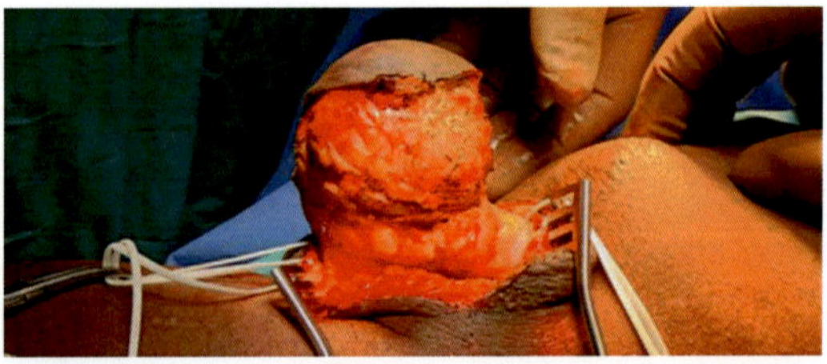

Fig. 10. Aneurysm of AVF dissected circumferentially with proximal and distal control, overlying ellipsed soft tissue.

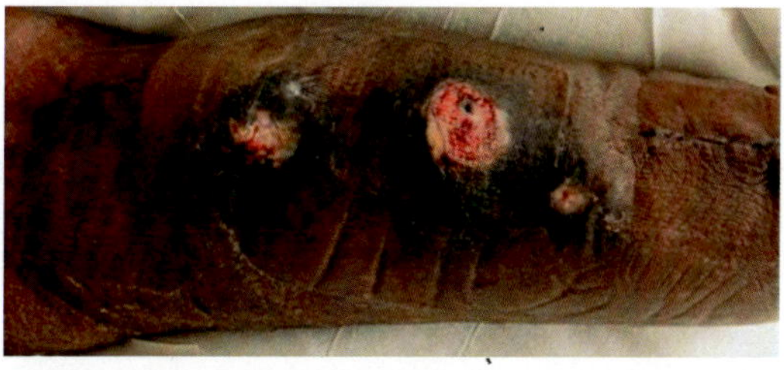

Fig. 11. AVF with overlying soft tissue erosions.

deep tendon reflex [72]. These neuropathies are not caused by access creation in hemodialysis patients, thus it is important to differentiate these neuropathies from those that are caused by the access itself.

Compressive neuropathies secondary to access creation include carpal tunnel syndrome (CTS), Guyton tunnel syndrome, and sometimes cutaneous nerve compression from the access itself. CTS is the most common compressive neuropathy seen and occurs 10 times more frequently in hemodialysis patients [73]. Two theories for increased CTS in hemodialysis patients exist. The first is venous hypertension and congestion causing edema and with median nerve compression in the tunnel [74]. The second is chronic irritation to the carpal tunnel ligament secondary to amyloid deposition [75]. CTS is clinically diagnosed with weakness, pain, and paresthesias in the median nerve distribution, confirmed by electromyogram and treated with decompression of the carpal tunnel. Other compressive neuropathies are treated in a similar fashion with surgical decompression of the affected nerve. These must be differentiated from ischemic symptoms.

An unpredictable and much less common condition, ischemic monomyelic neuropathy (IMN), occurs in less than 0.5% of patients after access creation. This can result in significant and irreversible deficits, especially if there is a delay in diagnosis. IMN is observed most often in brachial access creation, typically in patients with diabetes. It is theorized that access creation results in decreased perfusion to already compromised perfusion of peripheral nerves, at a microvascular level. It is different than ischemic steal syndrome, because, in IMN, the hand remains warm and has distal pulses by palpation or Doppler examination. Pain, weakness, and hyperesthesia is out of proportion to physical findings, and usually is noted within hours of access creation. This can affect one or all of the ulnar, radial, or median nerves. Many believe treatment should be urgent ligation of the access, as symptoms rarely reverse without eliminating the shunt. Even with urgent ligation, permanent deficits may persist [76].

High flow states

High-output congestive heart failure (CHF) may occur in a high flow access. This is diagnosed clinically with the Nicoladoni-Branham sign, where temporary occlusion of the access causes slowing of the heart rate. Flow rates causing CHF are typically greater than 2.5 L/min and divert 25% or more of cardiac output. High flow states causing symptoms are usually seen in brachial-based access. Banding or ligation may be used for surgical correction [77,78].

SUMMARY

The demand for hemodialysis access is increasing and many challenges remain. Improvements in prevalence of autogenous access has not reduced the need for improvements in maintenance and treatment of complications of hemoaccess. The usefulness of endovascular technologies has increased, but surgical therapies will remain important for the foreseeable future.

References

[1] Collins AJ, Foley RN, Chavers B, et al. US renal data system 2013 annual data report. Am J Kidney Dis 2014;63(1):A7.

[2] DeSilva RN, Patibandla BK, Vin Y, et al. Fistula first is not always the best strategy for the elderly. J Am Soc Nephrol 2013;24(8):1297–304.

[3] Fry AC, Stratton J, Farrington K. Factors affecting long-term survival of tunneled haemodialysis catheters—a prospective audit of 812 tunneled catheters. Nephrol Dial Transplant 2008;23:275–81.

[4] Şanal B, Nas ÖF, Doğan N, et al. Safety and functionality of transhepatic hemodialysis catheters in chronic hemodialysis patients. Diagn Interv Radiol 2016;22(6):560–5.

[5] Liu F, Bennett S, Arrigain S, et al. Patency and complications of translumbar dialysis catheters. Semin Dial 2015;28(4):E41–7.

[6] Brescia MJ, Cimino JE, Appel K, et al. Chronic hemodialysis using venipuncture and a surgically created arteriovenous fistula. N Engl J Med 1966;275:1089–92.

[7] Dageforde LA, Harms KA, Feurer ID, et al. Increased minimum vein diameter on preoperative mapping with duplex ultrasound is associated with arteriovenous fistula maturation and secondary patency. J Vasc Surg 2015;61:170–6.

[8] Ghaffarian AA, Driffin CL, Kraiss LW, et al. Comparative effectiveness of one-stage versus two-stage basilic vein transposition arteriovenous fistulas. J Vasc Surg 2018;67:529–35.

[9] Chan MR, Young HN, Becker YT, et al. Obesity as a predictor of vascular access outcomes: analysis of the USRDS DMMS Wave II study. Semin Dial 2008;21:274–9.

[10] Bourquelot P, Rawa M, Van Laere O, et al. Long-term results of femoral vein transposition for autogenous arteriovenous hemodialysis access. J Vasc Surg 2012;56:440–5.

[11] Mallios A, Jennings WC, Boura B, et al. Early results of percutaneous arteriovenous fistula creation with the Ellipsys Vascular Access System. J Vasc Surg 2018;68:1150–6.

[12] Liechty JM, Fisher T, Davis W, et al. Experience with chest wall arteriovenous grafts in hemodialysis patients. Ann Vasc Surg 2015;29(4):690–7.

[13] Hurt AV, Batello-Cruz M, Skipper BJ, et al. Prosthetic thigh arteriovenous access: outcome with SVS/AAVS reporting standards. J Vasc Surg 2004;39(2):381–6.

[14] Miller CD. Comparison of arteriovenous grafts in the thigh and upper extremities in hemodialysis patients. J Am Soc Nephrol 2003;14(11):2942–7.

[15] III. NKF-K/DOQI clinical practice guidelines for vascular access: update 2000. Am J Kidney Dis 2001;37(1); https://doi.org/10.1016/s0272-6386(01)70007-8.

[16] Chintz JL, BJ, et al. Bovine carotid artery heterografts versus polytetrafluoroethylene grafts: a prospective, randomized study. Am J Surg 1983;6:844–7.

[17] Kennealey PT, Elias N, Hertl M, et al. A prospective, randomized comparison of bovine carotid artery and expanded polytetrafluoroethylene for permanent hemodialysis vascular access. J Vasc Surg 2011;53(6):1640–8.

[18] Pineda DM, Dougherty MJ, Wismer MC, et al. Bovine carotid artery xenografts for hemodialysis access. J Vasc Surg 2017;65:1729–34.
[19] Arhuidese I, Reifsnyder T, Islam T, et al. Bovine carotid artery biologic graft outperforms expanded polytetrafluoroethylene for hemodialysis access. J Vasc Surg 2017;65(3): 775–82.
[20] Abdoli S, Mahajan A, Han SM, et al. Early cannulation of bovine carotid artery grafts (Artegraft) after primary vascular access and fistula revision procedures. J Vasc Surg 2018;68(6):1865–71.
[21] Gage SM, Lawson JH. Bioengineered hemodialysis access grafts. J Vasc Access 2017;18(1_suppl):56–63.
[22] Sgroi MD, Patel MS, Wilson SE, et al. The optimal initial choice for permanent arteriovenous hemodialysis access. J Vasc Surg 2013;58:539–48.
[23] Woo K, Ulloa J, Allon M, et al. Establishing patient-specific criteria for selecting the optimal upper extremity vascular access procedure. J Vasc Surg 2017;65(4):1089–103.e1.
[24] Lok CE, Oliver MJ, Su J, et al. Arteriovenous fistula outcomes in the era of the elderly dialysis population. Kidney Int 2005;67:2462–9.
[25] Lazarides MK, Georgiadis GS, Antoniou GA, et al. A meta-analysis of dialysis access outcome in elderly patients. J Vasc Surg 2007;45:420–6.
[26] Johnasen KL, Dalrymple LS, Glidden D, et al. Association of performance-based and self-reported function-based definitions of frailty with mortality among patients receiving hemodialysis. Clin J Am Soc Nephrol 2016;11:626–32.
[27] Tamura MK, Tan JC, O'Hare AM. Optimizing renal replacement therapy in older adults: a framework for making individualized decisions. Kidney Int 2012;82:261–9.
[28] Letourneau I, Ouimet D, Dumont M, et al. Renal replacement in end-stage renal disease patients over 75 years old. Am J Nephrol 2003;23:71–7.
[29] Han A, Min S-K, Kim M-S, et al. A prospective, randomized trial of routine duplex ultrasound surveillance on arteriovenous fistula maturation. Clin J Am Soc Nephrol 2016;11(10): 1817–24.
[30] Dougherty MJ, Calligaro KD, Raviola CA, et al. Endovascular vs. surgical treatment for thrombosed hemodialysis grafts: a prospective, randomized study. J Vasc Surg 1999;30(6):1016–23.
[31] Marston WA, Criado E, Jaques PF, et al. Prospective randomized comparison of surgical versus endovascular management of thrombosed dialysis access grafts. J Vasc Surg 1997;26(3):373–80.
[32] Bittl JA. Catheter interventions for hemodialysis fistulas and grafts. JACC Cardiovasc Interv 2010;3(1):1–11.
[33] Kolakowski S, Dougherty MJ, Calligaro KD. Salvaging prosthetic dialysis fistulas with stents: forearm versus upper arm grafts. J Vasc Surg 2003;38(4):719–23.
[34] Quinn SF, Schuman ES, Demlow TA, et al. Percutaneous transluminal angioplasty versus endovascular stent placement in the treatment of venous stenoses in patients undergoing hemodialysis: intermediate results. J Vasc Interv Radiol 1995;6(6):851–5.
[35] Hoffer EK, Sultan S, Herskowitz MM, et al. Prospective randomized trial of a metallic intravascular stent in hemodialysis graft maintenance. J Vasc Interv Radiol 1997;8(6):965–73.
[36] Vesely T, Davanzo W, Behrend T, et al. Balloon angioplasty versus Viabahn stent graft for treatment of failing or thrombosed prosthetic hemodialysis grafts. J Vasc Surg 2016;64(5); https://doi.org/10.1016/j.jvs.2016.04.035.
[37] Falk A, Maya ID, Yevzlin AS. A prospective, randomized study of an expanded polytetrafluoroethylene stent graft versus balloon angioplasty for in-stent restenosis in arteriovenous grafts and fistulae: two-year results of the RESCUE study. J Vasc Interv Radiol 2016;27(10): 1465–76.
[38] Khawaja AZ, Cassidy DB, Shakarchi JA, et al. Systematic review of drug eluting balloon angioplasty for arteriovenous haemodialysis access stenosis. J Vasc Access 2016;17(2): 103–10.

[39] Kitrou PM, Katsanos K, Spiliopoulos S, et al. Drug-eluting versus plain balloon angioplasty for the treatment of failing dialysis access: final results and cost-effectiveness analysis from a prospective randomized controlled trial (NCT01174472). Eur J Radiol 2015;84(3): 418–23.
[40] Illig KA. Management of central vein stenoses and occlusions: the critical importance of the costoclavicular junction. Semin Vasc Surg 2011;24:113–8.
[41] Davis KL, Gurley JC, Davenport DL, et al. The use of HeRo catheter in catheter-dependent dialysis patients with superior vena cava occlusion. J Vasc Access 2016;17(2):138–42.
[42] Freeman BM, Tingen JS, Hale AL, et al. The inside-out technique: a vascular surgeon's guide to complex catheter placement. J Vasc Surg 2018;67:e6.
[43] Butterly DW, Schwab SJ. Dialysis access infections. Curr Opin Nephrol Hypertens 2000;9: 631–5.
[44] Saad TF. Bacteremia associated with tunneled, cuff hemodialysis catheters. Am J Kidney Dis 1999;34:1114–24.
[45] Antoniou GA, Lazarides MK, Georgiadis GS, et al. Lower-extremity arteriovenous access for haemodialysis: a systematic review. Eur J Vasc Endovasc Surg 2009;38:365–72.
[46] Labriola L, Crott R, Desmet C. Infectious complications following conversion to buttonhole cannulation of native arteriovenous fistulas: a quality improvement report. Am J Kidney Dis 2011;57:442–8.
[47] Turmel-Rodrigues L1, Mouton A, Birmelé B, et al. Salvage of immature forearm fistulas for haemodialysis by interventional radiology. Nephrol Dial Transplant 2001;16(12): 2365–71.
[48] Dixon B. Why don't fistulas mature? Kidney Int 2006;70(8):1413–22.
[49] Scali ST, Huber TS. Treatment strategies for access-related hand ischemia. Semin Vasc Surg 2011;24(2):128–36.
[50] Suding PN, Wilson SE. Strategies for management of ischemic steal syndrome. Semin Vasc Surg 2007;20(3):184–8.
[51] Roddy SP. Treatment strategies of arterial steal after arteriovenous access. J Vasc Surg 2011;54(1):278.
[52] Valentine R, Bouch CW, Scott DJ, et al. Do preoperative finger pressures predict early arterial steal in hemodialysis access patients? A prospective analysis. J Vasc Surg 2002;36(2): 351–6.
[53] Lazarides MK. Onset of arterial steal following proximal angioaccess: immediate and delayed types. Nephrol Dial Transplant 2003;18(11):2387–90.
[54] Schanzer A, Nguyen LL, Owens CD, et al. Use of digital pressure measurements for the diagnosis of AV access-induced hand ischemia. Vasc Med 2006;11(4):227–31.
[55] Mascia S, Spiezia S, Assanti A, et al. Ischemic steal syndrome in a hemodialysis patient: the roles of Doppler ultrasonography and dynamic Doppler studies in diagnosis and treatment selection. J Ultrasound 2010;13(3):104–6.
[56] Plumb TJ, Lynch TG, Adelson AB. Treatment of steal syndrome in a distal radiocephalic arteriovenous fistula using intravascular coil embolization. J Vasc Surg 2008;47(2):457–9.
[57] Jean-Baptiste E, Hassen-Khodja R, Haudebourg P, et al. Axillary loop grafts for hemodialysis access: midterm results from a single-center study. J Vasc Surg 2008;47(1):138–43.
[58] Miller GA, Goel N, Friedman A, et al. The MILLER banding procedure is an effective method for treating dialysis-associated steal syndrome. Kidney Int 2010;77:359–66.
[59] Leake AE, Winger DG, Leers SA, et al. Management and outcomes of dialysis access-associated steal syndrome. J Vasc Surg 2015;61(3):754–61.
[60] Scali ST, Chang CK, Raghinaru D, et al. Prediction of graft patency and mortality after distal revascularization and interval ligation for hemodialysis access related hand ischemia. J Vasc Surg 2013;57(2):451–8.
[61] Minion DJ, Moore E, Endean E. Revision using distal inflow: a novel approach to dialysis-associated steal syndrome. Ann Vasc Surg 2005;19(5):625–8.

[62] Misskey J, Yang C, MacDonald S, et al. A comparison of revision using distal inflow and distal revascularization-interval ligation for the management of severe access-related hand ischeia. J Vasc Surg 2016;63(6):1574–81.
[63] Zanow J, Kruger U, Scholz H. Proximalization of the arterial inflow: a new technique to treat access-related ischemia. J Vasc Surg 2006;43(6):1216–21.
[64] Shah AS, Valdes J, Charlton-Ouw KM, et al. Endovascular treatment of hemodialysis access pseudoaneurysms. J Vasc Surg 2012;55:1058–62.
[65] Hossny A. Partial aneurysmectomy for salvage of autogenous arteriovenous fistula with complicated venous aneurysms. J Vasc Surg 2014;59:1073–7.
[66] Vo T, Tumbaga G, Aka P, et al. Staple aneurysmorrhapy to salvage autogenous arteriovenous fistulas with aneurysm-related complications. J Vasc Surg 2015;61:457–62.
[67] Barshes NR, Annambhotla S, Bechara C, et al. Endovascular repair of hemodialysis graft-related pseudoaneurysm: an alternative treatment strategy in salvaging failing dialysis access. Vasc Endovascular Surg 2008;42:228–34.
[68] Ayarragaray JE. Surgical treatment of hemodialysis-related central venous stenosis or occlusion: another option to maintain vascular access. J Vasc Surg 2003;37(5):1043–6.
[69] van Loon MM, Goovaerts T, Kessels AG, et al. Buttonhole needling of haemodialysis arteriovenous fistulae results in less complications and interventions compared to the rope-ladder technique. Nephrol Dial Transplant 2010;25(1):225–30.
[70] Ellingson KD, Paledkar RS, Lucero CA, et al. Vascular access hemorrhages contribute to deaths among hemodialysis patients. Kidney Int 2012;82:686–92.
[71] Ndip A, Lavery LA, Boulton AJ. Diabetic foot disease in people with advanced nephropathy and those on renal dialysis. Curr Diab Rep 2010;10(4):283–90.
[72] Pirzada NA, Morgenlander JC, et al. Peripheral neuropathy in patients with chronic renal failure: a treatable source of discomfort and disability. Postgrad Med 1997;102:249–61.
[73] Burn DJ, Bates D. Neurology and the kidney. J Neurol Neurosurg Psychiatry 1998;65: 810–21.
[74] Kocyigit I, Unal A, Guney A, et al. Carpal tunnel release surgery and venous hypertension in early hemodialysis patients without amyloid deposits. ScientificWorldJournal 2013;2013: 481348.
[75] Borman H, Akinbingol G, Maral T, et al. Entrapment neuropathy of the upper extremity in hemodialysis patients. Plast Reconstr Surg 2002;109:2598–9.
[76] Wilbourn AJ, Furlan AJ, Hulley W, et al. Ischemic monomelic neuropathy. Neurology 1983;33:447–51.
[77] Ahearn DJ, Maher JF. Heart failure as a complication of hemodialysis arteriovenous fistula. Ann Intern Med 1972;77(2):201–4.
[78] Anderson CB, Etheredge EE, Harter HR, et al. Blood flow measurements in arteriovenous dialysis fistulas. Surgery 1977;81(4):459–61.

Advances in Surgery 53 (2019) 103–115

ADVANCES IN SURGERY

Has Personalized Medicine for Pancreatic Cancer Arrived?

Ashley Krepline, MD, Susan Tsai, MD, MHS*

Department of Surgery, Medical College of Wisconsin, 8701 West Watertown Plank Road, Milwaukee, WI 53226-3596, USA

Keywords

• Pancreatic cancer • Precision medicine • Personalized medicine
• Next-generation sequencing • Clinical trial

Key points

- Next-generation DNA and RNA sequencing methodologies have enabled scientists to discriminate several molecular subtypes of pancreatic cancer.
- Up to a quarter of all pancreatic cancers may have a highly actionable mutation for which targeted therapies may be available.
- The translation of sequencing methodologies into clinical practice in a clinically relevant time frame remains challenging and requires a dedicated clinical infrastructure.
- Early studies utilizing molecular profiling to guide treatment have been associated with encouraging results.

INTRODUCTION

In 1990, when the Human Genome Project was initiated, the objective was to sequence the entire human genome, and, although the project was met with initial skepticism, it ushered in a new era of clinical medicine whereby the genetic basis of disease could be leveraged to inform clinical care [1]. At the core of this revolution is a belief that a deeper understanding of the genetic basis of disease will result in the development of better targeted therapies, as highlighted by President Barack Obama in his 2015 State of the Union Address, when he laid out a vision for a national Precision Medicine Initiative in the United States [2]. The combination of rapidly declining costs for genomic

Disclosure Statement: The authors have nothing to disclose.

*Corresponding author. *E-mail address:* stsai@mcw.edu

https://doi.org/10.1016/j.yasu.2019.04.006
0065-3411/19/

technologies and the explosion of direct-to-consumer companies has made the promise of precision medicine accessible to the public and has irrevocably changed the landscape of oncology for patients and their families.

The terms, *precision medicine* and *personalized medicine*, although closely related, are subtly distinct. The US National Research Council has championed the development of a new taxonomy of human disease based on molecular biology and has defined precision medicine as a population-based approach of classifying individuals through genomic, environmental, or social characteristics, with the goal of identifying effective therapeutics based on a combination of these factors [3]. The report envisioned a comprehensive disease classification that combines information from biomedical research, public health, and health care–delivery communities to advance understanding of disease pathogenesis and improve health. In contrast, personalized medicine implies the development of therapeutics for specific individuals. Ideally, all patients receive personalized medicine, while precision medicine would serve as the foundation for the application of population-based observations at an individual level. Ultimately, the promise of precision medicine is captured in the ubiquitous phrase, "The right treatment for the right patient at the right time."

Coincident with the rapid advances in genomic sequencing technology, significant gains have been achieved in the development of effective therapeutics for pancreatic cancer. As one of the most challenging human malignancies to treat, pancreatic cancer currently is the third leading cause of cancer-related deaths in the United States [4]. Over the past decade, the chemotherapeutic options for patients with pancreatic cancer have evolved from single-agent gemcitabine to multiagent regimens, such as 5-fluorouracil, irinotecan, & oxaliplatin (FOLFIRINOX) and gemcitabine/nab-paclitaxel, which have produced significant gains in overall survival [5,6]. In addition, with the multiagent regimens, exceptional responders have been reported, notably among patients with genetic defects in the homologous recombination DNA repair pathway [7]. The molecular basis for these exceptional responders was uncovered when these patients received poly(ADP-ribose) polymerase (PARP) inhibitor–based and/or platinum-based therapies. Platinum-based agents cause DNA cross-linking and induce DNA strand breaks, which are unable to be repaired in cells with deficient DNA repair mechanisms, such as BRCA1 and BRCA2. In addition to platinum-based therapy, tumors with deficient DNA repair mechanisms also have increased sensitivity to PARP inhibitors, which target the ribosylation of ADP necessary for DNA repair pathways and apoptosis. In a study by O'Reilly and colleagues [8], 9 patients with BRCA mutations received PARP inhibitor in combination with gemcitabine and cisplatinum; 5 of 9 patients demonstrated a partial response and the remaining 4 patients demonstrated stable disease. These early observations reinforced the hypothesis that histopathologic similarities among pancreatic cancers belied an underlying genomic diversity, which, if fully understood, could be used to better stratify subgroups of patients for specific targeted agents.

EVOLUTION OF THE MOLECULAR CLASSIFICATION OF PANCREATIC CANCER

Over the past 10 years, important advances in large sequencing efforts have culminated in a series of comprehensive integrated genomic analyses, summarized in Table 1. For several decades, it has been well established that pancreatic cancer was the product of the accumulation of successive genetic mutations. The progression from dysplasia to invasive carcinoma is paralleled by a series of genetic mutations that include the activation of the KRAS oncogene and the inactivation of the tumor suppressors genes, CDKN2A, TP53, and SMAD4 [9]. These 4 genetic alterations were confirmed in a seminal report by Jones and colleagues [10] in 2008, which sequenced a total of 114 metastatic pancreatic cancers. In addition, the sequencing revealed a diverse genetic mutations. Given that most cellular pathways and processes involve multiple proteins that function in a concerted manner, the investigators identified 12 core signaling pathways, which were altered in most pancreatic cancer specimens. Unfortunately, many of the pathways were not targetable, and no tumors carried mutations in homologous recombination deficiency. This study laid the framework, however, for future studies categorizing pancreatic cancer into subtypes and ignited the search for new therapeutic options for pancreatic cancer.

In 2011, Collisson and colleagues [11] performed a combined analysis of the transcriptional profiles of 27 resected tumor specimens, as well as those of human and mouse pancreatic cancer cell lines. By applying global gene expression analysis, they identified a 62-gene signature that could classify pancreatic cancers into 3 specific subtypes, which they defined as classical, quasimesenchymal, and exocrine-like. The classical subtype had genes that expressed high levels of epithelial and cell adhesion molecules and were phenotypically more well-differentiated. In contrast, the quasimesenchymal subtype demonstrated high levels of mesenchymal-associated genes and correlated with a more poorly-differentiated phenotype. The exocrine-like subtype had relatively high expression of tumor cell-derived digestive enzyme genes. Importantly, the genetic subtypes had prognostic significance, with patients with classical tumors having the most favorable survival. In the analysis of murine pancreatic cancer cell lines, the classical subtype was observed to be KRAS-dependent and, therefore, more susceptible to KRAS-targeted therapies. Similarly, knockdown of GATA6 expression reduced the growth of classical cell lines but not quasimesenchymal cell lines. Finally, the 62-gene signature has been validated in other published expression data sets, demonstrating the robust nature of the subtype classification [12].

In 2012, Biankin and colleagues [13] utilized whole-exome sequencing and copy number analysis of resected pancreatic cancer. A total of 99 samples were sequenced and, similar to other studies, common mutations were identified in: KRAS, TP53, CDKN2A, SMAD4, MLL3, TGFBR2, ARID1A, and SF3B1.

Table 1
Comparison of recent large-scale genomic studies in pancreatic cancer

Study	Type of Tissue Utilized	Methodology	Classification
Jones et al [10], 2008	114 pancreatic cancers—metastatic patients	Sequencing of protein-coding exons with polymerase chain reaction	Identification of 12 core signaling pathways
Collison et al [11], 2011	27 microdissected tumors from surgical specimens + human and murine pancreatic cancer cell lines	Gene expression microarrays	Three subtypes identified Classical: associated with adhesion and epithelial genes Quasimesenchymal: mesenchyme-associated genes Exocrine-like: associated with digestive enzyme genes
Biankin et al [13], 2012	142 primary resected pancreatic cancers	Exon sequencing and copy number analysis	Multiple core signaling pathways, including new subgroups involving: G1/S checkpoint, apoptosis, angiogenesis, transforming growth factor β signaling, and axon guidance
Waddell et al [14], 2015	142 primary resected pancreatic cancers	Whole-genome sequencing and copy number analysis	Subtypes Stable: ≤50 structural variation events Locally rearranged: significant focal event on 1 or 2 chromosomes Scattered: moderate nonrandom chromosomal damage and <200 structural variations Unstable: >200 structural variation events; defects in DNA maintenance.

(*continued on next page*)

Table 1
continued

Study	Type of Tissue Utilized	Methodology	Classification
Moffitt et al [15], 2015	357 primary and metastatic pancreatic cancers, normal tissue, pancreatic cancer cell lines.	Virtual microdissection with microarrays and RNA sequencing	Two subtypes of tumors Classical: high adhesion associated, ribosomal, and epithelial gene expression, elevated GATA-6 Basal-like: laminin and keratins Two subtypes of stroma Normal: markers for pancreatic stellate cells Activated: genes associated with macrophages and tumor promotion
Bailey et al [16], 2016	456 primary resected pancreatic cancers	Integrated genomic analysis	Four subtypes Squamous: enriched for integrin signaling and activated EGF signaling. ADEX: transcriptional networks in later stages of pancreatic development and differentiation; genes associated with endocrine differentiation Pancreatic progenitor: genes regulated pancreatic development, fatty acid oxidation, steroid hormone biosynthesis, pancreatitis and regeneration Immunogenic: immune infiltrate; B-cell signaling pathways, antigen presentation, T-cell and Toll-like receptor signaling pathways

In addition, they identified novel mutations in chromatin modification (EPC1 and ARID2) and DNA repair (ATM), which represent additional targetable mutations. The investigators also identified mutations in tumor cell invasion and metastases (SLIT2, ROBO2, SEMA3A, SEMA3E, and PLXNA1).

In 2015, 2 large-scale genomic studies were reported. Waddell and colleagues [14] utilized whole-genome sequencing in 100 patients with resected pancreatic cancer and identified 4 distinct subtypes: (1) stable subtype, which contained fewer than 50 structural variations and represented 20% of the samples, (2) locally rearranged subtype, in which the genetic abnormality was limited to one or two chromosomes, and represented 30% of the sample, (3) scattered subtype, which harbored a moderate number (<200) of structural variation events and represented 36% of the sample, and (4) unstable subtype which had a large number of structural variations, suggesting a defect in DNA maintenance.

The unstable subtypes were more likely to have mutations in BRCA1, BRCA2, PALB2, ATM, FANCM, XRCC4, and XRCC6 and were more likely to be responsive to platinum-based therapies. This was the first report to demonstrate that variation in chromosomal structure as an important mechanism of DNA damage in pancreatic carcinogenesis. Moffitt and colleagues [15] extended the work from Collison and colleagues by defining 2 tumor subtypes and 2 stromal subtypes, using a wide range of pancreatic cancer samples, including 145 primary tumors and 61 metastatic samples with adjacent normal controls. Unique to this analysis, the investigators performed a digital separation of gene expression between tumor, stroma, and adjacent normal tissue. Two tumor-specific subtypes were identified (classical and basal-like) and 2 stroma subtypes (normal and activated). An activated stroma was associated with significantly worse prognosis, and specific combinations of tumor and stroma subtypes had a cumulative effect on prognosis, with those patients with classical tumors and normal stroma having the best outcome. Overall, the Moffitt classical subtype overlapped with the Collison classical subtype and was characterized by high adhesion-associated proteins, ribosomal and epithelial gene expression, and elevated GATA6 expression.

Finally, in 2016, Bailey and colleagues [16] reported on 456 resected pancreatic cancers that underwent whole-exome sequencing and copy number analysis. Analysis included differential expression of transcription factors and downstream targets. The RNA analysis revealed clustering into 4 distinct subtypes: squamous, pancreatic progenitor, immunogenic, and aberrantly differentiated endocrine exocrine (ADEX). The squamous subtype harbored the greatest number of mutations in TP53 and KDM6A and had the poorest prognosis. The pancreatic progenitor subtype expressed genes involved in pancreatic development, with an enrichment in inactivating mutation of TGFBR2. The immunogenic subtype was characterized by pathway-mediated acquired immune suppression. These tumors had significant immune infiltration and up-regulation of inhibitory immune checkpoint pathways. The ADEX subtype was characterized by expression of genes involved in later stages of both pancreatic exocrine and endocrine cell development. When this transcriptome classification is compared with the Collison classification, there is significant overlap except for the addition of the immunogenic subtype. The Collison quasimesenchymal corresponds to the squamous subtype, classical corresponds to the pancreatic progenitor, and the exocrine-like to the ADEX. There was less similarity between the Moffitt and Bailey subtypes, likely due to the reduced stromal content in the latter study.

Overall, these studies demonstrate that reproducible biologic subgroups exist in pancreatic cancer. There are strong biologic similarities between the Collison, Moffitt, and Bailey classifications. In general, the prognosis of quasimesenchymal/squamous/basal-like subtypes is worse than that of the classical/pancreatic progenitor subtypes and may be more responsive to chemotherapy. The clinical utility of molecular subtyping is only realized if the information provided has an impact on treatment selection. The Know Your Tumor Initiative was developed as a joint collaboration between the Pancreatic Cancer Action Network and Perthera, with the goal of offering patients with pancreatic cancer multi-omic molecular profiling [17]. The study recruited patients from 44 states, including academic and community practices. Next-generation sequencing and immunohistochemical (IHC) profiling were performed in commercial laboratories (Foundation Medicine [Cambridge, MA], PGDX [Baltimore, MD], Caris Life Sciences [Dallas, TX], and NeoGenomics [Fort Myers, FL]). An online tumor board reviewed the molecular profiling results, and a report with treatment options was created for the treating oncologists. In total, 640 tumor specimens were sent for next-generation sequencing and IHC, 591 of which were pancreatic adenocarcinoma. After obtaining tissue from a local pathologist, the median time to report delivery was 30 days. Of 640 patients, 458 (72%) had metastatic disease, 137 (21%) had locally advanced disease, and 45 (7%) had resectable disease or borderline resectable disease. Of 640 patients, at least 1 mutation was identified in 616 samples (median 4 mutations per sample). The tumor board identified actionable genomic alterations in 50% of patients (with 27% highly actionable) and actionable proteomic alterations (excluding chemopredictive markers) in 5%. Highly actionable mutations were identified as those in the homologous recombinant DNA repair pathway (15%), cell cycle genes (11%), and AKT/mTOR (19%) pathways. As a result of the molecular profiling, 156 (24%) of 640 patients were transitioned to a new treatment regimen, 173 (27%) remained on their treatment started prior to sequencing, 111 (17%) passed away prior to transitioning to a new treatment based on tumor sequencing, and 200 (31%) patients were lost to follow-up. A subset analysis of patients with highly actionable biomarkers who received profile-directed therapy ($n = 17$) demonstrated a significantly longer median progression-free survival than those with unmatched therapy ($n = 18$) (hazard ratio 0.47; $P = .003$).

TRANSLATING MOLECULAR PROFILING INTO CLINICAL RELEVANCE

Although the ability to characterize pancreatic cancers into molecular subtypes has evolved substantially over the past decade, its translation into clinical practice has been markedly slower. One of the first reported precision medicine trials for patients with pancreatic cancer was the individualized molecular pancreatic cancer therapy (IMPaCT) trial [18]. This was a pilot study of 76 patients with metastatic or recurrent pancreatic cancer who underwent targeted sequencing of BRCA1, BRCA2, PALB2, ATM, or KRAS genes as well as an assessment of HER2 amplification from formalin-fixed paraffin-embedded samples. Patients then were randomized to single-agent gemcitabine or target-specific therapy (patients deficient in the homologous recombinant DNA repair pathway received 5-fluorouracil and mitomycin C, patients with HER2 amplification received gemcitabine and trastuzumab, patients with wild-type KRAS received gemcitabine and erlotinib). A genetic target was identified in 22 (28%) patients (14 wild-type KRAS, 5 HER2 amplification, 2 BRCA2, and 1 ATM). The median time from enrollment to relay of test results was 21.5 days, but no patient was successfully treated on trial. The investigators recognized that rapid disease progression made the return of genomic results in a meaningful time frame challenging.

Another clinical trial designed to provide comprehensive real-time genomic analysis for patients with advanced pancreatic cancer was the comprehensive molecular characterization of advanced pancreatic ductal adenocarcinoma for better treatment selection (COMPASS) trial [19]. In this trial, 63 patients underwent tumor biopsy and whole-genome sequencing, and RNA sequencing was performed from the fresh tumor tissue. The primary endpoint of the trial was the feasibility of reporting the sequencing results prior to 8 weeks. Overall, 18 (28%) patients were identified with actionable mutations: 5, ARID1A; 1, BRAF; 4, CDK4/6; 4, PIK3CA; 3, PTEN; and 2, FNG43. Genomic results were reported at a median of 35 days from biopsy. In 5 patients, the second-line therapy was based on the COMPASS results. The investigators categorized the tumors based on the Moffitt classical and basal-like subtypes and compared responses to first-line chemotherapy based on molecular subtype. They observed improved progression-free survival among patients with the classical subtype who were treated with FOLFIRINOX. Importantly, GATA6 protein expression was found a robust surrogate biomarker for differentiating classical and basal-like subtypes, suggesting that simple proteomic correlates may be identified as surrogates of genomic subtyping.

Although the clinical value of genetic sequencing from these early experiences is mixed, the necessity of a robust clinical infrastructure to support the acquisition and analysis of biospecimens for next-generation sequencing within a reasonable timeframe was unquestionable. The investigators of the IMPaCT trial summarized the need for programmatic infrastructure including: (1) a sufficient volume of patients, (2) the ability to acquire suitable tumor specimens for the testing platform, (3) a clinically acceptable turnaround time, and (4) an attractive clinical trial design for patients. [18]

Implicit in these requirements is a cooperative and integrated relationship between the molecular laboratories, clinical staff, and a variety of clinical disciplines, with dedicated resources to expedite the molecular profiling services. As previous studies have suggested, higher levels of physician engagement in multidisciplinary teams are associated with more rapid initiation of treatment and increased enrollment of patients in clinical trials [20,21].

An alternative approach to molecular profiling is the use of IHC protein expression rather than next-generation sequencing. This approach has several advantages over next-generation sequencing in that IHC profiling already is performed ubiquitously in pathologic laboratories, has a rapid turnaround time, and is relatively cost-effective. One of the first studies to utilize molecular profiling of tumors to guide treatment regimens was the Bisgrove study [22]. This study enrolled patients with a variety of refractory metastatic cancers and utilized IHC and flourescence in situ hybridization assays to assess 11 proteins and performed oligonucleotide microarray gene expression of an additional 51 genes. The goal of the study was to compare the progression-free survival for each patient using a treatment regimen selected by molecular profiling as compared with the prior progression-free survival on the most recent regimen prior to enrollment on the trial. In this study design, each patient served as his/her own control. In total, 86 patients enrolled in the study, and a molecular target was identified in 84 (98%). Of the 84 patients, 66 (79%) received profile-directed therapy, and 18 (27%) of the 66 patients had a progression-free survival, which exceeded the most recent regimen on which the patient had experienced progression (progression-free survival ratio $\geq$1.3).

The first molecular profiling trial in patients with localized pancreatic cancer recently was reported [23]. The trial utilized 6 putative biomarkers of chemotherapeutic responsiveness, including nucleoside transporter hENT1 and ribonucleotide reductase M1 for gemcitabine responsiveness, secreted protein acidic and rich in cysteine for nab-paclitaxel responsiveness, thymidylate synthase for 5-fluorouracil responsiveness, excision repair cross-complementing protein for platinum sensitivity, and topoisomerase 1 for irinotecan resistance. Biopsies from endoscopic ultrasound–guided fine-needle aspirates and surgical specimens underwent molecular profiling to guide neoadjuvant therapy and adjuvant therapy, respectively. The primary endpoint of the trial was to improve the rate of surgical resection after neoadjuvant therapy from 80% to 90% in patients with resectable pancreatic cancer and from 50% to 70% in patients with borderline resectable pancreatic cancer. In total, 130 patients were enrolled at 2 institutions, 61 (47%) with resectable disease and 69 (53%) with borderline resectable disease. Adequate cellularity for molecular profiling of the endoscopic ultrasound–guided fine-needle aspirate specimens was present in 95 (73%) patients, and the median time to reporting of the molecular profiling was 5 days. Of the 130 patents, 107 (82%) completed all intended neoadjuvant therapy and surgery–56 (92%) patients with resectable disease and 51 (74%) patients with borderline resectable disease. The median overall survival of all patients was 38 months, 45 months among patients who completed all neoadjuvant therapy and surgery and 11 months for patients who were not resected. As alluded to from the IMPaCT study, the investigators noted that the inclusion of advanced gastroenterologists and integrated molecular pathology services was essential to developing a comprehensive pipeline to screen and enrolling patients with localized pancreatic ductal adenocarcinoma. The presence of on-site cytopathologists expedited the pathologic evaluation of the biopsy specimen and increased the yield of available tissue for molecular profiling [24]. In contrast to clinical trials utilizing next-generation sequencing, the rapid turnaround time utilizing IHC greatly improved the ability to place patients on molecular profiled therapy as the first line of therapy. Furthermore, close communication with the trial coordinators and the molecular pathology laboratory allowed for rapid reporting of results in a median of 5 days. In contrast, with next-generation sequencing the sample preparation, sequencing, and bioinformatic analysis can take up to 21 days. This study demonstrated the feasibility of utilizing molecular profiling to guide treatment selection and emphasized the need to identify rapid molecular assays to reduce patient attrition during molecular profiling [18].

MOVING FROM PRECISION MEDICINE TO PERSONALIZED MEDICINE

With the exception of a small subset of patients with microsatellite instability, homologous recombinant DNA repair pathways, or potentially targetable KRAS mutations, the therapeutic implications of pancreatic cancer subtypes remain largely unknown. To better understand the biologic consequences of these subtypes, both patient-derived xenografts and patient-derived organoids offer an opportunity to test potential biomarkers and refine therapeutic interventions.

Patient-derived xenografts are generated directly from engraftment of individual human tumor tissue into severely immunocompromised mice to allow for the efficient engraftment of the tumor. These have been shown to faithfully recreate the genomic and histopathologic characteristics of the human tumor, including tumor heterogeneity, at least in early passages [25]. Generation of patient-derived xenografts may provide a renewable and valuable resource with which multiple treatments may be studied with the ultimate goal of determining the best therapeutic option for the patient. Clinical studies have demonstrated remarkable correlations between drug activity in the xenograft model and patient outcome [26]. Although patient-derived xenografts have yielded important insights into pancreatic cancer, their generation often requires a large amount of tissue, multiple months to establish, and serial passaging results in replacement of human stroma with murine components. An alternative to patient-derived xenografts is the creation of 3-D cell cultures of dissociated tumors, also termed organoids. Patient-derived organoids have been established from surgical resection specimens, as well as fine-needle biopsy [27]. In a recent report, 66 patient-derived organoid cultures underwent molecular characterization using whole-genome and RNA sequencing, which recapitulated the molecular characteristics of the primary tumor [27]. The organoids were then subjected to the 5 chemotherapeutic agents most commonly used to treat patients with pancreatic cancer, with marked variability in response to therapy. Furthermore, the drug sensitivity of the organoid cultures reflected the clinical outcomes of the patients. These results suggest a broad range of intrinsic drug sensitivity to conventional chemotherapeutic agents and interpatient diversity to chemotherapeutic drug responses. The biologic basis of drug responsiveness currently is under investigation and may involve drug transport, metabolism, and/or response to cell damage. Importantly, such responses currently are not reflected in the models of pancreatic cancer subtyping and reveal the opportunity to further develop a complementary pharmacogenomic classification of drug response.

SUMMARY

The era of next-generation sequencing has shepherded a new molecular taxonomy of pancreatic cancer, which may better inform our understanding disease pathogenesis. It will become important for surgeons to become familiar with these subtypes, especially how molecular genotypes are related to therapeutic vulnerabilities. Although the clinical impact of these advances is yet to be fully realized, there is a powerful momentum toward precision medicine for pancreatic cancer. In the future, streamlining clinical infrastructure and reducing turnaround time for genomic sequencing will be paramount, and these obstacles may be overcome with technological advancements or through the development of surrogate proteomic markers. Although advances in genomic classification have opened the door to precision medicine for pancreatic cancer, additional models, such as patient-derived organoids, may be necessary to fully realize a personalized approach for individual patients.

Acknowledgments

This article received funds from WeCare Fund for Medical Innovation and Research, Advancing a Healthier Wisconsin, Batterman Foundation Fund.

References

[1] Lander ES, Linton LM, Birren B, et al. Initial sequencing and analysis of the human genome. Nature 2001;409(6822):860–921.

[2] Collins FS, Varmus H. A new initiative on precision medicine. N Engl J Med 2015;372(9):793–5.

[3] National Research Council (US) Committee on A Framework for Developing a New Taxonomy of Disease. Toward precision medicine: building a knowledge network for biomedical research and a new taxonomy of disease. Washington, DC: National Academies Press (US); 2011.

[4] Howlander N, NA, Krapcho M, et al. SEER cancer statistics review, 1975-2012 2015. Available at: http://seer.cancer.gov/csr/1975_2012/. Accessed November 19, 2018.
[5] Conroy T, Desseigne F, Ychou M, et al. FOLFIRINOX versus gemcitabine for metastatic pancreatic cancer. N Engl J Med 2011;364(19):1817–25.
[6] Von Hoff DD, Goldstein D, Renschler MF. Albumin-bound paclitaxel plus gemcitabine in pancreatic cancer. N Engl J Med 2014;370(5):479–80.
[7] Kaufman B, Shapira-Frommer R, Schmutzler RK, et al. Olaparib monotherapy in patients with advanced cancer and a germline BRCA1/2 mutation. J Clin Oncol 2015;33(3): 244–50.
[8] O'Reilly EM, Lowery MA, Segal MF, et al. Phase IB trial of cisplatin (C), gemcitabine (G), and veliparib (V) in patients with known or potential BRCA or PALB2-mutated pancreas adenocarcinoma (PC). J Clin Oncol 2014;32(15):4023.
[9] Feldmann G, Beaty R, Hruban RH, et al. Molecular genetics of pancreatic intraepithelial neoplasia. J Hepatobiliary Pancreat Surg 2007;14(3):224–32.
[10] Jones S, Zhang X, Parsons DW, et al. Core signaling pathways in human pancreatic cancers revealed by global genomic analyses. Science 2008;321(5897):1801–6.
[11] Collisson EA, Sadanandam A, Olson P, et al. Subtypes of pancreatic ductal adenocarcinoma and their differing responses to therapy. Nat Med 2011;17(4):500–3.
[12] Balagurunathan Y, Morse DL, Hostetter G, et al. Gene expression profiling-based identification of cell-surface targets for developing multimeric ligands in pancreatic cancer. Mol Cancer Ther 2008;7(9):3071–80.
[13] Biankin AV, Waddell N, Kassahn KS, et al. Pancreatic cancer genomes reveal aberrations in axon guidance pathway genes. Nature 2012;491(7424):399–405.
[14] Waddell N, Pajic M, Patch AM, et al. Whole genomes redefine the mutational landscape of pancreatic cancer. Nature 2015;518(7540):495–501.
[15] Moffitt RA, Marayati R, Flate EL, et al. Virtual microdissection identifies distinct tumor- and stroma-specific subtypes of pancreatic ductal adenocarcinoma. Nat Genet 2015;47(10): 1168–78.
[16] Bailey P, Chang DK, Nones K, et al. Genomic analyses identify molecular subtypes of pancreatic cancer. Nature 2016;531(7592):47–52.
[17] Pishvaian MJ, Bender RJ, Halverson D, et al. Molecular profiling of patients with pancreatic cancer: initial results from the know your tumor initiative. Clin Cancer Res 2018;24(20): 5018–27.
[18] Chantrill LA, Nagrial AM, Watson C, et al. Precision medicine for advanced pancreas cancer: the individualized molecular pancreatic cancer therapy (IMPaCT) trial. Clin Cancer Res 2015;21(9):2029–37.
[19] Aung KL, Fischer SE, Denroche RE, et al. Genomics-driven precision medicine for advanced pancreatic cancer: early results from the COMPASS trial. Clin Cancer Res 2018;24(6): 1344–54.
[20] McNair AG, Choh CT, Metcalfe C, et al. Maximising recruitment into randomised controlled trials: the role of multidisciplinary cancer teams. Eur J Cancer 2008;44(17):2623–6.
[21] Onukwugha E, Petrelli NJ, Castro KM, et al. ReCAP: impact of multidisciplinary care on processes of cancer care: a multi-institutional study. J Oncol Pract 2016;12(2):155–6, e157-68.
[22] Von Hoff DD, Stephenson JJ Jr, Rosen P, et al. Pilot study using molecular profiling of patients' tumors to find potential targets and select treatments for their refractory cancers. J Clin Oncol 2010;28(33):4877–83.
[23] Tsai S, Christians KK, George B, et al. A phase II clinical trial of molecular profiled neoadjuvant therapy for localized pancreatic ductal adenocarcinoma. Ann Surg 2018;268(4): 610–9.
[24] Mehmood S, Jahan A, Loya A, et al. Onsite cytopathology evaluation and ancillary studies beneficial in EUS-FNA of pancreatic, mediastinal, intra-abdominal, and submucosal lesions. Diagn Cytopathol 2015;43(4):278–86.

[25] Kim MP, Evans DB, Wang H, et al. Generation of orthotopic and heterotopic human pancreatic cancer xenografts in immunodeficient mice. Nat Protoc 2009;4(11):1670–80.
[26] Byrne AT, Alferez DG, Amant F, et al. Interrogating open issues in cancer precision medicine with patient-derived xenografts. Nat Rev Cancer 2017;17(4):254–68.
[27] Tiriac H, Belleau P, Engle DD, et al. Organoid profiling identifies common responders to chemotherapy in pancreatic cancer. Cancer Discov 2018;8(9):1112–29.

Advances in Surgery 53 (2019) 117–129

ADVANCES IN SURGERY

Is Hyperthyroidism Diagnosed and Treated Appropriately in the United States?

Ammar Asban, MD, Sophie Dream, MD,
Brenessa Lindeman, MD, MEHP*

Department of Surgery, The University of Alabama at Birmingham, Birmingham, AL, USA

Keywords

• Hyperthyroidism • Thyroid stimulating hormone • Underdiagnosis • Undertreatment • Thyroidectomy

Key points

- Recent studies suggest that hyperthyroidism is underdiagnosed and undertreated in the United States.
- Thyroid hormone has important effects on many organ systems and untreated hyperthyroidism can result in severe complications including cardiovascular disease and increased mortality.
- Hyperthyroidism should be suspected in patients with any clinical manifestations of the disease and screened for by obtaining a thyroid-stimulating hormone level.
- Hyperthyroidism can be readily treated through use of antithyroid drugs and more definitive therapies, such as radioactive iodine and total thyroidectomy.
- Diagnosis and treatment of hyperthyroidism warrant further study to understand the overall burden of cost to the US economy and health care system.

INTRODUCTION

Hyperthyroidism is a clinical condition that results from excessive levels of circulating thyroid hormone (thyroxine [T4] and tri-iodothyronine [T3], the active form). The prevalence of hyperthyroidism is 1.2% in the United States (0.5% overt and 0.7% subclinical) and 0.8% in Europe [1]. Worldwide, the

Disclosure Statement: The authors have nothing to disclose.

*Corresponding author. 1808 7th Avenue South, BDB 603, Birmingham, AL 35294. *E-mail address:* blindeman@uabmc.edu

https://doi.org/10.1016/j.yasu.2019.04.007
0065-3411/19/

most common etiologies are Graves' disease, followed by toxic multinodular goiter, and single toxic adenoma [2].

Although clinicians may suspect hyperthyroidism based on a wide variety of clinical signs and symptoms, the diagnosis is biochemical and made through demonstration of a suppressed thyroid-stimulating hormone (TSH) and/or elevated free T4 or T3. Further laboratory tests or imaging studies may be obtained for confirmation of the diagnosis and delineation of the etiology, such as the thyroid-stimulating immunoglobulin (TSI), thyrotropin receptor antibody (TRAb), and radiologic evaluation of the thyroid gland using radioactive iodine uptake (RAIU) scanning. Once the diagnosis of hyperthyroidism has been established, the key to definitive treatment lies in identification of the underlying cause of thyrotoxicosis. The 3 mainstays of therapy for hyperthyroidism are antithyroid drugs (ATDs), radioactive iodine (RAI), and surgery.

However, recent evidence suggests that hyperthyroidism may not be appropriately diagnosed and treated in the United States. In 1 study that identified all patients found to have a suppressed TSH at a large academic center, only 33% received further evaluation (including a repeat TSH), and 37% remained undiagnosed after further evaluation of their suppressed TSH [3]. Additionally, of those with an established diagnosis of hyperthyroidism, only 55% were referred for definitive therapy (34% to RAI and 21% to surgery) [3].

Therefore, this article highlights the most recent updates concerning the diagnosis and management of hyperthyroidism in the United States, and discusses potential implications of widespread underdiagnosis and undertreatment of hyperthyroidism.

SIGNIFICANCE

Disease impact on multiple organ systems

The thyroid gland affects nearly every organ system in the body, and owing to the potentially wide-reaching morbidities of undiagnosed and untreated disease, health care providers should maintain a higher level of suspicion for hyperthyroidism in patients presenting with any of its clinical manifestations. In 2016, the American Thyroid Association published guidelines recommending a comprehensive history and physical examination, including pulmonary, cardiac, and neuromuscular function evaluation, for all patients with suspected or known hyperthyroidism [2]. Hyperthyroidism symptoms are attributed to elevated thyroid hormone levels, and the wide range of clinical manifestations among these patients depends on the severity and duration of disease, patient age, comorbidities, and the underlying cause of hyperthyroidism. Some common clinical manifestations are independent of the underlying etiology, including sweating, heat intolerance, irritability, decreased concentration, anxiety, weight loss, and fatigue. Table 1 summarizes symptoms and signs of hyperthyroidism [4]. Other signs and symptoms are related to a specific etiology of hyperthyroidism, particularly Graves' disease, in which patients may present with ophthalmopathy and an infiltrative dermopathy where the skin is raised, hyperpigmented, and like an orange peel, particularly in the pretibial region.

Table 1
Symptoms and signs of hyperthyroidism

	Symptoms	Signs
Constitutional	Weight loss despite increased appetite; heat-related symptoms (heat intolerance, sweating, and polydipsia)	Weight loss
Neuromuscular	Tremor; nervousness; anxiety; fatigue; weakness; disturbed sleep; poor concentration	Tremor of the extremities; hyperactivity; hyperreflexia; pelvic and girdle muscle weakness
Cardiovascular	Palpitations	Tachycardia; systolic hypertension; irregular heartbeat (atrial fibrillation)
Pulmonary	Dyspnea, shortness of breath	Tachypnoea
Gastrointestinal	Hyperdefecation; nausea, vomiting	Abdominal tenderness
Skin	Increased perspiration	Warm and moist skin
Reproductive	—	Menstrual disturbances
Ocular (Graves' disease)	Diplopia; sense of irritation in the eyes; eyelid swelling; retroorbital pain or discomfort	Proptosis; eyelid retraction and lag; periorbital edema; conjunctival injection and chemosis; ophthalmoplegia

Reprinted with permission from Elsevier De Leo S, Lee SY, Braverman LE. Hyperthyroidism. Lancet. 2016;388:906–18.

Unique presentations of hyperthyroidism can be observed in particular patient age groups. In the pediatric population, hyperthyroidism has a negative effect on growth, development, and neuropsychiatric skills [5,6]. About 3% of children are affected by hyperthyroidism, with an incidence of 4.6 in 100,000 person-years in a population-based study conducted in France in 2015 [7]. Compared with adults, children presented more often with voice problems and difficulty concentrating, which may more directly affect their intellectual and communication skills during an important period of growth and development. Therefore, it is essential for the pediatric population with hyperthyroidism to be diagnosed and treated at an early stage. Additionally, behavioral problems, a short attention span, mood swings, and hyperactivity tend to be more common in hyperthyroid children when compared with adults [8].

By contrast, older patients (>60 years) with hyperthyroidism more often lack the classic symptoms of sympathetic hyperactivity (heat intolerance, tremor, sweating, and bowel hyperactivity) compared with younger patients. They present more frequently with weight loss, decreased appetite, shortness of breath, apathetic thyrotoxicosis (weakness and asthenia), and cardiac manifestations such as atrial fibrillation (AF) and tachycardia [9–12]. In a cross-sectional study of 3000 patients with hyperthyroidism, older patients had significantly fewer classical signs and symptoms of hyperthyroidism [10]. A national study in Denmark showed that 3% of 145,623 patients with new onset AF were found to have hyperthyroidism, compared with 1% of the general population [13]. In addition, those who are older than 60 years were more likely to develop congestive heart failure and/or embolic stroke secondary to AF. Similarly, 17% patients with AF of unknown cause were found to have underlying undiagnosed hyperthyroidism [14]. In this group of patients, hyperthyroidism was found to be underdiagnosed and symptoms were sometimes misdiagnosed as depression [15].

Pregnant women with undiagnosed or untreated hyperthyroidism may present with pregnancy complications, such as spontaneous abortion, stillbirth, premature labor, low birth weight, preeclampsia, hypertension, or heart failure [16]. Last, patients may also present with thyroid storm, the most severe and life-threatening form of hyperthyroidism. Patients with untreated hyperthyroidism who subsequently have noncompliance with medications, infection, trauma, or any other form of stress are believed to be most at risk. Clinical manifestations of thyroid storm include cardiovascular complications such as severe tachycardia, AF, congestive heart failure, central nervous system alterations, gastrointestinal and hepatic disturbances, and death from cardiopulmonary and/or multiorgan failure [17]. Mortality from this rare syndrome was 10.7% to 25.0% in a case series that included 28 patients [17,18].

Physical examination of patients with hyperthyroidism should not be limited to just the neck. Evaluation of the neck should include inspection for distended neck veins as well as any asymmetry of the thyroid and palpation for enlargement, nodularity, fixation, and retrosternal extension. In some patients, a bruit may be auscultated over thyroid gland. Patients with hyperthyroidism will also express signs of a hyperactive sympathetic nervous system, including tremor, warm and sweaty hands, hyperreflexia, and occasionally muscle weakness. Cardiovascular examination often reveals tachycardia with elevated systolic blood pressure and hyperdynamic precordium, and patients with AF will have an irregularly irregular rhythm [11]. Patients may also demonstrate hyperactivity, rapid speech, anxiety, and a facial flushing. Finally, extrathyroidal features of Graves' disease such as ophthalmopathy (periorbital edema, lid lag and retraction, conjunctival redness and edema), dermopathy (as described), or pretibial myxedema may be prominent.

Laboratory and imaging evaluation

The first step in the evaluation for hyperthyroidism is measurement of serum TSH, because it has high sensitivity and specificity, and can also be used as a screening test [2]. Hyperthyroidism is routinely divided into 2 entities: overt and subclinical hyperthyroidism. In overt hyperthyroidism, TSH is usually suppressed to less than 0.04 mU/L (undetectable) with elevated T3 and/or T4. In subclinical hyperthyroidism, TSH is below the reference range, but T3 and T4 are within the normal range. Thus, an abnormally suppressed TSH should trigger further measurement of circulating thyroid hormones and total and free T4 and T3. Furthermore, in the majority of patients, the underlying etiology of hyperthyroidism is suspected based on the clinical presentation, with the triad of exophthalmos, palpitations and goiter first described by Robert James Graves (1796–1853) continuing to be seen commonly today.

In relatively asymptomatic patients, however, the underlying etiology of hyperthyroidism may be unknown until after the diagnosis of hyperthyroidism is established. Such further evaluation can be accomplished by laboratory tests including measurement of TSI or TRAb, and imaging studies such as RAIU scan or measurement of thyroid blood flow on ultrasound. In the absence of a nodular goiter on physical examination, a diagnosis of Graves' disease can be confirmed by measurement of TSI or TRAb, which has sensitivity and specificity of 97% and 99%, respectively [2,19]. In the United States, measurement of TRAb has not been preferred in routine practice, and is often only considered in situations where RAIU is contraindicated. This is in contrast to the practice in Europe, Korea, and Japan, where TRAb is preferred over RAIU [20–23]. Additionally, TRAb has been shown to decrease overall costs by 47%, with a 46% faster time to diagnosis in an evidence-based economic model study in the United States [24].

Ultrasound examination has the ability to assess thyroid blood flow and evaluate the gland for abnormal nodules that would warrant further testing such as fine needle aspiration biopsy. The 2016 American Thyroid Association guidelines recommend RAIU if the clinical presentation suggests toxic multinodular goiter or toxic adenoma, but thyroid Doppler ultrasound examination for pregnant and breastfeeding women or other patients for whom RAIU is contraindicated [2]. For Graves' disease, one cost-effectiveness study comparing ultrasound examination with RAIU found ultrasound examination to be more cost-effective and sensitive for diagnosis compared with RAIU, 97.2% versus 95.2%, respectively [25]. Additionally, ultrasound examination has the advantages of being inexpensive, noninvasive, and patients are not exposed to any ionizing radiation. Furthermore, the accuracy of ultrasound examination can be improved by using color flow Doppler techniques. Thyroid gland vascularity, especially flow through the inferior thyroid artery, can be diagnostic, with high flow consistent with Graves' disease and low flow more indicative of destructive thyroiditis [26–28]. Additionally, change in echogenicity across serial ultrasound examinations has been shown to predict both remission after initiation of ATDs and to identify patients at high risk for recurrence after ATD withdrawal. Ultrasound examination can also identify and characterize incidental thyroid nodules, which have been reported in 16% of Graves' disease patients in 1 series [25].

RAI I^{131} uptake is commonly used in the United States to identify the underlying etiology of hyperthyroidism. Hyperactive thyroid tissue will trap and organify the radiolabeled iodine, and this can be measured by a gamma camera after an interval of 24 hours. Pregnancy and breastfeeding are absolute contraindications to RAIU scanning. When obtained, RAIU scans show increased diffusely homogenous uptake in Graves' disease, asymmetric irregular uptake in toxic multinodular goiter, and an area of focally increased uptake in toxic adenoma. In contrast, normal to low RAI uptake will be observed in destructive conditions such as subacute, viral, and postpartum thyroiditis, and with exogenous thyroid hormone administration. Although RAIU is still considered by some to be a useful tool for calculating the dose of iodine for those opting to receive RAI therapy as definitive treatment, this is discouraged by the European guidelines for patients receiving RAI owing to its poor prognostic ability, higher cost, patient inconvenience, and radioactive isotope exposure [20,29,30]. Owing to its low sensitivity in detecting thyroid nodules as well as higher cost compared with ultrasound examination, the usefulness of RAIU scans for patients with hyperthyroidism is limited and can be reserved for selected cases where the diagnosis cannot be clearly established by laboratory evaluation and ultrasound examination [20,25,31].

Treatment of hyperthyroidism

Antithyroid drugs

ATDs may be used to achieve a euthyroid state for remission of thyrotoxicosis or before a more definitive treatment such as RAI or surgery. The 2 major ATDs used in the United States are methimazole (MMI) and propylthiouracil (PTU). Both drugs are absorbed by the thyroid and bind to thyroid peroxidase, preventing the coupling of iodide to the tyrosyl residues of thyroglobulin, inhibiting the synthesis of T3 and T4. PTU additionally acts on peripheral tissues to inhibit tetraiodothyronine 5′ deiodinase from converting T4 to T3. The use of PTU in the first trimester of pregnancy is preferred over MMI as protein binding decreases its ability to cross the placenta. Both PTU and MMI have been associated with adverse effects, including rash, hepatotoxicity, and agranulocytosis, in up to 13% of patients in 1 study [32]. Of these patients, those treated with MMI experienced adverse effects more often than those taking PTU (14.9% vs 6.9%; odds ratio, 2.3; 95% confidence interval [CI], 1.80–3.06), however, hepatotoxicity was more common with PTU administration (2.7% vs <1.0%) [32]. Agranulocytosis was similarly rare with both medications, occurring in less than 1% of patients on ATDs [32]. Therefore, before the initiation of ATDs, patients should have a complete blood count and liver function tests, and receive education about the symptoms of allergic reaction, hepatotoxicity, and agranulocytosis. They should be instructed to stop these medications and call their prescribing physician if they have any symptomatology. When evaluating the use of ATDs in Graves' disease, the rate of relapse for both high- and low-dose regimens are 51% and 54%, respectively [33]. The optimal duration of treatment of Graves' disease with ATD is 12 to 18 months; use beyond 18 months has not demonstrated benefit [33]. Regarding cost, the use of ATDs for more than 12 months has been shown to have a higher cost of therapy when compared with patients undergoing RAI, without a difference in achieving a euthyroid state [34].

Radioactive iodine ablation

The oral administration of I^{131} results in uptake of radioiodine by thyroid follicular cells, which results in the release of β-ray emission and subsequent follicular cell destruction. Although this is the most common method of definitive treatment for hyperthyroidism in the United States, it is suboptimal for patients needing rapid control of symptoms or those with organ dysfunction secondary to hyperthyroidism, as the treatment effect takes 6 to 8 weeks on average, and can be as long as 6 months. After an initial dose of RAI, 86% of patients achieve a euthyroid or hypothyroid state [35]. An additional dose of RAI may be given to patients that have persistent hyperthyroidism after 4 to 6 months. A second dose is more likely necessary in patients who have received lower doses of RAI (185 MBq) when compared with patients receiving higher doses (370 MBq) [36].

RAI is contraindicated in patients who are pregnant, breastfeeding, or plan to become pregnant within 6 months after therapy, because it crosses the placenta and may be concentrated within the fetal thyroid at 10 to 12 months of gestation [37]. Owing to concerns for thyroid cancer later in life as well as precipitation of other secondary neoplasms, RAI is relatively contraindicated in children and those in close contact with children. Patients who undergo RAI for multinodular goiter have been shown to have increased risk of thyroid cancer mortality [38]. RAI has also been linked to an increased incidence of cancers in organs that concentrate I^{131} (salivary glands, kidneys, bladder), as well as those in the breast, digestive, and respiratory tracts [39–42]. Severe ophthalmopathy may be worsened with the use of RAI in approximately 15% of patients; therefore, it is a relative contraindication. Tallstedt and colleagues [43] performed a randomized, controlled trial of patients receiving RAI for Graves' disease compared with patients receiving MMI for 18 months or subtotal thyroidectomy. They demonstrated that patients who underwent RAI had statistically significant worsening of their ophthalmopathy compared with patients treated with MMI or surgery (33% vs 10% and 13%, respectively; $P = .02$) [44]. When comparing 2793 patients undergoing RAI with age- and gender-matched controls, Metso and colleagues [45] found that there was an increase in all-cause mortality (rate ratio, 1.12; 95% CI, 1.03–1.20). This increased mortality rate was found to be due to cerebrovascular disease and cancer. Additionally, the risk of mortality increased with rising RAI dose in patients with nodular thyroid disease, but not Graves' disease [45]. Franklyn and colleagues [46] found significantly increased mortality in 7209 patients treated with RAI for hyperthyroidism owing to all causes (standardized mortality ratio [SMR], 1.1; 95% CI, 1.1–1.2; $P < .001$), cardiovascular disease (SMR, 1.2; 95% CI, 1.2–1.3), and cerebrovascular disease (SMR, 1.4; 95% CI, 1.2–1.5), and fracture (SMR, 2.9; 95% CI, 2.0–3.9) when compared with population age-matched controls. Mortality increase in this study was the most apparent in the year after RAI administration.

Surgery

Surgery is the preferred treatment for thyrotoxicosis in patients with compressive symptoms, thyroid nodule(s) concerning for malignancy, contraindication to RAI, children, severe Graves' orbitopathy, and patient preference. Owing to the risk of thyroid storm, patients should be relatively euthyroid before undergoing surgery. This may be achieved with ATDs or inorganic iodide. Symptomatic control of thyrotoxicosis may be achieved with the use of beta-blockade while ATDs take effect, which may take several weeks. Inorganic iodide may be administered as oral saturated potassium iodide (Lugol's solution), or intravenous sodium iodide. Iodide acts through the Wolff-Chaikoff effect, which inhibits the organification of iodine in the thyroid, inhibits the production of thyroid hormone, and prevents the release of thyroid hormone. The mainstay of surgical treatment for hyperthyroidism is total thyroidectomy, and is indicated in toxic multinodular goiter and amiodarone-induced thyrotoxicosis poorly managed with medication. For patients with Graves' disease, total thyroidectomy is also the treatment of choice owing to risk of recurrence, which has been shown to be 7.9% to 23.8% with subtotal thyroidectomy [47–49]. The risk of recurrence of Graves' disease after surgery is nearly 0% for total thyroidectomy [49]. The only indication for subtotal thyroidectomy in patients with hyperthyroidism is that owing to a solitary toxic nodule, when the contralateral thyroid lobe is without abnormality. Thyroidectomy, when performed by a surgeon who performs 25 or more thyroidectomies a year, carries a low risk of complications [50,51]. The risk of permanent hypoparathyroidism is less than 2%, permanent recurrent laryngeal nerve injury is less than 1%, and need for reoperation owing to bleeding 0.3% to 0.7% [52,53]. These risks are slightly increased in patients with Graves' disease, with rates of permanent hypoparathyroidism being 1.8%, permanent recurrent laryngeal nerve injury being 1.8%, and immediate postoperative bleeding being 1.0% [54]. More recently, evidence has shown that thyroidectomy can be safe and effective, even if it is done in an outpatient setting for patients with Grave's disease [55].

Treatment of thyroid storm

Treatment of thyroid storm requires supportive therapy, reduction of thyroid hormone levels, and treatment of the underlying cause, including the definitive management of hyperthyroidism. Reduction of thyroid hormone should be achieved with PTU, because it not only blocks the synthesis of thyroid hormone, but also the peripheral conversion of T4 to T3. Inorganic iodide may be used to stun the thyroid and prevent further production and release of thyroid hormone. The systemic effects of thyroid storm should additionally be managed with the administration of beta-blocker (propranolol), steroids, intravenous fluids, and external cooling, among other potential therapies. Although these patients are not ideal operative candidates, they often require surgery to achieve immediate and definitive management of their thyrotoxicosis.

DISCUSSION (PRESENT RELEVANCE AND FUTURE AVENUES)

Underdiagnosis of hyperthyroidism

In the United States, despite widespread availability of thyroid function laboratory assessment, as well as an increasing number of people with access to health care, a large number of patients with both overt and subclinical hyperthyroidism remain undiagnosed [3]. A recently published, large, retrospective study of 3336 patients with suppressed TSH revealed that 67% did not undergo further evaluation for their suppressed TSH (T3, T4, thyroid peroxidase antibodies, TSI, or RAIU) and hyperthyroidism remained undiagnosed in 37% of patients who had the appropriate workup [3]. Contrary to the conventional approach, thyroid peroxidase antibody evaluation was more frequently obtained (51%) in this study compared with T3 (20%) and T4 (22%). Interestingly, patient age group, race, and presentation symptoms were associated with an increased likelihood of hyperthyroidism diagnosis. Asban and colleagues [3] found that patients who are younger, African American, present with ophthalmopathy or weight loss, have no medical comorbidities, have private commercial insurance, lower TSH, and are in the outpatient setting were more likely to be recommended for further workup and evaluation among all patients with suppressed TSH. The authors attributed these findings to both a failure of the system to recognize a suppressed TSH as the first clinical finding for hyperthyroidism and alert health care providers, as well as to a knowledge gap among health care providers in understanding the gravity of untreated hyperthyroidism and the need for urgency in further work up and potential treatment [56,57]. To mitigate the system factors, some institutions have implemented algorithms to trigger an automatic serum free T3 and T4 in cases with a suppressed TSH [58]. Although this approach has a significant upfront cost, it likely pales in comparison to the costs of undiagnosed hyperthyroidism and its subsequent complications, especially cardiovascular disease, the leading cause of mortality in hyperthyroid patients [59]. Ongoing research into the prevalence and cost effectiveness of hyperthyroidism diagnostic algorithms is needed.

Undertreatment of hyperthyroidism

Sundaresh and colleagues [32] performed a metaanalysis of 8 studies including 1402 patients undergoing treatment for Graves' hyperthyroidism. Their findings demonstrated that patients treated with ATDs (52%) had higher relapse rates than RAI (15%) and surgery (10%). When comparing treatment modalities for Graves' disease across multiple studies, patients treated surgically consistently have the lowest recurrence rates. Torring and colleagues [60] performed a randomized, controlled trial of 179 patients undergoing treatment for Graves' disease where younger patients (18–34 years) were randomized to treatment with ATDs for 18 months versus subtotal thyroidectomy, and older patients (35–55 years) were randomized to receive ATDs, RAI, or subtotal thyroidectomy. Their results demonstrated relapse of 42% and 34% in both young and older medically treated groups, respectively, and those treated with RAI had a relapse rate of 21%. Patients in the surgical treatment group had the lowest rate of relapse, 3% and 8% for young and older patients, respectively. Palit and colleagues [48] performed a metaanalysis of 35 studies including 538 patients who underwent total thyroidectomy for Graves' disease, and their results demonstrated that all patients (100%) achieved hypothyroidism, with low rates of permanent complications: 0.9% recurrent laryngeal nerve injury and 1.6% hypoparathyroidism.

Despite the demonstrated safety and efficacy of total thyroidectomy for the treatment of hyperthyroidism, patients in the United States are most often treated with RAI. At our institution, only 21% of patients were referred to a surgeon for thyroidectomy despite evidence demonstrating lower relapse rates with surgical intervention when compared with alternative treatments [3]. In the hands of an experienced surgeon, the risks of thyroidectomy for Graves' disease are low (permanent hypoparathyroidism, <2%; permanent recurrent laryngeal nerve injury, 1.8%; and immediate postoperative bleeding, 1%) [54], particularly when compared with the 13% rate of adverse effects from ATD administration and complications of RAI, which include worsening orbitopathy, increased mortality rates, and increased risk of thyroid cancers and secondary malignancies. Further evaluation of the current treatment practices in the United States should be conducted to determine if hyperthyroidism patients broadly are receiving the most efficacious and cost-effective care, which will likely include surgical therapy for a larger population than that identified in current studies.

SUMMARY

To date, hyperthyroidism remains largely underdiagnosed and undertreated in the United States. Although thyroidectomy is the most effective definitive treatment modality, it is still underused despite the increasing evidence for its safety, efficacy, and long-term cost reduction. Underdiagnosis and undertreatment of hyperthyroidism could harbor a significant impact on health care costs in the United States, as well as directly impacting the outcomes of patients who suffer from the disease, given the vast effect of thyroid hormone on multiple tissues and organ systems. Therefore, future research should be directed toward identifying the most effective approaches to early detection of disease both by educating health care providers to have a high index of suspicion to further investigate patients with disease manifestations, and the institution of systems to automatically evaluate further all patients with a suppressed TSH. Finally, more definitive and effective treatment options, including total thyroidectomy, should be adopted by endocrinologists as well as primary care providers.

References

[1] Garmendia Madariaga A, Santos Palacios S, Guillen-Grima F, et al. The incidence and prevalence of thyroid dysfunction in Europe: a meta-analysis. J Clin Endocrinol Metab 2014;99:923–31.

[2] Ross DS, Burch HB, Cooper DS, et al. 2016 American Thyroid Association guidelines for diagnosis and management of hyperthyroidism and other causes of thyrotoxicosis. Thyroid 2016;26:1343–421.

[3] Asban A, Chung SK, Tresler MA, et al. Hyperthyroidism is underdiagnosed and undertreated in 3336 patients: an opportunity for improvement and intervention. Ann Surg 2018;268:506–12.

[4] De Leo S, Lee SY, Braverman LE. Hyperthyroidism. Lancet 2016;388:906–18.

[5] Cassio A, Corrias A, Gualandi S, et al. Influence of gender and pubertal stage at diagnosis on growth outcome in childhood thyrotoxicosis: results of a collaborative study. Clin Endocrinol (Oxf) 2006;64:53–7.
[6] Segni M, Leonardi E, Mazzoncini B, et al. Special features of Graves' disease in early childhood. Thyroid 1999;9:871–7.
[7] Simon M, Rigou A, Le Moal J, et al. Epidemiology of childhood hyperthyroidism in France: a nationwide population-based study. J Clin Endocrinol Metab 2018;103:2980–7.
[8] Loomba-Albrecht LA, Bremer AA, Styne DM, et al. High frequency of cardiac and behavioral complaints as presenting symptoms of hyperthyroidism in children. J Pediatr Endocrinol Metab 2011;24:209–13.
[9] Trivalle C, Doucet J, Chassagne P, et al. Differences in the signs and symptoms of hyperthyroidism in older and younger patients. J Am Geriatr Soc 1996;44:50–3.
[10] Boelaert K, Torlinska B, Holder RL, et al. Older subjects with hyperthyroidism present with a paucity of symptoms and signs: a large cross-sectional study. J Clin Endocrinol Metab 2010;95:2715–26.
[11] Woeber KA. Thyrotoxicosis and the heart. N Engl J Med 1992;327:94–8.
[12] Smith TJ, Hegedus L, Douglas RS. Role of insulin-like growth factor-1 (IGF-1) pathway in the pathogenesis of Graves' orbitopathy. Best Pract Res Clin Endocrinol Metab 2012;26:291–302.
[13] Selmer C, Hansen ML, Olesen JB, et al. New-onset atrial fibrillation is a predictor of subsequent hyperthyroidism: a nationwide cohort study. PLoS One 2013;8:e57893.
[14] Bruce SA, Rangedara DC, Lewis RR, et al. Hyperthyroidism in elderly patients with atrial fibrillation and normal thyroid hormone measurements. J R Soc Med 1987;80:74–6.
[15] Vitti P, Hegedüs L. Thyroid diseases: pathogenesis, diagnosis, and treatment. Cham, Switzerland: Springer International Publishing; 2018.
[16] Luewan S, Chakkabut P, Tongsong T. Outcomes of pregnancy complicated with hyperthyroidism: a cohort study. Arch Gynecol Obstet 2011;283:243–7.
[17] Swee du S, Chng CL, Lim A. Clinical characteristics and outcome of thyroid storm: a case series and review of neuropsychiatric derangements in thyrotoxicosis. Endocr Pract 2015;21:182–9.
[18] Akamizu T. Thyroid storm: a Japanese perspective. Thyroid 2018;28:32–40.
[19] Barbesino G, Tomer Y. Clinical review: clinical utility of TSH receptor antibodies. J Clin Endocrinol Metab 2013;98:2247–55.
[20] Kahaly GJ, Bartalena L, Hegedus L. The American Thyroid Association/American Association of Clinical Endocrinologists guidelines for hyperthyroidism and other causes of thyrotoxicosis: a European perspective. Thyroid 2011;21:585–91.
[21] Burch HB, Burman KD, Cooper DS. A 2011 survey of clinical practice patterns in the management of Graves' disease. J Clin Endocrinol Metab 2012;97:4549–58.
[22] Yamashita S, Amino N, Shong YK. The American Thyroid Association and American Association of Clinical Endocrinologists hyperthyroidism and other causes of thyrotoxicosis guidelines: viewpoints from Japan and Korea. Thyroid 2011;21:577–80.
[23] Moon JH, Yi KH. The diagnosis and management of hyperthyroidism in Korea: consensus report of the korean thyroid association. Endocrinol Metab (Seoul) 2013;28:275–9.
[24] McKee A, Peyerl F. TSI assay utilization: impact on costs of Graves' hyperthyroidism diagnosis. Am J Manag Care 2012;18:e1–14.
[25] Cappelli C, Pirola I, De Martino E, et al. The role of imaging in Graves' disease: a cost-effectiveness analysis. Eur J Radiol 2008;65:99–103.
[26] Vitti P, Rago T, Mazzeo S, et al. Thyroid blood flow evaluation by color-flow Doppler sonography distinguishes Graves' disease from Hashimoto's thyroiditis. J Endocrinol Invest 1995;18:857–61.
[27] Kurita S, Sakurai M, Kita Y, et al. Measurement of thyroid blood flow area is useful for diagnosing the cause of thyrotoxicosis. Thyroid 2005;15:1249–52.

[28] Hari Kumar KV, Pasupuleti V, Jayaraman M, et al. Role of thyroid Doppler in differential diagnosis of thyrotoxicosis. Endocr Pract 2009;15:6–9.
[29] de Bruin TW, Croon CD, de Klerk JM, et al. Standardized radioiodine therapy in Graves' disease: the persistent effect of thyroid weight and radioiodine uptake on outcome. J Intern Med 1994;236:507–13.
[30] Okosieme OE, Chan D, Price SA, et al. The utility of radioiodine uptake and thyroid scintigraphy in the diagnosis and management of hyperthyroidism. Clin Endocrinol (Oxf) 2010;72:122–7.
[31] Torizuka T, Kasagi K, Hatabu H, et al. Clinical diagnostic potentials of thyroid ultrasonography and scintigraphy: an evaluation. Endocr J 1993;40:329–36.
[32] Sundaresh V, Brito JP, Wang Z, et al. Comparative effectiveness of therapies for Graves' hyperthyroidism: a systematic review and network meta-analysis. J Clin Endocrinol Metab 2013;98:3671–7.
[33] Abraham P, Avenell A, McGeoch SC, et al. Antithyroid drug regimen for treating Graves' hyperthyroidism. Cochrane Database Syst Rev 2010;(1):CD003420.
[34] Jayaraman M, Pawah AK, Narayanan CS. Antithyroid drugs in Graves' disease: are we stretching it too far? Indian J Endocrinol Metab 2016;20:600–4.
[35] Alexander EK, Larsen PR. High dose of (131)I therapy for the treatment of hyperthyroidism caused by Graves' disease. J Clin Endocrinol Metab 2002;87:1073–7.
[36] Allahabadia A, Daykin J, Sheppard MC, et al. Radioiodine treatment of hyperthyroidism-prognostic factors for outcome. J Clin Endocrinol Metab 2001;86:3611–7.
[37] Hodges RE, Evans TC, Bradbury JT, et al. The accumulation of radioactive iodine by human fetal thyroids. J Clin Endocrinol Metab 1955;15:661–7.
[38] Ron E, Doody MM, Becker DV, et al. Cancer mortality following treatment for adult hyperthyroidism. Cooperative Thyrotoxicosis Therapy Follow-up Study Group. JAMA 1998;280:347–55.
[39] Goldman MB, Maloof F, Monson RR, et al. Radioactive iodine therapy and breast cancer. A follow-up study of hyperthyroid women. Am J Epidemiol 1988;127:969–80.
[40] Hoffman DA, McConahey WM, Fraumeni JF Jr, et al. Cancer incidence following treatment of hyperthyroidism. Int J Epidemiol 1982;11:218–24.
[41] Hall P, Berg G, Bjelkengren G, et al. Cancer mortality after iodine-131 therapy for hyperthyroidism. Int J Cancer 1992;50:886–90.
[42] Vanderpump M. Cardiovascular and cancer mortality after radioiodine treatment of hyperthyroidism. J Clin Endocrinol Metab 2007;92:2033–5.
[43] Tallstedt L, Lundell G, Torring O, et al. Occurrence of ophthalmopathy after treatment for Graves' hyperthyroidism. The Thyroid Study Group. N Engl J Med 1992;326(26):1733–8.
[44] Marcocci C, Bruno-Bossio G, Manetti L, et al. The course of Graves' ophthalmopathy is not influenced by near total thyroidectomy: a case-control study. Clin Endocrinol (Oxf) 1999;51:503–8.
[45] Metso S, Jaatinen P, Huhtala H, et al. Increased cardiovascular and cancer mortality after radioiodine treatment for hyperthyroidism. J Clin Endocrinol Metab 2007;92:2190–6.
[46] Franklyn JA, Maisonneuve P, Sheppard MC, et al. Mortality after the treatment of hyperthyroidism with radioactive iodine. N Engl J Med 1998;338:712–8.
[47] Sugino K, Mimura T, Ozaki O, et al. Early recurrence of hyperthyroidism in patients with Graves' disease treated by subtotal thyroidectomy. World J Surg 1995;19:648–52.
[48] Palit TK, Miller CC 3rd, Miltenburg DM. The efficacy of thyroidectomy for Graves' disease: a meta-analysis. J Surg Res 2000;90:161–5.
[49] Hermann M, Roka R, Richter B, et al. Early relapse after operation for Graves' disease: postoperative hormone kinetics and outcome after subtotal, near-total, and total thyroidectomy. Surgery 1998;124:894–900.
[50] Sosa JA, Bowman HM, Tielsch JM, et al. The importance of surgeon experience for clinical and economic outcomes from thyroidectomy. Ann Surg 1998;228:320–30.

[51] Adam MA, Thomas S, Youngwirth L, et al. Is there a minimum number of thyroidectomies a surgeon should perform to optimize patient outcomes? Ann Surg 2017;265:402–7.
[52] Abbas G, Dubner S, Heller KS. Re-operation for bleeding after thyroidectomy and parathyroidectomy. Head Neck 2001;23:544–6.
[53] Roher HD, Goretzki PE, Hellmann P, et al. Complications in thyroid surgery. Incidence and therapy. Chirurg 1999;70:999–1010 [in German].
[54] Guo Z, Yu P, Liu Z, et al. Total thyroidectomy vs bilateral subtotal thyroidectomy in patients with Graves' diseases: a meta-analysis of randomized clinical trials. Clin Endocrinol (Oxf) 2013;79:739–46.
[55] Mallick R, Asban A, Chung S, et al. To admit or not to admit? Experience with outpatient thyroidectomy for Graves' disease in a high-volume tertiary care center. Am J Surg 2018;216: 985–9.
[56] Abe E, Marians RC, Yu W, et al. TSH is a negative regulator of skeletal remodeling. Cell 2003;115:151–62.
[57] Meikle AW. The interrelationships between thyroid dysfunction and hypogonadism in men and boys. Thyroid 2004;14(Suppl 1):S17–25.
[58] Davey RX, Clarke MI, Webster AR. Thyroid function testing based on assay of thyroid-stimulating hormone: assessing an algorithm's reliability. Med J Aust 1996;164:329–32.
[59] Selmer C, Olesen JB, Hansen ML, et al. Subclinical and overt thyroid dysfunction and risk of all-cause mortality and cardiovascular events: a large population study. J Clin Endocrinol Metab 2014;99:2372–82.
[60] Torring O, Tallstedt L, Wallin G, et al. Graves' hyperthyroidism: treatment with antithyroid drugs, surgery, or radioiodine–a prospective, randomized study. Thyroid Study Group. J Clin Endocrinol Metab 1996;81:2986–93.

Advances in Surgery 53 (2019) 131–143
ADVANCES IN SURGERY

How Do We Prevent Burnout in Surgery?

Gerard M. Doherty, MD
Department of Surgery, Brigham and Women's Hospital, Harvard Medical School, Brigham Health & Dana-Farber Cancer Institute, 75 Francis Street, Boston, MA 02115, USA

Keywords

• Burnout • Surgery • Professional satisfaction

Key points

- Our profession should fit our lives, rather than the contrary approach as designed into the monastic surgeon paradigm.
- Improving professional satisfaction and decreasing the high rate of burnout among surgeons is a critical task facing all of us in surgery, but especially those of us who have chosen to assume some administrative responsibility for the field.
- The list of potential interventions here is long, and can include everything from simple ways to better respect surgeons' time off, such as email-free weekends, to employment policies that provide for temporary or permanent part-time work, parental leaves, and intermittent retraining opportunities to acquire new skills.

INTRODUCTION

Burnout among attending surgeons in and out of academic settings is a prevalent condition, and its treatment and prevention are a societal imperative if we are to maintain an optimal surgical workforce. Intervention requires understanding the causes of burnout, and how we came to be in this position, before we can make plans to alleviate or preclude it. The premise of this article, based on the personal and managerial experience of the author, is that surgery is young, the visionary leaders who created the field were fully engaged in surgery as their life's passion, and they came from a social era different than the current. The professional structures and expectations that they erected reflected themselves. Over the past 30 years, surgery has changed, and surgeons

Disclosure Statement: The author has nothing to disclose.

E-mail address: gmdoherty@bwh.harvard.edu

https://doi.org/10.1016/j.yasu.2019.04.017

have changed, but the professional orthodoxies have not. This has created discordance in surgeons' satisfaction with their professional and personal lives, leading to the constellation of symptoms that we reflect as burnout. Alleviating this requires changes in what we expect from ourselves, our colleagues, and our employers.

HOW DID WE COME TO BE WHERE WE ARE AS A PROFESSION?

Although the arc of surgery as a modern therapeutic endeavor is short, it has spanned several generations of careers, which makes it difficult for new trainees to form a perspective on the pace of change. The dependence of surgical education on mentor/mentee relationships, and the transfer of clinical management skills as a complex and habit-based craft, contribute to the sense that surgeons are entrusted with special knowledge. They must behave in exceptional ways to maintain the line of continuity from year to year, chief class to intern class, and senior surgeon to junior partner. All of this is true and useful; surgical problems happen at inconvenient times, discipline around details of care affect patient outcomes, and the judgment and skills of master surgeons are highly valuable. However, the model surgeon developed in this developing field to address these truths (the monastic surgeon) may not be the only, or best, way forward.

Surgery is a young field in the midst of transition

To those who enter surgery, whether in training or for treatment, it likely seems as though this is a mature field, and that our predecessors have tried all potential arrangements and settled on our current plan as the best. Many lectures on surgery begin with our ancestry tying back to ancient Egyptian surgeons and before, through the barber surgeon era, and so forth. However, surgery as a modern discipline, reflecting the wide application of operations to correct ills, is a new phenomenon, dating to the late nineteenth century at the earliest. Only with the introduction of general anesthesia and principles of antisepsis could surgical technique be developed to the point that it could be applied routinely. Even then, it started slowly. The Peter Bent Brigham Hospital (PBBH) was founded in 1913, and the first surgeon-in chief was Harvey Cushing, a surgical pioneer who helped to develop neurosurgery. In the first full year of operative statistics, 1915, PBBH surgeons performed 1526 operations on 1328 patients, a number that would now be a busy fortnight for the successor institution, Brigham and Women's Hospital (BWH). This did not change quickly. By 1935, PBBH surgeons performed 2135 operations on 1838 patients. In 2018, BWH surgeons performed 41,275 operations. Just this growth implies that the field changed dramatically over less than 100 years.

Other data also reveal this change. We have a human tendency to expand the history that has occurred during our memories, and to compress what preceded us. Dr Cushing appears from that lens to be ancient history: an established icon who developed entire fields of surgery, and established a premiere hospital and surgical training program based on the Johns Hopkins model from which he was recruited. However, there have been just five surgeons-in-chief at the Brigham (PBBH or BWH) since Dr Cushing, including the incumbent (and author). This is clearly too few principals for us to assume that every recommendable arrangement has been trialed, and that the current one is clearly best. This also allows for the idea that each of these people capably addressed the changing field of surgery and hospitals as appropriate for their time, but that none of those constructs are relevant to our current circumstance. Although we may believe as we enter surgery that the field is fixed and optimized, in fact, the field is young and still in significant flux.

Training in surgery, as developed in improved form for this modern era under Dr Halsted at Johns Hopkins in the late nineteenth century, is based on an extended period of committed didactic and practical study of the field after medical school. As originally arranged and often recounted, these house officers were nearly always unmarried men who lived in the hospital for a period of years, and served to support the 24/7 needs of the hospitalized and ambulatory patients (or out-door patients, as they are termed in the early PBBH reports). Once they had completed this training, under the observation of equally devoted mentors who were simultaneously developing surgery, they joined the practice of surgery with the same expectations of devoted service. Our historic ideal of the monastic surgeon, completely committed to their profession with all other obligations being secondary if acknowledged, I believe, descends from these beginnings.

Over time, we have improved many aspects of this training to reflect current expectations of a field that has become more routine. Recent examples include the work-hour changes developed through the Accreditation Council on Graduate Medical Education over the past two decades, and the standardized expectations of training program experience. These reflect an institutionalization of a field that has become less idiosyncratic as it has matured. The challenge now is to reflect that change across the arc of a surgical career.

Surgery has changed

Over the past 30 years, surgery has also changed. Medical care has advanced in many ways, nearly always to the benefit of patients. Disruptive technologies have been introduced that changed our practices. These include the advent of camera-based laparoscopy, allowing multiple operating room personnel to observe the intracorporeal contents, and for the surgeon to use two hands and multiple ports to perform more complex procedures. Imaging has changed the evaluation of trauma patients and eliminated the need for many laparotomies. Acid-suppression therapy and *Helicobacter pylori* treatment has virtually eliminated the need for ulcer operations, just as sentinel lymph node biopsy has greatly reduced the indications for lymph node dissections in melanoma or patients with breast cancer. Percutaneous vascular interventions have changed coronary and peripheral revascularization procedures, and cardiac valve procedures.

These advances have been accompanied by a blurring of boundaries among specialties. Previously, intervention for many conditions had required the involvement of those with surgical training. Novel approaches disrupted that, and have led to nonsurgeon interventionalists, rare 30 years ago, but integral to high-quality care now. Some of these specialists even work in the operating room, with the support of anesthesiologists and specialized nurses, but without training in surgery, something that essentially never happened not so long ago. The differentiating features of surgeons, interventions and the operating room, are no longer entirely exclusive. Thus, surgery has changed, and "outsiders" have demonstrated that they can participate, and effectively so, in the territory previously only accessible to the monastic surgeon.

The effects of these changes have been varied. In some cases, as surgeons have developed or adopted new techniques, as in vascular surgery, the surgeons have migrated to new sites of practice, and incorporated new approaches. In other areas, as for many cardiac procedures, surgeons have struggled to remain involved in the care for problems that were once solely in their domain.

In general, these approaches have involved less intensive care for patients, including shorter or no hospital stay, limited wounds that do not often require the specialized care learned in surgical training, and care for fewer complications that have occupied so much attention from surgeons and training programs. This has led to significant change in surgical practice, as many more patients and their conditions are managed outside of the hospital, or with limited stays. That has enabled many more patients to cycle through the same number of hospital beds, and increased the need for outpatient operating room facilities. With many of the previously low-acuity hospitalized patients now at home, the patients who are in the hospital are much more precarious, or in need of more laborious care. At the same time, the patients at home require more contact and ambulatory follow-up than previously.

This process has created increased productivity; more patients and more conditions treated in the same span of time and space. However, it has taken the busy surgeon or surgical service, and hustled it to an unsustainable pace, without redesign of the care team and system. Although some groups have been successful by changing their approach, others have struggled with the process changes necessary. And a major reason may be that persistent paradigm of the monastic surgeon: always personally available, with no inviolable commitments outside of patient care.

Pellegrini has delivered a characteristically useful analogy for the current state of change in surgery [1]:

> For many years, however, the pace at which innovation occurred allowed for intervals of time to test and validate the new idea and, when useful, to design educational and training methods that ensured its safe adoption. In some ways it resembled a trip down a river with rapids interspersed with waters of relative tranquility in which to recover. The pace of change has

> increased substantially over the last few years, and I predict that this pace will only accelerate in the future: the equivalent of navigating permanently in white waters.

This analogy may serve equally well for the pace of innovation and the pace of practice. As it has become possible to be more efficient at patient care, that increase in efficiency has also become expected. The only way to exceed last year's standard is to do even more next year. As we measure clinical productivity with ever increasing precision, we steadily increase the expectations of improvement.

Surgeons have changed

Over those same 30 years, surgeons have also changed. The prototypical surgeon then was a partnered male surgeon in a single-income household. Of course, there were exceptions, and the prevalence of the prototype was inconsistent around the country, but that was the prototype on which the medical system, and the life of the surgical attendings and residents, was built. By 2010, for male surgeons, 47% were in dual-income households, and 83% of female surgeons had a partner working outside of the home [2]. There are also more female surgeons overall compared with previously, and currently about half of surgery residents are women. This change in who we are as surgeons must affect our expectations of what we want from our profession. Our system, built for that previous archetype, the prototypical male, monastic surgeon, was not designed for the diversity of our current or future surgical workforce.

Finally, those surgeons from 30 years ago often came from privileged backgrounds. Even for those of us from comfort but not wealth benefitted from an era with lower tuitions and favorable student loan terms. In 1986, when I graduated from medical school, the mean student loan debt of a graduating medical student was $36K ($70K in 2018 USD) [3]. I personally had $43K in student loan debt, which seemed daunting then. In 2016, the median student loan debt for a graduating student from a US medical school was $197K. For general surgery-bound interns, 61% owed more than $100K in student loan debt. In addition, the terms of the current student loan debt are generally less favorable than what we faced 30 years ago, often with interest that accumulates during training.

Today's surgeons are different and in dissimilar circumstances than were faced previously; there are more women, with more partners in the workforce, and the student loan burden is substantially greater. These conditions may lead them to have different expectations of their professional lives.

Our career structure and expectations have been static

Although the practice of surgery has changed substantially, and surgeons have changed who we are, the structure of surgery and our expectations of ourselves have remained settled. This may be understandable. The attributes that contribute to a highly functional surgeon include diligence, commitment, maybe even some stubbornness to give up in difficult circumstances. Those behaviors are rewarded with better outcomes for patients. Why would these same people behave in a more agile way with respect to their career environment? Added to that is the length of training in surgery, typically 5 years minimum, but often 7 to 10 years by the end of research and specialty training. By that point, the trainee may be so invested in the current system, that their propensity to change is limited.

Surgery has changed, and in important ways, such as the Accreditation Council on Graduate Medical Education duty hours renovation. In fact, however, that was a change mandated by the threat from an outside agency as external forces planned imposition of work rules for residents. Internally driven change has been more limited. We have few features of a professional employment model. Options for part-time employment, on-going training to develop new opportunities, or clear career-planning through retirement are often limited. Our approaches to the increased number of female surgeons have been erratic, including our provisions for childbirth, nursing, and child-rearing for parents of both genders [4–7].

BURNOUT IS A PREVALENT AND THREATENING ISSUE

Our awareness of burnout among physicians and surgeons has become more widespread and more acute over the last several years. The measurements seem clear and consistent across institutions. Tait Shanafelt, now at Stanford University, has been a pioneer in these measurements. He and his group have surveyed US physicians nationally, and compared them with the general US population, regarding evidence of burnout and professional satisfaction as measured by the Maslach Burnout scale [8]. They have demonstrated that more than half of US physicians show evidence of burnout, and that those symptoms became more prevalent between 2011 and 2014 (Fig. 1). The prevalence also varies by specialty. Subsequent evaluations at the institutional level, including our own institution, shows that burnout is more prevalent, and professional satisfaction is lower, than one would expect or prefer in such a highly educated, well-compensated group.

How does this affect us? Clearly, it makes us less happy with our professional choices than we should be. It also makes us less effective in our roles as clinicians, teachers, mentors, and role models. The Shanafelt data show us that some specialties in particular have high levels of burnout, and low levels of professional satisfaction, and some of those are surgical specialties for which we must bear some personal responsibility to address. Our institutional data also show that women experienced symptoms of burnout at a higher rate than men at each phase of career, whether grouped by age or academic rank. We clearly have a burning platform that must be addressed. These findings have also been extended to the experience of residency training.

As Dr Pellegrini has described, there have always been times when professional demands were "over the top," causing stress with the clash between personal relationships and professional demands (the "rapids"), but these periods

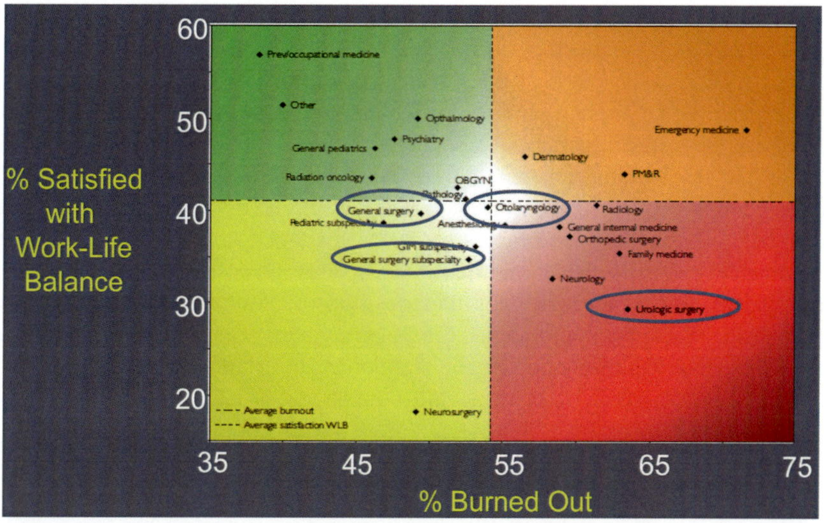

Fig. 1. Physician burnout, by specialty, as measured through surveys in 2014. (*Adapted from* Shanafelt TD, Changes in burnout and satisfaction with work-life balance in physicians and the general US working population between 2011 and 2014. Mayo Clin Proc 2015;90(12):1600–13; with permission.)

were separated by intervals of relative calm and routine, which provided space for recovery (the tranquil water of Pellegrini's metaphor). Now, however, the pace of practice has increased to approach continuous whitewater.

In the worst case, this has led to surgical practice assessment being reduced to its most basic revenue-producing essence: the surgeon as technician, functioning as a cog-in-a-wheel, reduced to a set of operative productivity numbers. The corporatization of medicine, with the frequent focus on measuring surgical productivity, hospital supply chain costs, revenue cycle performance, and relative surgeon efficiency, is necessary in our complex environment for us to meet all of our institutional goals. However, that emphasis and effort in measuring these items can leave the impression that efficient clinical productivity is the only important ambition. One can imagine the pinnacle of this as the surgeon who has determined how to practice with the utmost efficiency, year after year, and increasing by 3% per annum. This can inevitably lead to professional dissatisfaction for many who were attracted to the profession by the joy of forming therapeutic relationships with patients and families, the prospect of multidisciplinary interaction and decision-making to optimize patient care, and the opportunity to provide their best to each situation, all of which may be placed at jeopardy by the productivity demands of the corporate approach.

The key question is why? Why do our administrative systems place such emphasis on surgeon productivity? In the answer to that lies a key to addressing the burnout and professional satisfaction challenge facing our profession.

Interventional activity, and surgical activity in particular, is critical to hospital and health system financial performance. Not only is interventional work reimbursed at high rates, but also the infrastructure costs to enable interventional activity are high. Surgeons influence the use of these resources directly, and so we are measured precisely because we should be; our work has a direct effect on the institutional financial performance. As surgeons have increasingly become employed by the institution, directly, or indirectly through institutional subsidies, we too have become assets to be managed and optimized. To be responsible stewards of all of their human and physical resources, health care systems should measure and manage our work. But we as administrators must also take responsibility for the care and maintenance of our surgical workforce. The recent illumination of the state of burnout and workforce satisfaction should tell us that we have room to improve.

The impetus to address this is enhanced by an impending imbalance between the supply of surgeons in the workforce, and the demand for surgical services in the United States over the coming decade. As our population grows and ages, there will be substantially more demand for surgeons, but less supply growth compared with other specialties [9]. Although the overall supply of physicians will increase, as projected by the American Association of Medical Colleges, the projections for surgeon supply is flat across a variety of modeling scenarios. These scenarios include the projected retirement dates for surgeons, and the effect of slightly earlier or later retirements, and the anticipation that younger surgeons may choose to work at a slower productivity pace than their predecessors (millennial hours in based on some survey data of younger physicians. Finally, there is little opportunity for graduate medical education expansion to affect this by 2030 given the length of time required to fully train a surgeon.

At the same time, the demand for surgical services will increase, and there is little if any opportunity to replace surgeon work with alternative workers (nurses, nurse practitioners, or physician assistants). The projected shortfall of surgeons in 2030 in the United States will likely fall at about 25,000 full time equivalents. Thus, although current surgeons are showing symptoms of burnout that may be related in part to the pace of our required work, our future surgeons will be faced with even more work to be done, and no additional surgeons with whom to share it. Thus, our motivation to address burnout and professional satisfaction is only amplified by the anticipated future state. This increased demand also creates our opportunity; we as a profession and as health care institutions have no choice but to address this.

WHAT AFFECTS PHYSICIAN SATISFACTION?

Our plans should be guided by what we know about physician satisfaction. In 2013, the RAND Corporation prepared a report sponsored by the American Medical Association, to define the factors that affect physician satisfaction in the United States (factors affecting physician professional satisfaction and their implications for patient care, health systems, and health policy) [10]. The report addresses professional satisfaction broadly across specialties, geography, practice settings, and physician demographics. This may provide us some guidance as to where we can effectively change to address surgeon burnout. The full report contains substantial detail, but some common themes of what affects physician satisfaction can be gleaned, and can be ordered by their influence (Box 1).

The most impactful feature affecting physician satisfaction was their self-perception of the opportunity to provide high-quality care. This is reassuring, and indicates that the humanitarian values that attracted many to medical practice continue to be influential during practice. Conversely, barriers to providing high-quality care were strongly perceived as professional dissatisfiers, and included an unsupportive practice environment, blockages to preferred care by payors, and too high of a practice pace.

The electronic health record (EHR) was a complex issue. Physicians recognize the value of the EHR as a concept, and some of the ways that it improves professional practice and patient care, mainly around the immediacy of access to information. However, the execution of the EHR is perceived as flawed, and the input and curation of data in the EHR as a barrier to quality care and satisfaction. In particular, the EHR was perceived to clutter the patient record with notes that are not helpful for care, introducing a lot of material that is useful for billing, but that obscures the information needed for patient care.

Physician autonomy was an important satisfier. Not all physicians want to lead a practice but all want to be heard, and want to believe that their input impacts their environment. Conversely, the absence of this input leads to feeling helpless and disgruntled. In a related item, alignment of the physician goals with the practice leadership goals is important to the satisfaction with the professional setting. It seems straightforward to imagine that the opportunity to influence the practice, and the alignment of one's goals with the practice goals, must be related.

People are social by nature, and the opportunity to experience a positive social environment at work has a positive effect on physician satisfaction. Expressed as collegiality, this includes affirmative interactions in multiple

Box 1: Determinates of physician satisfaction

- Quality of care
- Electronic health records management
- Autonomy and work control
- Practice leadership
- Collegiality, fairness, and respect
- Work quantity and pace
- Work content, allied health professionals, and staff
- Payment, income, and practice finances

relationships, such as within the practice itself, but also including the relationships with patients and with referring physicians.

Work quantity affects all physicians, but in different ways for varied specialties. Surgeons and other procedural specialties tend to have the most complex relationship with work quantity, because they prefer too much work to too little work. For too little work, surgeons are concerned about practice viability and stability, which tends to be less of an issue with a practice that is too busy and can be expanded. For nonprocedural specialties, the relationship was generally simpler, with less work being preferable.

The content of the clinical practice is an important professional satisfaction actor. Physicians prefer to do work that is "top of license," that is, work that can only be done by physicians. They prefer to develop patient relationships that enable continuity in their practice. It seems that this is a particular dissatisfier for groups that have contact through limited episodes without reaching resolution, such as emergency medicine, or primary care practices that exclude management input during acute issues, such as hospitalizations. For specialists, the development of some niche of expertise supports physician satisfaction with their practice. Finally, for all groups, the opportunity to work with trusted staff is critical.

Practice finances are important to physician satisfaction. This includes their personal compensation, but also includes their perception of the stability of practice finances. Personal compensation satisfaction is affected by the stability of compensation over time, the compensation compared with the expectations of the individual, and the perception of fairness of compensation compared with others in the practice. Overall, there was decreased stress regarding compensation for employed physicians.

WHAT WE SHOULD DO TO ALLEVIATE AND PREVENT BURNOUT

Knowledge of our past including how we came to be where we are, and information about the present including what physicians tell us is important, should inform our plans for the future of our profession. We have an obligation to approach this thoughtfully to protect our surgeon workforce, and its important service to society.

We face some issues that are systemic and some that are self-inflicted. In the author's opinion, we must eliminate the latter, and position ourselves to best accommodate the former; we should fix what we can control and advocate for the rest. Synthesizing the information presented here into one plan is difficult, and we should anticipate that we will make changes that will work, and some that will not. Fear of the few failures should not stop us from action, because the status quo is untenable. Some suggestions are shown in Table 1.

Align with patients

The most important professional satisfier is the ability to provide high-quality care. Fortunately, that is also what patients prefer. We should align our goals of

Table 1
The way forward

- Align with patients
  - Use patient-reported outcome measurements to guide care
  - Promote quality = professional satisfaction
  - Support universal health care access to eliminate barriers to quality care
- Develop expertise in diseases, not techniques
  - Discipline of surgery not operating
  - Be adaptable and valuable
  - Find and develop a niche of expertise
- Practice redesign
  - Surgeon supply prevents us from doing clerical work
  - Care redesign with allied health care professionals to extend us
  - EHR customization to support work
  - Scribes or other documentation enhancement
  - Do not cede role of primary patient advisor or perioperative care to others
- Progressive employment policies
  - Profession needs to fit life
  - Respect time away from work: build "calm between the rapids" (eg, email-free weekends)
  - Part-time work
  - Parental leaves
  - Mid-career retraining opportunities
  - End-of-career practice adjustment
  - Focus on career development; support our professional talent as in other industries
- Respect choices
  - More than one definition of success
  - Space for different paths

providing care directly with what patients perceive as high-quality, and doing so requires knowing what that is. The emerging science of measuring patient-reported outcomes should dominate our judgment regarding the quality of our care. As with the business-related metrics that we commit so many resources to measuring, giving primacy of place to patient-reported measures will signal the importance of patients, and enable us to optimize the system for this metric in addition to the financial ones.

Develop expertise in diseases, not techniques

We have pursued the discipline of surgery, not the discipline of operating. We must resist the tides that might push surgeons toward financial optimization solutions that decrease our patient interactions. The discipline of surgery includes the operative and nonoperative management of a spectrum of diseases. Obvious examples include trauma care, but less obvious examples might be cancer care or heart disease. We must not cede our role as a primary advisor to patients and families in the care of these issues. Helping patients and families work through the options for management of their complex vascular disease, for example, might result in a plan to pursue nonoperative therapy. The professional satisfaction that comes with this level of involvement is important to us; however, to preserve that we must make sure that the service that we provide is also important to the patient and the care team. We need to maintain and value that decision-making, and patient-advisory expertise that makes our involvement useful. In short, remain an expert in the management of the disease, with a deep understanding of the operative issues, rather than becoming focused on merely the technical aspects of our craft.

Practice redesign

Surgeon supply and demand projections will prevent us from taking on clerical or administrative tasks, those that are away from the "top of license" tasks of counseling patients and performing operations. Care redesign will be critical, with allied health care professionals involved to extend our work, not to replace us in the patient counseling or technical tasks. Examples of this might be staffing a clinic to screen anorectal patient complaints to identify those who need our direct services, or engaging staff to perform portions of a visit that are important but clerical, such as medicine reconciliation. Management of the time spent documenting in the EHR can include such approaches as scribes to generate drafts of notes, or customization of the record entry with templates to abbreviate common tasks. However, these approaches should not include surrender of perioperative care to other specialists. For example, we should not move responsibility for postoperative care to specialties, such as anesthesiology or hospitalist medicine, because those maneuvers that separate the surgeons from the continuity of the patient recovery are dissatisfiers. Although those specialties may have important roles in the perioperative care, we would cede this responsibility at the risk of our own professional satisfaction.

Progressive employment policies

Our profession should fit our lives, rather than the contrary approach as designed into the monastic surgeon paradigm. Medicine in general and surgery in particular have been slow to adapt to modern concepts of work-life balance, and the employment compacts that underlie that. These compacts can be considered as ways to build "calm water between rapids." We cannot change surgical diseases, which in many cases arise at unpredictable times, and evolve over short cycles, but we can design our approach to providing the necessary availability and continuity of care in ways that provide individual surgeons with space to recover. The list of potential interventions here is long, and can include everything from simple ways to better respect surgeons' time off, such as email-free weekends, to employment policies that provide for temporary or permanent part-time work, parental leaves, and intermittent retraining opportunities to acquire new skills. These opportunities are common in other industries for professionals of our prominence. It is time for them to become common in surgery as well.

Respect our own choices

Finally, too often in surgery, we have valued one definition of success to the exclusion of others that might be more important to an individual. The monastic surgeon archetype of being singularly devoted to work, and for whom a career might not be defined as successful unless some position of administrative responsibility is obtained, does not sufficiently allow for many other paths to personal success. Those might include part-time work and focus on family or other pursuits, or an extended commitment to laboratory research, or a surgeon who wishes to practice full-time and not take up administrative roles. To the extent that we fail to respect these other choices as legitimate definitions of success, we hurt ourselves and our profession. We must allow space for people to follow different paths and to define success on their own terms.

Improving professional satisfaction and decreasing the high rate of burnout among surgeons is a critical task facing all of us in surgery, but especially those of us who have chosen to assume some administrative responsibility for the field. We owe it to ourselves and our successors to make conscious changes to the ways that we live and work, and succeed or fail, as surgeons and as people. We owe it to ourselves, our patients, our trainees, and our families to choose our way forward carefully and wisely.

References

[1] Pellegrini CA. Presidential address: the surgeon of the future: anchoring innovation and science with moral values. Bull Am Coll Surg 2013;98(12):8–14.
[2] Dyrbye LN, Shanafelt TD, Balch CM, et al. Physicians married or partnered to physicians: a comparative study in the American College of Surgeons. J Am Coll Surg 2010;211(5): 663–71.
[3] Grischkan J, George BP, Chaiyachati K, et al. Distribution of medical education debt by specialty, 2010-2016. JAMA Intern Med 2017;177(10):1532–5.
[4] Rangel EL, Castillo-Angeles M, Changala M, et al. Perspectives of pregnancy and motherhood among general surgery residents: a qualitative analysis. Am J Surg 2018;216(4): 754–9.
[5] Rangel EL, Lyu H, Haider AH, et al. Factors associated with residency and career dissatisfaction in childbearing surgical residents. JAMA Surg 2018;153(11):1004–11.
[6] Rangel EL, Smink DS, Castillo-Angeles M, et al. Pregnancy and motherhood during surgical training. JAMA Surg 2018;153(7):644–52.
[7] Scully RE, Davids JS, Melnitchouk N. Impact of procedural specialty on maternity leave and career satisfaction among female physicians. Ann Surg 2017;266(2):210–7.
[8] Shanafelt TD, Hasan O, Dyrbye L, et al. Changes in burnout and satisfaction with work-life balance in physicians and the general US working population between 2011 and 2014. Mayo Clin Proc 2015;90:1600–13.
[9] IHS Markit, The Complexities of Physician Supply and Demand 2017 Update: Projections from 2015 to 2030. Washington, DC: American Association of Medical Colleges; 2017. Available at: https://aamc-black.global.ssl.fastly.net/production/media/filer_public/a5/c3/a5c3d565-14ec-48fb-974b-99fafaeecb00/aamc_projections_update_2017.pdf. Accessed May 13, 2019.
[10] Friedberg MW, Chen PG, Van Busum KR, et al. Factors affecting physician professional satisfaction and their implications for patient care, health systems, and health policy. RAND corporation research report series. American Medical Association; 2013. p. 1–122.

Advances in Surgery 53 (2019) 145–160

ADVANCES IN SURGERY

Elimination of Bile Duct Injury in Cholecystectomy

Maria S. Altieri, MD, MS, L. Michael Brunt, MD*

Section of Minimally Invasive Surgery, Department of Surgery, Washington University School of Medicine, 660 Euclid Avenue, Campus Box 8109, St Louis, MO 63110, USA

Keywords

• Bile duct injury • Cholecystectomy • Laparoscopy • Gallbladder disease

Key points

- Laparoscopic cholecystectomy has been a remarkable advance in surgical care that has positively benefited millions of patients over the past 30 years.
- Although overall it is a safe operation, opportunities exist to reduce bile duct injury, which remains a priority for surgical quality improvement.
- The collective efforts of surgical societies to address this issue and the dissemination of safe operative management strategies and the development of consensus conference guidelines have the potential to make this operation even safer in the future.

INTRODUCTION

Gallbladder disease is common in the general adult population [1,2], making cholecystectomy one of the most commonly performed procedures in the United States and worldwide [3]. Early after its introduction in the late 1980s, laparoscopic cholecystectomy became the standard of care due to its advantages of reduced pain and hospital length of stay, reduced general complications (wound and cardiopulmonary), faster return to activity, lower costs, and increased patient satisfaction [4–6]. Although it is considered a safe procedure, complications still occur in approximately 5% to 6% of patients [7].

Bile duct injury (BDI) remains the most dreaded complication after laparoscopic cholecystectomy. Previous data report an incidence of 0.2% of BDI during the era of open cholecystectomy [8] and significantly higher for

Disclosure Statement: The authors have nothing to disclose.

*Corresponding author. *E-mail address:* bruntm@wustl.edu

https://doi.org/10.1016/j.yasu.2019.04.018

laparoscopic cholecystectomy [9]. In 2001, a survey questionnaire from the American College of Surgeons completed by practicing surgeons reported 34% of the responders self-reported a BDI [9]. Although its incidence has improved since laparoscopy was first introduced, studies have described an incidence ranging from 0.08% to 0.4%, depending on the definition of BDI [10–13]. One of the largest studies examining BDI comes from prospectively collected data from the Swedish National Quality Registry of Gallstone Surgery and Endoscopic Retrograde Cholangiopancreatography (GallRiks), which was established in 2005. This registry, which captures approximately 90% of all cholecystectomies in Sweden, examined 51,041 cholecystectomies and reported an overall incidence of BDI incidence of 1.5% (including bile duct leaks) and 0.4% incidence of major BDIs that required reconstruction [13]. Other administrative database studies and systematic reviews from the past 5 years have shown major BDI rates of 0.15% to 0.3% [10,14–17]. In the United States, where up to 1,000,000 cholecystectomies are performed annually, this translates into 2500 to 3000 BDIs per year.

BDI is a devastating and potentially life-threatening event that has been associated with other complications and the necessity for other procedures/interventions, lower quality of life, disability, higher mortality, and litigation [18,19]. Complications include biliary fistula, infection, and biliary obstruction. Studies have shown both increased short-term and long-term mortality due to BDI [20–23]. Pitt and colleagues [22] reviewed a single-institution experience of 528 patients with BDIs and reported a 2.4% mortality rate within 3 months of intervention after the injury. A study in 2013 examining 1083 cholecystectomies reported a BDI rate of 0.1% and an all-cause mortality rate of 0.8%. The attributed BDI mortality was 0.2% [21]. Halbert and colleagues [23] examined 156,958 laparoscopic cholecystectomies performed between 2005 and 2010. In this analysis, 125 patients with common bile duct (CBD) injury required further reconstruction. No 30-day mortality was observed; however, all-cause mortality was 20.8%, which was 8.8% above the cohort's expected age-adjusted rate of death. A more recent study examined 800 patients referred to a tertiary center after a BDI. The mean survival after BDI was 17.6 years and BDI-related mortality was 3.5% (28/800), because patients treated surgically had significantly higher survival. Finally, BDI patients reported a significantly worse physical quality of life, worse disease-specific quality of life, and higher loss of productivity compared with a control group and had a higher rate of disability [20].

BDI also has been associated with a significant economic health care burden, with reported total costs due to this complication surpassing $1 billion annually [19]. BDI remains a key source of malpractice claims against surgeons and is the most common reason for litigation against general surgeons [24]. Because BDI is associated with significant adverse effects on patient lives and is a contributor to increased health care costs, prevention of this complication is of high importance and strategies for minimizing BDIs have become a top priority for quality improvement in general surgery.

ETIOLOGY AND RISK FACTORS

BDIs can be classified as major and minor. Major injuries are those that require biliary reconstruction whereas minor injuries include bile leaks and tangential BDIs, most of which can be managed endoscopically. The GallRiks national registry for cholecystectomies in Sweden identified 747 BDIs among 51,041 patients performed between 2005 and 2010. A majority of the injuries were Hanover grade A1 (cystic duct leak, 35.5%), followed by a Hanover grade C1, C2, or C3 (tangential lesion in the CBD, 17.4%) [25].

One way to classify these injuries is by the Strasberg classification, which is a modification of the Bismuth classification and allows precise differentiation between small and serious injuries performed during laparoscopic cholecystectomy and the level of injury [26]. Types A, B, C, and D injuries are those that result in a bile leak without transection whereas type E injuries are those in which the main bile duct is completely transected and are classified by severity from E1 to E5. The etiology and mechanism of biliary injury may be multifactorial and includes aberrant biliary anatomy, acute or chronic inflammation in the hepatocystic triangle, technical factors, and misidentification of anatomy. Way and colleagues [27] in a landmark 2003 study evaluated the causes of BDI in 252 laparoscopic cholecystectomies. The investigators used operative, pathology and radiology reports and reviewed unedited videos of the procedures. BDIs were classified by the Stewart-Way classification. The primary cause was a visual perceptual illusion in which the surgeon believes the cystic duct is being dissected when in fact it is the CBD. Faults in technical skills were identified as the primary mechanism of injury in only 3% of cases.

Dissection during laparoscopic cholecystectomy should be performed gently and electrosurgery should be used carefully with short activations (2–3 s) to avoid thermal injuries. One common mistake is to start the dissection too low, which can endanger the bile duct and porta hepatis and can lead to misperception of biliary anatomy. In addition, retraction of the gallbladder is important because the fundus should be retracted cephalad, whereas the infundibulum should be retracted laterally and slightly caudal to avoid parallel alignment of the cystic duct with the CBD. The critical view of safety (CVS) is recommended for secure identification of structures to minimize the risk of a misidentification injury. Anatomic situational awareness also is important in limiting the risk of injury. Both of these aspects of safe cholecystectomy are discussed in further detail later.

CONDITIONS ASSOCIATED WITH THE DIFFICULT GALLBLADDER

Several conditions have been associated with increased difficulty of cholecystectomy that include acute cholecystitis, severe chronic cholecystitis (especially a shrunken, contracted gallbladder), obesity, Mirizzi syndrome, and cirrhosis. Obese patients may be more difficult due to difficulty in lifting the gallbladder to expose the hepatocystic triangle due to a bulky, fatty liver; omentum that hinders the exposure; and intrahepatic position of the GB. In such cases, placement of a fifth port in the right midabdomen for a retractor to displace the omentum inferiorly may be helpful. Both severe acute and/or chronic inflammation may obscure the anatomy and result in biliary inflammatory fusion of the cystic structures and neck of the gallbladder to the CBD and right hepatic artery, which can make it difficult or dangerous to obtain the CVS. Mirizzi syndrome consists of a large stone impacted in the gallbladder neck that causes partial obstruction of the CBD. In such cases, there often is considerable inflammation in the area, and surgeons should be aware of the potential for a fistula between the gallbladder and the bile duct. As a result, these patients are best managed in a center with expertise in difficult cholecystectomy and available interventional endoscopy.

Acute cholecystitis and timing of cholecystectomy

Acute cholecystitis is the most common condition that increases the difficulty of cholecystectomy. Several randomized controlled trials have examined the timing of surgery after presentation with acute cholecystitis with respect to early versus delayed cholecystectomy. In a study from Roulin and colleagues [28], early cholecystectomy was defined as performed after the index hospital admission, whereas delayed cholecystectomy was performed at least 6 weeks after initial antibiotic treatment. The investigators concluded that early cholecystectomy even beyond 72 hours of symptoms was safe and associated with less overall morbidity, cost, and hospital length of stay. Gutt and colleagues [29] in a study of 618 patients reported that morbidity was significantly lower in the immediate cholecystectomy group (11.8% vs 34.4%), although conversion rates and mortality did not differ between the 2 groups. Hospital costs and mean length of stay also were lower in the early group. A meta-analysis published in 2015 found that early laparoscopic cholecystectomy was associated with decreased wound infections, shorter length of stay and decreased costs, lower rates of BDIs and leaks, and lower rates of conversion to open cholecystectomy [30]. In none of these studies was the severity of the cholecystitis graded according to the Tokyo guidelines or other severity criteria. Nonetheless, it is generally recommended that in patients with acute cholecystitis who are acceptable risk candidates for surgery, laparoscopic cholecystectomy be performed early (<72 hours) after the onset of symptoms rather than later in the course.

STRATEGIES FOR REDUCING BILIARY INJURY

Despite description of the CVS more than 20 years ago and numerous publications on BDI and cholecystectomy, the problem continues to occur. In 2014, the Society of Gastrointestinal and Endoscopic Surgeons (SAGES) formed the Safe Cholecystectomy Task Force, with the goal of enhancing a culture of safety around this operation. A nominal group consensus technique was used to survey 160 surgeons to identify key domains important to safe dissection [31]. The result from this effort was development of a 6-step program of strategies that can be used by surgeons intraoperatively, described in detail later. SAGES also has recently published online a series of 12 educational modules that provide more depth to the topic and are freely available to the surgical community (fesdidactic.org).

Recently, a multisociety consensus conference sponsored by SAGES, the Americas Hepato-Pancreato-Biliary Association, International Hepato-Pancreato-Biliary Association, Society for Surgery of the Alimentary Tract, and European Association for Endoscopic Surgery on prevention of BDI in cholecystectomy was held to develop evidence-based practice recommendations and guidelines on this topic. In addition, priorities for future studies to address unanswered questions in the field also were formulated. The recommendations from the consensus meeting are available for viewing at www.preventbdi.org and will be published in the coming year.

The 6 steps in the SAGES program are as follows:

1. Use of the CVS for the identification of the cystic duct and artery
2. Awareness of the potential for aberrant anatomy
3. Liberal use of intraoperative cholangiography (IOC) or other methods for identification of structures
4. The use of an intraoperative time-out or pause during the procedure prior to clipping, cutting, or transecting the cystic duct or cystic artery to verify the anatomy
5. Recognizing when it is not safe to proceed if the dissection is entering a zone of danger and considering the need to alter the approach
6. Getting help from another surgeon if needed

Step 1: use of the critical view of safety

The CVS, first introduced in 1995 by Strasberg and colleagues [26], has 3 requirements (Fig. 1).

1. The hepatocystic triangle, which is defined as the triangle formed by the cystic duct, the common hepatic duct (CHD), and the inferior edge of the liver, should be cleared of fat and fibrous tissue.
2. The cystic plate should be exposed in such a manner that the lower third of the gallbladder is separated from the liver.
3. Only 2 structures, the cystic duct and cystic artery, should be visualized to enter the gallbladder.

The CVS method of identification has been the approach most accepted by surgeons around the world during laparoscopic cholecystectomy [32,33]. Although there are no direct comparisons or randomized controlled trials of using the CVS versus other methods, such as the infundibular or top-down techniques, several lines of indirect evidence suggest that the use of the CVS reduces BDI. Several large cohort studies have reported no or lower BDIs while using the CVS, [32,34,35]. The largest study, by Palanivelu and colleagues [34], examined a total of 9864 laparoscopic cholecystectomies and reported a BDI rate of 0.07%. In addition, case series studies of BDIs with analysis of the mechanism of injury using either intraoperative reports or video review indicate that the method of anatomic identification was nearly always something other than the use of the CVS [36–38]. The largest such study [39] comes from the Netherlands and encompasses 800 BDIs, of which 528

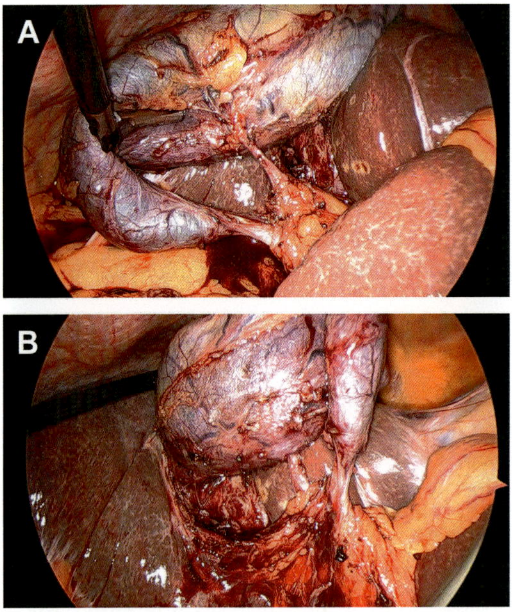

Fig. 1. Operative photograph of the CVS during laparoscopic cholecystectomy. Shown are the (*A*) anterior view and (*B*) posterior lateral view. Confirmation of the CVS should be made from both viewpoints.

operative reports were available. The CVS technique was reported in only 33 patients (6.3%) [39].

In another study of 1108 cases of laparoscopic cholecystectomy [37], 65 cases with complications underwent video review. Operative notes in these cases stated that the CVS was achieved in 80% when in fact it was reached in only 10.8%. Importantly, the CVS was not used in any of the cases of identified BDIs. In addition, because this technique was been introduced in 1995, only 1 report of a BDI using this technique has reported; however, the exact mechanism of BDI was unclear [37]. The Dutch Society of Surgery has now recommended that all surgeons use the CVS method of identification routinely during cholecystectomy [39]. Studies also suggest that the CVS is incompletely understood or not applied appropriately in many circumstances. Deal and colleagues [40] extracted 160 video cases of laparoscopic cholecystectomy from the internet and scored them both by expert surgeons and crowd workers according to published criteria for achievement of the CVS. They found an average CVS score of 3.6 (1–6 scale) and only 12.5% of videod cases achieved a CVS score greater than or equal to 5, which indicates considerable room for improvement [40].

Step 2: understanding normal and aberrant anatomy

Variations in biliary anatomy are common and are important considerations in reducing the risk of biliary injury. The hepatocystic triangle is bounded by the cystic duct, CHD, and the liver. Most commonly, the cystic artery is medial to the cystic duct and arises from the right hepatic artery, which commonly crosses posteriorly to the bile duct. The right hepatic artery may have a hump, which lies close to the gallbladder wall and may be vulnerable to injury if the dissection is too posterior. The cystic duct can be short due to inflammation and fibrosis and can have a variable course and path of entry into the CBD.

Variations in right hepatic duct anatomy are especially common and include separate entries of the anterior and posterior sectoral ducts into the CHD, low insertion of the right posterior duct on the CHD, and insertion of the cystic duct directly into the right hepatic duct (2%). The cystic duct may have a lateral, medial, or posterior entry into the CHD and may run parallel to it for a variable distance before entering it (Fig. 2). Rouviere sulcus is a fissure in the right lobe of the liver in which the right port pedicle runs and which demarcates the plane of the porta hepatis (Fig. 3). The dissection, therefore, always should stay anteriorly to Rouviere sulcus. The CBD also has an epicholedochal plexus on it which can help distinguish it from the cystic duct. Finally, a clue that the dissection may be on the CBD instead of the cystic duct is when the dissection is taking place in close proximity to the duodenum. A more detailed review of anatomy is available in the SAGES safe cholecystectomy modules (www.fesdidactic.org).

Step 3: role of intraoperative imaging to enhance identification of structures (cholangiogram, ultrasound, and intraoperative cholangiography)

IOC should be considered an integral tool in a surgeon's armamentarium when undertaking cholecystectomy, whether laparoscopic or open. Surgeons should

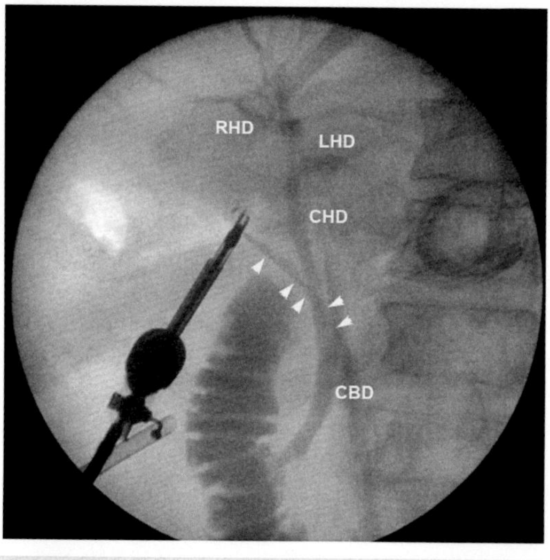

Fig. 2. IOC with parallel cystic duct (*arrowheads*). LHD, left hepatic duct; RHD, right hepatic duct. Note no filling defects and normal filling of duodenum with contrast.

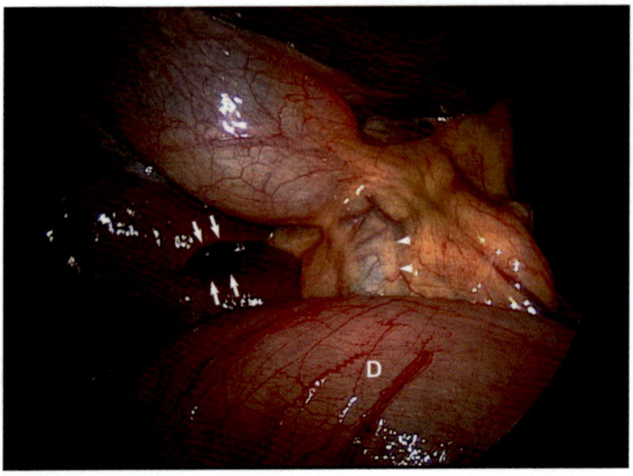

Fig. 3. Laparoscopic view of the gallbladder and Rouviere sulcus (*arrows*), which marks the plane of the porta hepatis. Note also the CBD (*arrowheads*) with epicholedochal plexus and proximity of duodenum (D) to the CBD.

be comfortable not only with the technique of IOC but also with the ability to accurately interpret the images. Since its introduction in the 1930s [41], the benefits of IOC have been debated. Many investigators advocate the routine use of IOC [11,42,43], although selective use has been advised as well and is practiced more commonly [44]. A study in 2002 reported a use of IOC during laparoscopic cholecystectomy in 44.6% of cases [45] and more recently a population study showed a decreasing rate of use of IOC with rates of utilization of IOC of 10% to 12% per year. This decrease in utilization of IOC raises the issue of adequacy of training in residency with its use and interpretation [25,43].

The use of IOC is controversial, because opponents consider it time consuming, cumbersome, and subject to misinterpretation or false-positive findings regarding the presence of CBD stones and without a clear impact of the risk of biliary injury [46,47]. Evidence from several large administrative database studies suggest, however, a benefit of reduction in BDI with IOC use [13,25,43,48–50] whereas others do not [15,46]. These studies are limited by a lack of detail regarding the reasons for IOC use and other variables, which make them at high risk of bias. When properly interpreted, however, IOC has been associated with increased intraoperative recognition of injury, which may decrease the severity of injury and avoid transection or excision of a portion of the duct. A systematic review of 8 randomized controlled trials showed no level 1 evidence for or against the use of IOC. Most of these trials were small, however, with few biliary injuries and were not sufficiently powered to answer the question in terms of biliary injury [51].

Buddingh and colleagues [39] performed a systematic review of articles examining several imaging techniques for prevention of BDI during laparoscopic cholecystectomy. The investigators concluded that IOC or laparoscopic ultrasound is recommended to be performed routinely. In the GallRiks Swedish database of 51,404 cholecystectomies, multivariable analysis showed that use of IOC was protective for BDI in acute cholecystitis and a history of acute cholecystitis only [13]. Another study from GallRiks found that routine IOC use was associated with a reduction in mortality during cholecystectomy [13] These findings highlight the importance of intraoperative imaging in potentially difficult cases.

Laparoscopic ultrasonography and fluorescent cholangiography are other methods for visualization during laparoscopic cholecystectomy. Compared with IOC, laparoscopic ultrasonography is not associated with radiation and is less time consuming. Studies have shown good fidelity with laparoscopic intraoperative ultrasound in identification of biliary anatomy. A disadvantage is that most surgeons have not been adequately trained with its use and interpretation, so its value is highly operator dependent [52,53].

Near-infrared fluorescent cholangiography was first described in 2009. It uses an injection of indocyanine green, which is excreted into bile and emits light with a peak wavelength of 830 nm when illuminated with near-infrared light (Fig. 4). This technique has reported rates of visualization of 71.4% to 100% for the cystic duct, 33.3% to 100% for the CHD, 25% to 100% for the cystic duct/CHD junction, and 50% to 100% for the CBD [47]. An advantage of this modality is that it can be used repeatedly throughout the procedure, that is, continuously mapping biliary anatomy, and is easy to perform technically. Although it can potentially help with identification of structures during laparoscopic cholecystectomy, data are insufficient to assess its role in higher risk patients (eg obesity and acute cholecystitis) and regarding its impact on biliary injury. Two prospective trials (NCT02558556 and NCT02702843) currently are ongoing to assess its value during cholecystectomy.

Step 4: intraoperative time-out

Intraoperative time-out or a stop point should be considered at any point in the dissection if the anatomy is unclear and before clipping or cutting of the cystic duct and artery. The purpose of this step is to encourage a mindful pause, to step back and take a fresh look at the field and verify that the anatomic perceptions of the anatomy is accurate. Although there are no data to support this

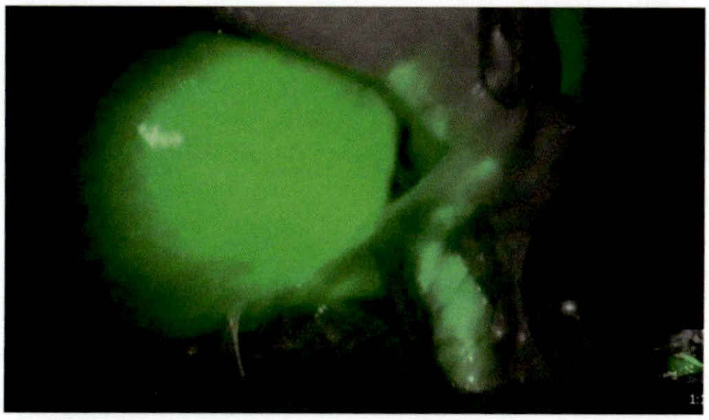

Fig. 4. The use of indocyanine green showing the CBD with the bright green fluorescence background of the liver. Some fluorescence also is seen in the cystic duct. (*Courtesy of* A. Pryor, MD, Centereach, NY.)

approach specifically in laparoscopic cholecystectomy, this step is in alignment with principles that have derived from studies of surgical checklists and the time-out done to minimize wrong site surgery and other safety checks in the operative environment.

Step 5: bailout options (when the dissection and conditions in the hepatocystic triangle are difficult and potentially dangerous)

Surgical decision making plays a critically important role in managing difficult gallbladder scenarios. In those cases in which the dissection has stalled, the CVS cannot be obtained because of severe inflammation, or the anatomy is uncertain, consideration should be given to one of several alternative or bailout options, as listed in Box 1.

Conversion to open cholecystectomy

Historically, conversion to open cholecystectomy has been the default bailout option because it may allow for better exposure and enhanced ability to palpate, or feel, the tissues. The decision to convert to open should factor in background and experience performing open cholecystectomy as well as comfort with laparoscopic bailout options. It also should be noted that a difficult laparoscopic cholecystectomy usually remains a difficult open cholecystectomy, and there are instances of biliary injuries that have occurred after conversion from laparoscopic to open [54]. Moreover, many of the recent generation of trainees have had limited experience with open cholecystectomy, especially in difficult cases.

There are several situations where conversion to open may be appropriate besides a difficult dissection. These include hemodynamic instability due to pneumoperitoneum (a rare event), inability to visualize the anatomy through a laparoscopic approach, uncontrolled bleeding, adherent colon or duodenum to gallbladder, suspected gallbladder cancer, and management of numerous bile duct stones that are not amenable to endoscopic retrograde cholangiopancreatography.

Aborting the operation

Rarely, it may be necessary or advisable to abort the operation altogether. Such circumstances include instability of the patient or hemodynamic instability or inability to identify the gallbladder, due to inflammation or dense omental pack or adhesions. This setting also is a situation in which calling for help would be advisable.

Box 1: Bailout options for difficult anatomy

Conversion to open cholecystectomy
Aborting the operation
Cholecystostomy tube drainage (surgical or percutaneous)
Subtotal cholecystectomy
Help from another surgeon/transfer to tertiary center

Cholecystostomy tube drainage

Percutaneous cholecystostomy tube (PCT) is a minimally invasive procedure that can be used as the initial treatment in the critically ill, elderly, or high-risk patients presenting with acute cholecystitis who are not candidates for surgery or those with severe cholecystitis. It can be definitive management in some cases or as a bridging procedure to eventual cholecystectomy. Yeo and colleagues [55] examined 103 patients who received PCT; 41% underwent eventual cholecystectomy with a conversion rate of 15%. Major postoperative complications were described in 5% of the patients, with the investigators reporting 1 BDI. Another study using the New York SPARCS administrative database examined outcomes of 9738 patients. The rate of cholecystectomy after PCT increased from 25% in 2000 to 31.7% in 2012. Of the patients who underwent cholecystectomy after PCT, 47 experienced a major BDI requiring intervention (1.57%), which is significantly higher than the reported rate of BDI during laparoscopic cholecystectomy of 0.2% to 0.4% [56]. Thus, it is important to recognize that subsequent cholecystectomy after PCT often is a more technically challenging procedure. Surgical cholecystostomy tube drainage also may be used intraoperatively if on exploration conditions are deemed too difficult to proceed safely with the dissection. A Foley-type catheter may simply be placed in the dome of the gallbladder and secured in place with a purse-string suture.

Subtotal cholecystectomy

Subtotal cholecystectomy is another bailout method that is gaining interest and can be done laparoscopically or open. Indications to consider subtotal cholecystectomy are a densely inflamed or fused hepatocystic triangle and inability to obtain the CVS (Fig. 5). In this procedure, the gallbladder is opened just above

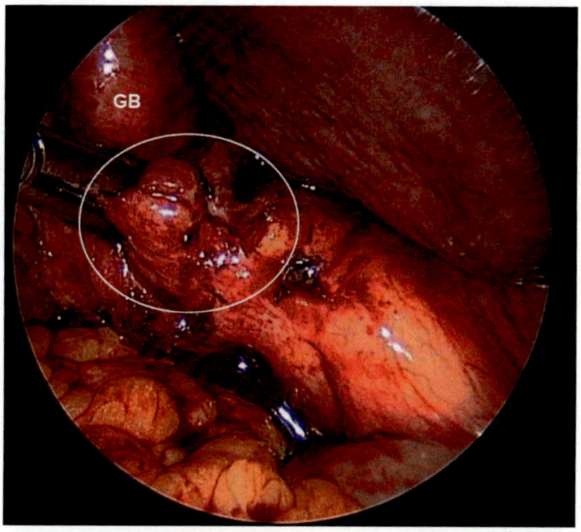

Fig. 5. Difficult inflamed gallbladder with inflammatory fusion of the hepatocystic triangle (circled). In this scenario, a bailout option should be considered (eg, fenestrating subtotal cholecystectomy). GB, body of gallbladder.

the neck, which allows a shield or cuff of gallbladder to protect the critical structures in the area of dense inflammation in the hepatocystic triangle. All stones are removed along with the front and side walls of the gallbladder. If deemed feasible, the entire back wall of the gallbladder can be removed as well. A cholangiogram may be done through the cystic duct orifice to confirm the anatomy and exclude residual cystic or CBD stones. If visible, the cystic duct orifice may be closed from the inside the gallbladder with a suture.

Recently, subtotal cholecystectomy has been defined into 2 subtypes: fenestrating subtotal cholecystectomy and reconstituting subtotal cholecystectomy [57]. In fenestrating subtotal cholecystectomy, the neck of the gallbladder is left open whereas in the reconstituting method it is closed either by suturing or stapling across it, which reconstitutes a small gallbladder remnant [57]. As a result, the reconstituting type is associated with an increased risk of recurrent stones, symptoms, and reoperation. For this reason, fenestrating subtotal cholecystectomy is the preferred procedure although it is associated with a higher rate of bile leakage; however, the bile leaks usually either resolve or can be managed by endoscopic retrograde cholangiopancreatography and stent placement [58]. Regardless of the approach, a closed suction drain should be left in place until the drainage is clear and the patient is tolerating a diet. Several systematic reviews describe these techniques as safe procedure [59,60]. Surgeons should consider their own expertise, however, in deciding which of these bailout options to use in a given patient.

Step 6: getting help from another surgeon when conditions are difficult

Another principle of safe cholecystectomy is that surgeons should have a low threshold for calling for help from another surgeon when feasible to do so. Conditions in which help might be called for are similar to those under which conversion to open operation or another bailout option is considered, as described previously, or when an experienced or higher-level assistant is needed. Calling for help is a sign of good judgment and should be considered liberally, especially early in a practice. In many practices, calling another surgeon is not always feasible and depends on the local hospital and surgical environment. Another help option if a surgeon is uncertain what to do and no immediate help is available is to call a referral center to discuss the operative scenario with an experienced surgeon in the field.

SUSPECTED BILE DUCT INJURY

If a BDI is suspected or confirmed in the operating room, it is critical to minimize the consequences and avoid extending the injury. If the anatomy is unclear, consideration should be given to performing an IOC or other imaging modality (US or near-infrared cholangiography). The IOC can be done through the neck of the gallbladder or putative cystic duct or divided ductal structure if present. Converting to open operation should be avoided unless there is local expertise to repair the injury or associated bleeding that cannot be controlled because this may complicate subsequent repair. Calling for help from another surgeon not only may help clarify the situation but also provide an unbiased perspective on the circumstances at hand.

If a major BDI is evident, it is important to acknowledge that the best outcomes of repair are by surgeons experienced in biliary reconstruction [61,62]. If such expertise is not locally available, it is best to leave a closed suction drain in place to control bile leakage and expeditiously transfer the patient to a center with advanced hepato-pancreato-biliary surgeons. The role of advanced endoscopic and interventional radiology support is also crucial to a successful outcome in this setting.

SUMMARY

Laparoscopic cholecystectomy has been a remarkable advance in surgical care that has benefited millions of patients positively over the past 30 years. Although overall it is a safe operation, opportunities exist to reduce BDI, which remains a priority for surgical quality improvement. The collective efforts of surgical societies to address this issue and the dissemination of safe operative management strategies and development of consensus conference guidelines have the potential to make this operation even safer in the future.

References

[1] Teilum D. The prevalence of gallstones in autopsies from a Danish urban area.Frederiksberg 1914–1955. Acta Chir Scand 1989;155(2):103–6.
[2] Schirmer BD, Winters KL, Edlich RF. Cholelithiasis and cholecystitis. J Long Term Eff Med Implants 2005;15(3):329–38.
[3] Truven Health Analytics (Thomson/Solucient), USA Procedure Volumes 2014.
[4] Calland JF, Tanaka K, Foley E, et al. Outpatient laparoscopic cholecystectomy: patient outcomes after implementation of a clinical pathway. Ann Surg 2001;233(5):704–15.
[5] Shea JA, Berlin JA, Bachwich DR, et al. Indications for and outcomes of cholecystectomy: a comparison of the pre and postlaparoscopic eras. Ann Surg 1998;227(3): 343–50.
[6] Lillemoe KD, Lin JW, Talamini MA, et al. Laparoscopic cholecystectomy as a "true" outpatient procedure: initial experience in 130 consecutive patients. J Gastrointest Surg 1999;3(1):44–9.
[7] Giger UF, Michel JM, Opitz I, et al. Risk factors for perioperative complications in patients undergoing laparoscopic cholecystectomy: analysis of 22,953 consecutive cases from the Swiss Association of Laparoscopic and Thoracoscopic Surgery database. J Am Coll Surg 2006;203(5):723–8.
[8] Morgenstern L, Wong L, Berci G. Twelve hundred open cholecystectomies before the laparoscopic era. Arch Surg 1992;127:400–3.
[9] Archer SB, Brown DW, Smith CD, et al. Bile duct injury during laparoscopic cholecystectomy: results of a national survey. Ann Surg 2001;234(4):549–58.
[10] Barrett M, Asbun HJ, Chien HL, et al. Bile duct injury and morbidity following cholecystectomy: a need for improvement. Surg Endosc 2018;32(4):1683–8.
[11] Buddingh KT, Weersma RK, Savenije RA, et al. Lower rate of major bile duct injury and increased intraoperative management of common bile duct stones after implementation of routine intraoperative cholangiography. J Am Coll Surg 2011;213(2): 267–74.
[12] Halbert C, Pagkratis S, Yang J, et al. Beyond the learning curve: incidence of bile duct injuries following laparoscopic cholecystectomy normalize to open in the modern era. Surg Endosc 2016;30(6):2239–43.

[13] Törnqvist B, Strömberg C, Persson G, et al. Effect of intended intraoperative cholangiography and early detection of bile duct injury on survival after cholecystectomy: population based cohort study. BMJ 2012;345:e6457.
[14] Schwaitzberg SD, Scott DJ, Jones DB, et al. Threefold increased bile duct injury rate is associated with less surgeon experience in an insurance claims database: more rigorous training in biliary surgery may be needed. Surg Endosc 2014;28(11):3068–73.
[15] Lilley EJ, Scott JW, Jiang W, et al. Intraoperative cholangiography during cholecystectomy among hospitalized medicare beneficiaries with non-neoplastic biliary disease. Am J Surg 2017;214(4):682–6.
[16] Pucher PH, Brunt LM, Davies N, et al. Outcome trends and safety measures after 30 years of laparoscopic cholecystectomy: a systematic review and pooled data analysis. Surg Endosc 2018;32(5):2175–83.
[17] Fong ZV, Pitt HA, Strasberg SM, et al. Diminished survival in patients with bile leak and ductal injury: management strategy and outcomes. J Am Coll Surg 2018;226(4):568–76.
[18] Kern KA. Malpractice litigation involving laparoscopic cholecystectomy. Cost, cause, and consequences. Arch Surg 1997;132:392–7.
[19] Carroll BJ, Birth M, Phillips EH. Common bile duct injuries during laparoscopic cholecystectomy that result in litigation. Surg Endosc 1998;12(4):310–3.
[20] Booij KAC, de Reuver PR, van Dieren S, et al. Long-term impact of bile duct injury on morbidity, mortality, quality of life, and work related limitations. Ann Surg 2018;268(1):143–50.
[21] Udekwu PO, Sullivan WG. Contemporary experience with cholecystectomy: establishing 'benchmarks' two decades after the introduction of laparoscopic cholecystectomy. Am Surg 2013;79:1253–7.
[22] Pitt HA, Sherman S, Johnson MS. Improved outcomes of bile duct injuries in the 21st century. Ann Surg 2013;258(3):490–9.
[23] Halbert C, Altieri MS, Yang J, et al. Long-term outcomes of patients with common bile duct injury following laparoscopic cholecystectomy. Surg Endosc 2016;30(10):4294–9.
[24] Roy PG, Soonawalla ZF, Grant HW. Medicolegal costs of bile duct injuries incurred during laparoscopic cholecystectomy. HPB (Oxford) 2009;11(2):130–4.
[25] Törnqvist B, Strömberg C, Akre O, et al. Selective intraoperative cholangiograpy and risk of bile duct injury during cholecystectomy. Br J Surg 2015;102:952–8.
[26] Strasberg SM, Hertl M, Soper NJ. An analysis of the problem of biliary injury during laparoscopic cholecystectomy. J Am Coll Surg 1995;180:101–25.
[27] Way LW, Stewart L, Gantert W, et al. Causes and prevention of laparoscopic bile duct injuries: analysis of 252 cases from a human factors and cognitive psychology perspective. Ann Surg 2003;237(4):460–9.
[28] Roulin D, Saadi A, Di Mare L, et al. Early versus delayed cholecystectomy for acute cholecystitis, are the 72 hours still the rule?: A randomized trial. Ann Surg 2016;264(5):717–22.
[29] Gutt CN, Encke J, Köninger J, et al. Acute cholecystitis: early versus delayed cholecystectomy, a multicenter randomized trial (ACDC study, NCT00447304). Ann Surg 2013;258(3):385–93.
[30] Cao AM, Eslick GD, Cox MR. Early cholecystectomy is superior to delayed cholecystectomy for acute cholecystitis: a meta-analysis. J Gastrointest Surg 2015;19(5):848–57.
[31] Pucher PH, Brunt LM, Fanelli RD, et al. SAGES expert Delphi consensus: critical factors for safe surgical practice in laparoscopic cholecystectomy. Surg Endosc 2015;29(11):3074–85.
[32] Yegiyants S, Collins JC. Operative strategy can reduce the incidence of major bile duct injury in laparoscopic cholecystectomy. Am Surg 2008;74:985–7.
[33] Auyang ED, Hungness ES, Vaziri K, et al. Natural orifice translumenal endoscopic surgery (NOTES): dissection for the critical view of safety during transcolonic cholecystectomy. Surg Endosc 2009;23:1117–8.

[34] Palanivelu C, Jani K, Maheshkumar GS. Single-center experience of laparoscopic cholecystectomy. J Laparoendosc Adv Surg Tech A 2007;17(5):608–14.
[35] Avgerinos C, Kelgiorgi D, Touloumis Z, et al. One thousand laparoscopic cholecystectomies in a single surgical unit using the "critical view of safety" technique. J Gastrointest Surg 2009;13(3):498–503.
[36] Booij KA, de Reuver PR, Nijsse B, et al. Insufficient safety measures reported in operation notes of complicated laparoscopic cholecystectomies. Surgery 2014;155(3):384–9.
[37] Nijssen MA, Schreinemakers JM, Meyer Z, et al. Complications after laparoscopic cholecystectomy: a video evaluation study of whether the critical view of safety was reached. World J Surg 2015;39(7):1798–803.
[38] Strasberg SM, Eagon CJ, Drebin JA. The "hidden cystic duct" syndrome and the infundibular technique of laparoscopic cholecystectomy–the danger of the false infundibulum. J Am Coll Surg 2000;191(6):661–7.
[39] Buddingh KT, Nieuwenhuijs VB, van Buuren L, et al. Intraoperative assessment of biliary anatomy for prevention of bile duct injury: a review of current and future patient safety interventions. Surg Endosc 2011;25(8):2449–61.
[40] Deal SB, Stefanidis D, Telem D, et al. Evaluation of crowd-sourced assessment of the critical view of safety in laparoscopic cholecystectomy. Surg Endosc 2017;31(12):5094–100.
[41] Mirizzi PL. Operative cholangiography. Surg Gynecol Oncol 1937;65:702–10.
[42] Soper NJ, Brunt LM. The case for routine operative cholangiography during laparoscopic cholecystectomy. Surg Clin North Am 1994;74:953–9.
[43] Flum DR, Dellinger EP, Cheadle A, et al. Intraoperative cholangiography and risk of common bile duct injury during cholecystectomy. JAMA 2003;289(13):1639–44.
[44] Ladocsi LT, Benitez LD, Filippone DR, et al. Intraoperative cholangiography in laparoscopic cholecystectomy: a review of 734 consecutive cases. Am Surg 1997;63:150–6.
[45] Slater K, Strong RW, Wall DR, et al. Iatrogenic bile duct injury: the scourge of laparoscopic cholecystectomy. Aust N Z J Surg 2002;72:83–8.
[46] Sheffield KM, Riall TS, Han Y, et al. Association between cholecystectomy with vs without intraoperative cholangiography and risk of common duct injury. JAMA 2013;310: 812–20.
[47] Hope WW, Fanelli R, Walsh DS, et al. SAGES clinical spotlight review: Intraoperative cholangiography. Surg Endosc 2017;31(5):2007–16.
[48] Ludwig K, Bernhardt J, Steffen H, et al. Contribution of intraoperative cholangiography to incidence and outcome of common bile duct injuries during laparoscopic cholecystectomy. Surg Endosc 2002;16(7):1098–104.
[49] Hobbs MS, Mai Q, Knuiman MW, et al. Surgeon experience and trends in intraoperative complications in laparoscopic cholecystectomy. Br J Surg 2006;93(7):844–53.
[50] El-Dhuwaib Y, Slavin J, Corless DJ, et al. Bile duct reconstruction following laparoscopic cholecystectomy in England. Surg Endosc 2016;30(8):3516–25.
[51] Ford JA, Soop M, Du J, et al. Systematic review of intraoperative cholangiography in cholecystectomy. Br J Surg 2012;99(2):160–7.
[52] Biffl WL, Moore EE, Offner PJ, et al. Routine intraoperative laparoscopic ultrasonography with selective cholangiography reduces bile duct complications during laparoscopic cholecystectomy. J Am Coll Surg 2001;193(3):272–80.
[53] Machi J, Johnson JO, Deziel DJ, et al. The routine use of laparoscopic ultrasound decreases bile duct injury: a multicenter study. Surg Endosc 2009;23(2):384–8.
[54] Navez B, Ungureanu F, Michiels M, et al. Surgical management of acute cholecystitis: results of a 2-year prospective multicenter survey in Belgium. Surg Endosc 2012;26(9): 2436–45.
[55] Yeo CS, Tay VW, Low JK, et al. Outcomes of percutaneous cholecystostomy and predictors of eventual cholecystectomy. J Hepatobiliary Pancreat Sci 2016;23(1):65–73.

[56] Altieri MS, Bevilaqua L, Yang J, et al. Cholecystectomy following percutaneous cholecystostomy tube placement leads to higher rate of CBD injuries. Surg Endosc 2018. [Epub ahead of print].
[57] Strasberg SM, Pucci MJ, Brunt LM, et al. Subtotal cholecystectomy-"fenestrating" vs "reconstituting" subtypes and the prevention of bile duct injury: definition of the optimal procedure in difficult operative conditions. J Am Coll Surg 2016;222(1):89–96.
[58] van Dijk AH, Donkervoort SC, Lameris W, et al. Short- and long-term outcomes after a reconstituting and fenestrating subtotal cholecystectomy. J Am Coll Surg 2017;225(3):371–9.
[59] Elshaer M, Gravante G, Thomas K, et al. Subtotal cholecystectomy for "difficult gallbladders": systematic review and meta-analysis. JAMA Surg 2015;150(2):159–68.
[60] Henneman D, da Costa DW, Vrouenraets BC, et al. Laparoscopic partial cholecystectomy for the difficult gallbladder: a systematic review. Surg Endosc 2013;27(2):351–8.
[61] Perera MT, Silva MA, Hegab B, et al. Specialist early and immediate repair of post-laparoscopic cholecystectomy bile duct injuries is associated with an improved long-term outcome. Ann Surg 2011;253(3):553–60.
[62] Thomson BN, Parks RW, Madhavan KK, et al. Early specialist repair of biliary injury. Br J Surg 2006;93(2):216–20.

Advances in Surgery 53 (2019) 161–177

ADVANCES IN SURGERY

Surgical Emergencies in the Pregnant Patient

Don J. Selzer, MD, MS[a,*], Dimitrios Stefanidis, MD, PhD[b]

[a]Division of General Surgery, Indiana University School of Medicine, 545 Barnhill Drive, Emerson Hall 509, Indianapolis, IN 46202, USA; [b]Department of Surgery, Minimally Invasive and Bariatric Surgery, Indiana University School of Medicine, 545 Barnhill Drive, Emerson Hall 125, Indianapolis, IN 46202, USA

Keywords

• Pregnancy • Emergency • Abdominal • Appendicitis • Cholecystitis • Trauma

Key points

- One in 500 to 700 pregnancies in the United States present with an abdominal emergency requiring surgery.
- Treatment of the mother is the focus, but consideration of the impact on the fetus should be weighed.
- When indicated, timely operative intervention is better than delaying care.
- During pregnancy, diagnostic radiologic tests should enlist ultrasound first and foremost.

INTRODUCTION

One in 500 to 700 pregnancies in the United States are complicated by an abdominal emergency [1,2]. Several indications can present that necessitate operative intervention in 2% of cases. The most common developments include appendicitis, acute cholecystitis, ovarian torsion, small bowel obstruction, and traumatic injury (Table 1). Other less common etiologies include hepatic lesions, worsening inflammatory bowel disease, vascular pathology including splenic artery aneurysm, and urolithiasis with renal colic [1]. The dilemma of addressing these ailments can present challenges in any patient;

Disclosure Statement: Dr D.J. Selzer is on the Medical Advisory Board at Cook Biotech Inc, is a consultant and receives consulting fees at PolyNovo Inc, and has research support from Bard/ Davol, Inc. Dr D. Stefanidis has research support from Explorer Surgical and Johnson & Johnson.

*Corresponding author. *E-mail address:* dselzer@iupui.edu

https://doi.org/10.1016/j.yasu.2019.04.008

Table 1
Incidence of abdominal emergencies during pregnancy

Pathology	Incidence
Acute appendicitis	1 in 500–2000 pregnancies
Acute cholecystitis	1 in 1000 pregnancies
Ovarian torsion	1 in 1000–2500 pregnancies
Bowel obstruction	1 in 1500–16,000 pregnancies
Abdominal trauma	1.5%–5% of traumas in women
Abdominal wall hernias	1 in 500 pregnancies
Hepatic adenoma	1 in 1,000,000 women
Inflammatory bowel disease	Prepregnancy disease status determines severity, new diagnosis consistent with general population
Renal colic	1 in 3300 pregnancies
Splenic artery aneurysm	1 in 1000 women

Data from Refs [1–3].

pregnancy adds to the complexity and commonly calls into question the appropriate approach for definitive care. In general, it is commonly considered that infectious or hematologic issues can threaten the fetus and the mother unless addressed in a timely manner. Advancements in radiologic tools and understanding of their impact on the fetus has altered diagnostic methodology and algorithm. Establishing best practices for the management of nonobstetric abdominal emergencies that occur during pregnancy is key to the goal of reaching term and the delivery of a healthy baby (see Table 1) [1–3].

EVALUATION

The diagnosis and evaluation of surgical emergencies requires an understanding of the typical physiologic changes associated with each trimester of pregnancy. Grasping these changes in a pregnant woman's anatomy helps provide a basis for comparison, reframe testing results, and avoid unnecessary invasive tests or procedures.

Physiology and physical examination

During pregnancy, the development of the fetus is associated with numerous physiologic changes of the mother in addition to the increasing size of the uterus. The cardiovascular system sees an overall increase in plasma volume, cardiac output, stroke volume, and heart rate. However, blood pressure dips during late second trimester and early third trimester before it returns to baseline.

There is an increase blood flow to several organs including the kidneys. Glomerular filtration rate increases along with the blood flow. Common laboratory tests shift during pregnancy including white blood cell count. There is also a decrease in the serum albumin concentration and a reduction in the oncotic pressure of the mother's serum. Liver oxidative enzymes including cytochrome P-450 are altered.

Pulmonary physiology demonstrates an increase in tidal volume and minute ventilation. This is largely related to increased oxygen needs of the fetus and commonly results in mild tachypnea (16 breaths per minute). Other gastrointestinal changes include an increase in gastric emptying and small intestinal transit times which can lead to nausea and vomiting and associated gastroesophageal reflux disease.

Naturally, the growth of the fetus is the most obvious change in physiology and physical examination. In general, the fundal height presents at predictable locations throughout the advancing pregnancy. Examples include breaching of the fundus above the symphysis pubis at 12 weeks. At 20 weeks, the fundal height commonly reaches the umbilicus. At term, the uterus is generally palpable and approaches the costal margin. As the uterine fundus grows, it exerts pressure to surrounding abdominal structures, which may affect their function. For example, mothers in the last trimester of pregnancy are advised to avoid lying supine to prevent complete occlusion of the inferior vena cava. It is important for the general surgeon to recognize the changes that occur in the mother's anatomy by the expanding uterus because they impact placement of incisions and positioning on the operating table if an operative intervention is warranted.

Laboratory

In addition to anatomic changes, physiologic changes during pregnancy are also reflected in common laboratory tests (Table 2) [1,4]. Hematologic tests including the complete blood count commonly demonstrate changes beginning at the end of the first trimester. Erythropoietin leads to increased red blood cell mass and red blood cell volume. However, an increase in plasma volume that also accompanies pregnancy leads to hemodilution that generates a common picture of anemia most pronounced in the second trimester. In the third trimester, HELLP syndrome (hemolysis, elevated liver enzymes, low platelet count) can present and is associated with 10% to 15% of preeclampsia cases. As a result of increased polymorphonuclear cells, leukocytosis is also associated with pregnancy, particularly during the second semester where the white blood cell count may reach 16,000 white blood cells/mm^2. Coagulation indices are commonly altered during pregnancy with the development of a hypercoagulable state reflected by increased coagulation factors and reduced coagulation inhibitors.

Changes are also commonly seen in chemistry tests. The increase in plasma volume leads to a hemodilutional effect on serum creatinine and serum urea nitrogen. This is compounded by an increase in creatinine clearance and glomerular filtration rate. Similar hemodilutional effects are commonly seen in levels of albumin, bilirubin, and transaminases. However, alkaline phosphatase, produced by the placenta, is commonly elevated from 2 to 15 times normal values. In addition, the sedimentation rate is consistently elevated throughout pregnancy.

Table 2
Common laboratory changes during pregnancy

	1st trimester	2nd trimester	3rd trimester
Complete blood count			
Hemoglobin (g/dL)	11.7–13.7	9.7–11.5	9.8–12.3
Hematocrit (%)	36	33	34
Leukocytes (1000/mm^3)	3.2–15.3	6.3–16.1	5.0–16.6
Platelet count (per mm^3)	Unchanged	Unchanged	Unchanged
Liver function tests			
AST/ALT (μmol/L)	Unchanged	Unchanged	Unchanged
Bilirubin (μmol/L)	Unchanged	Unchanged	Unchanged
Alkaline phosphatase (IU/L)	Unchanged	2–15 × normal	2–15 × normal
Chemistries			
Na+ (mmol/L)	140 ± 5	Stable	Stable
K+ (mmol/L)	3.5–4.5	Stable	Stable
BUN (g/L)	Decreased	Decreased	Decreased
Creatinine (μmol/L)	Decreased	Decreased	Decreased
Lipase (IU/L)	Decreased	Stable	Stable
Inflammatory indicators			
C-reactive protein (mg/L)	Unchanged	Unchanged	Unchanged
Sedimentation rate (mm/h)	Very high	Very high	Very high

Abbreviations: ALT, alanine aminotransferase; AST, aspartate aminotransferase; BUN, serum urea nitrogen.

Data from Bouyou J, Gaujoux S, Marcellin L, et al. Abdominal emergencies during pregnancy. *J Visc Surg* 2015;152(6 Suppl):S105-115 and Cunningham FG, Leveno KJ, Bloom SL, et al. Williams obstetrics. 25th edition. Ed.

Radiology

Radiologic diagnostic tests have become a hallmark of modern medical evaluation. X-ray exposure to the developing fetus is unwanted in all phases of pregnancy, but it is most impactful during the first trimester where teratogenic effects are the most significant [5]. Fortunately, x-ray-based technology has improved dramatically in recent years yielding a lower amount of radiation exposure to all patients. As a result, these tests remain available, but they are commonly used only after alternatives that do not expose the patient to radiation have been considered and either proven ineffective or unavailable.

It is helpful to consider the amount of radiation exposure provided by each x-ray-based examination (Table 3) and the risks. Current guidelines recommend a cumulative exposure of less than 100 mGy of x-ray radiation to the fetus to limit teratogenic risk [3]. In addition to concerns regarding teratogenesis, studies raise concerns for the development of childhood cancer especially when radiation exposure occurs during the first trimester at a level greater than 50 mGy [6]. Generally, the risks for teratogenesis and childhood cancer fall significantly when exposure occurs in the second or third trimester. Limiting the radiation dose is key. This is commonly done with efficient use of computed tomography (CT) studies and algorithms, and the application of a lead apron over the fetus when the abdomen and pelvis are not actively being

Table 3
Radiation exposure to fetus from common radiating tests

Test/procedure	Fetal absorbed dose (mGy)[a]
Background	0.5–1
Abdomen radiograph	1–3
Abdominal CT	4
Abdominal and pelvic CT	25
Chest CT	0.02

Abbreviation: CT, computed tomography.
[a]Radiation shield placed over abdomen when not in the test field.

examined. Ultimately, in the later phases of pregnancies, CT, even with intravenous contrast, is considered an acceptable tool if other options have proven ineffective and it prevents delay in diagnosis and the eventual management of the patient [3].

During pregnancy and especially the first trimester, ultrasound is generally considered the first choice for the evaluation of the abdomen based on its lack of radiation exposure to the patient, its common use by obstetricians, rapid turnaround time, and overall availability in multiple health care environments including outpatient clinics. In addition, ultrasound is effective at evaluating solid organs and several common areas of concern in the gastrointestinal track including the gallbladder and appendix. Finally, obstetricians are able to use ultrasound to evaluate the status of the fetus to determine the impact of maternal maladies on it.

Second to ultrasound, MRI is often called on to evaluate pregnant patients with potential surgical emergencies. Currently, the American College of Radiology recommends MRI over CT for the evaluation of pregnant patients. Although iodinated contrasts used in CT seem to have limited impact of fetal development, gadolinium crosses the placenta into the fetal circulation and may result in nephrogenic systemic fibrosis. So, its use is limited to a select group of circumstances including placenta percreta [3].

COMMON EMERGENCIES

Appendicitis

Presentation

Among nonobstetric surgical emergencies, acute appendicitis is clearly the most common representing about 25% of cases with an incidence of 0.5 to 2 per 1000 pregnancy women [1]. Although it occurs most commonly during the second trimester, its incidence is roughly the same as in the general population.

Pain in the right lower quadrant remains the most common presenting symptom, but the movement of the appendix as a result of displacement by the enlarging uterus can lead to pain in right upper quadrant, flank, or even back. Physical examination findings of peritoneal signs including guarding and rebound tenderness can still occur, but they may also be impacted by the displacement of the appendix. Complaints of anorexia and nausea are also common, but these issues are common for all pregnant women, especially those in the first trimester. History and physical examination, although suggestive, are typically not adequate to secure the diagnosis in the pregnant patient.

Evaluation

With regard to laboratory blood tests, the presence of a leukocytosis, the hallmark of acute appendicitis, is an unreliable tool in the evaluation of pregnant women as a result of the physiologic leukocytosis of pregnancy. Given the limitations of history and physical examination and laboratory analysis in the pregnant patient, diagnosis of acute appendicitis relies mainly on radiologic tests. In order of preference, modalities commonly relied on include ultrasound, MRI, and CT. Earlier in pregnancy, before the displacement of the appendix and small intestine, ultrasound performed by a skilled technician is usually effective in securing the diagnosis. However, later in pregnancy, at locations where ultrasound is unavailable, or ultrasound findings are equivocal, MRI provides exceptional sensitivity and specificity for the diagnosis of acute appendicitis [7]. Nevertheless, MRI may also provide challenges based on availability and practicality, rendering CT the remaining modality that is equally sensitive for the diagnosis in pregnant patients as in the general population. When other diagnostic modalities are unavailable or inconclusive, concerns regarding radiation exposure by CT independent of trimester have to be balanced with the impact on the mother and fetus of a delayed or missed diagnosis. It is important for the surgeon to recognize that appendiceal perforation resulting from a diagnostic delay is associated with premature uterine contractions, preterm labor (in the third trimester), and fetal loss.

Treatment

Although nonoperative treatment of acute appendicitis continues to be explored within the general population, appendectomy remains the mainstay of treatment of acute appendicitis in pregnant women [8,9]. Laparoscopic appendectomy is the preferred approach for the treatment of acute appendicitis in the pregnant patient [3,10,11]. Initial port placement should consider the uterine fundal height, and the surgeon should rely on the entry technique with which he or she is most experienced and comfortable.

When an open technique is used the incision location should be determined by the point of greatest tenderness [12]. Reliably, in the first trimester, a classic right lower quadrant incision proves effective. As pregnancy progresses, however, the best location for the incision rises higher on the right side. In the third trimester, some surgeons prefer an upper midline incision to provide better access and exposure. A periumbilical midline incision is used effectively in cases of diffuse peritonitis.

Acute cholecystitis

Presentation

Biliary track disease, specifically acute cholecystitis, is the second most common nonobstetric surgical emergency occurring at a rate of 1 per 1600 to

10,000 pregnancies. The most common cause of acute cholecystitis in this setting is gallstones.

Presentation commonly follows classical teaching with nausea with or without vomiting, fatty food intolerance, and colicky right upper quadrant pain. Although this pattern of symptoms is similar to presentation among the general population, the differential diagnosis generated by this pattern of presenting complaints is much wider in the pregnant patient and has potentially greater impact if incorrect. A differential diagnosis mainly includes pancreatitis, hepatitis, peptic ulcer disease, pneumonia, and pyelonephritis. In addition, because of its shifting location, appendicitis may also present with a similar pattern of signs and symptoms. Obstetric diseases including fatty liver disease of pregnancy resulting from preeclampsia with HELLP syndrome must also be considered.

Evaluation

Laboratory blood tests are helpful in focusing the differential diagnosis, but physiologic leukocytosis and an elevated alkaline phosphatase associated with pregnancy render these specific tests less reliable. As a result, radiologic tests are relied on commonly to provide definitive diagnosis of acute cholecystitis. As in the general population, ultrasound remains the main modality for the evaluation of the biliary track including the gallbladder. The presence of gallstones, gallbladder wall thickening, and pericholecystic fluid in a pregnant patient with suggestive symptoms confirm the diagnosis similar to the general population. When the diagnosis is uncertain, a radionucleotide examination performed through nuclear medicine is generally considered safe and can be adjusted to limit radiation exposure to the fetus [3].

Treatment

Although nonoperative management has been the traditional approach in the pregnant patient out of fear for spontaneous abortion or premature delivery after surgery, surgical intervention is currently the treatment of choice for numerous reasons. When delaying treatment, recurrent gallbladder symptoms have been reported to occur in 44% to 92% of patients depending on pregnancy trimester, half of which require hospitalization [13] and up to 23% develop acute cholecystitis, cholangitis, or gallstone pancreatitis [13,90]. Importantly, depending on severity, complicated gallstone disease has been reported to lead to preterm labor in up to 20% of cases and fetal loss in 10% to 60% of cases [13].

For these reasons laparoscopic cholecystectomy is the treatment modality of choice for pregnant patients in the setting of acute cholecystitis, regardless of trimester [3,13,14]. Laparoscopic cholecystectomy has been reported to lead to shorter length of stay, shorter operative times, fewer complications, and decreased rates of spontaneous abortion and preterm labor when compared with laparotomy [6,12]. When choledocholithiasis is suspected, intraoperative cholangiography is applied safely and effectively [3]. Endoscopic ultrasound and choledochoscopy are good alternatives in the presence of appropriate expertise and avoid patient exposure to radiation. Furthermore, choledochoscopy can also be therapeutic allowing removal of common bile duct stones. Given that laparoscopic choledochoscopy experience of general surgeons tends to be limited, endoscopic retrograde cholangiopancreatography is usually used for the treatment of choledocholithiasis in the pregnant patient similar to the general population. Endoscopic retrograde cholangiopancreatography during pregnancy has been shown to be safe and effective [13,63] and associated with low radiation exposure of the pregnant patient. Endoscopic ultrasound and stenting provide options to further limit radiation exposure when addressing common bile duct stones. Gallstone pancreatitis presents an even greater challenge for diagnosis and treatment. Although ultrasound may be of benefit, generally MRI and CT are relied on for diagnostic purposes. Initial management is mainly supportive with limited oral intake, intravenous fluids, and pain control as in the general population. Given that recurrent pancreatitis is of significant concern and much more common than in the general population, early laparoscopic cholecystectomy after the pancreatitis has resolved may also be the best approach independent of trimester [3].

Ovarian torsion

Presentation

Impacting approximately 1 in 1000 to 1 in 2500 pregnancies, ovarian torsion commonly presents with abdominal pain corresponding to the affected adnexa and nausea and vomiting [1,15]. Those patients who underwent fertility treatments are at greater risk for the development of ovarian torsion. In addition, torsion seems to occur more commonly during the first trimester and more commonly on the right side. It seems that the presence of the corpus luteum and an overall increased ovarian mass as a result of hormonal stimulation contribute to the development of torsion. The differential diagnosis for right-sided pain should always include appendicitis and other pathologies.

Evaluation

Physical examination demonstrates ipsilateral adnexal tenderness. However, examination of the ovary may become more difficult as the pregnancy progresses. Laboratory tests demonstrate a leukocytosis that is generally unhelpful in pregnancy when an increased white blood cell count is typical. Therefore, ultrasound is the tool of choice to confirm the diagnosis. During the first trimester, a multicystic ovary is commonly identified [16], whereas a normal-appearing ovary is commonly seen in the later stages of pregnancy. The corpus luteum is commonly present in the affected ovary. The diagnosis is confirmed when reduced or absence of blood flow to the affected ovary is detected by Doppler.

Treatment

Surgical detorsion with oophoropexy is the treatment of choice with less common cystectomy or oophorectomy [17]. In limited studies evaluating ovarian torsion, time from presentation to operative intervention was significantly less for those in the first trimester rather than later stages. Potential explanations include more challenging physical examination of the ovaries because of the larger uterus and a lower threshold to operate on patients in earlier stages of pregnancy when preterm labor is less likely. The time from presentation to operative intervention is less for those in the first trimester than the nonpregnant population. Perhaps, the presence of pain in this population more commonly leads to early presentation and an increased suspicion of an abdominal emergency despite the vague, nondescript symptoms that may accompany the development of torsion.

Diagnostic laparoscopy is used to confirm the diagnosis in settings of unclear pathology. Delays in diagnosis and treatment may result in tissue necrosis necessitating resection. Because torsion commonly involves the ovary containing the corpus luteum, progesterone therapy may be required for episodes of torsion occurring during the first trimester [3].

Bowel obstruction

Presentation

Occurring in 1 in 1500 to 16,000 pregnancies, bowel obstruction resulting predominantly from adhesions is the third most common nonobstetric surgical emergency [1]. Historically, these patients experience significant risks for morbidity and mortality of the fetus and the mother. As the uterus grows in size, cecal volvulus should be considered on the differential diagnosis. With a pattern of symptoms similar to the general population, bowel obstruction in the pregnant patient is associated with central colicky abdominal pain, bloating or distention, nausea and vomiting, and constipation and/or obstipation.

Evaluation

Some reports have demonstrated the benefits of ultrasound in the diagnosis of bowel obstruction [18]. However, x-ray-based tests, specifically plain radiographs of the abdomen, prove most effective in the analysis of the patient with small bowel obstruction. The addition of enteral contrast can provide further elucidating information. The addition of enteral ionic contrast has proven safe in the pregnant patient. When administered with a CT, it can provide diagnostic and therapeutic benefits [19,20].

Treatment

In the stable patient, initial supportive care and expectant management including nasogastric decompression and hydration is appropriate [21]. Similar to the nonpregnant patient, failure of nonoperative management to result in resolution of the obstruction requires operative intervention [22]. When clinical findings are concerning for ischemia, immediate operative intervention is indicated similar to the general population. The patient's surgical history and size of uterus may assist in the consideration for operative approach with the potential for laparoscopy offering a safe option and shorter convalescence.

Abdominal trauma

Presentation

Between 1.5% and 5% of women suffering traumatic injuries are pregnant [23]. Abdominal trauma during pregnancy most commonly results from motor vehicle accidents (34%–70%), falls (9%–26%), and physical assault (11%–12%) [24]. Although a limited number of patients require surgical intervention, trauma represents the most common cause of nonobstetric maternal death. Fetal death from trauma-related injury is estimated at 3.7 fetal deaths per 100,000 live births. Obtaining an accurate history is of key importance in determining the potential systems exposed to injury [25].

Evaluation

A full trauma survey including the initial assessment and the secondary survey are needed to identify areas of concern. These surveys proceed largely unchanged from those used for evaluation of a nonpregnant patient. However, the secondary survey should include a detailed obstetric history including last menstrual cycle, expected delivery date, and problems that have occurred to date during the pregnancy. During the secondary survey, the abdominal examination should also include an assessment of uterine size to help confirm estimated gestational age of the fetus; this is used to determine the predicted survival of the fetus if cesarean section is required. Uterine fundal height at or above the umbilicus suggests a fetus with potential extrauterine viability. The secondary survey should also include a direct fetal assessment including examination of fetal heart rate and the presence of movement.

Discrepancies between the stated gestational age and the estimated gestational age determined by physical examination could suggest uterine trauma. In addition, the presence of vaginal bleeding, membrane rupture, bulging perineum, and the presence of contractions should all raise concern for serious injury. Laboratory tests including a Kleihauer-Betke test performed in all women more than 12 weeks gestational age assesses the presence of fetal blood cells in the maternal blood stream and suggests trauma to the uterus and fetus. Although there is no clear correlation between the severity of trauma and the presence of fetal cells in maternal circulation, a positive test should raise concern for severe injury and consideration for the administration of Rho(D) immune globin to avoid Rh sensitization. Some argue that all Rh-negative pregnant women suffering severe trauma should receive Rho(D) immune globin within 72 hours of the traumatic event regardless of test results [26].

A focused assessment with sonography in trauma provides high sensitivity and specificity for detecting major abdominal trauma [27]. Although ultrasound and MRI are commonly preferred modalities, it is generally recommended that the treating surgeons use the appropriate radiologic tests for effective evaluation of traumatic injuries regardless of radiation exposure [6]. It is recommended that a limitation of radiation dose is coordinated with the radiology technician when multiple x-ray-based tests are needed [28].

Treatment

Prehospital management of pregnant trauma patients recommends supplemental oxygen and liberal use of intravenous fluids to prevent fetal hypoxia. However, the underlying modus operandi aim to address treatment of the mother over the treatment of the fetus. A tool used on a limited basis for management of severe blunt traumatic injury in the general population, military antishock trousers are contraindicated during pregnancy because they can exacerbate injury to uterus or fetus during the second and/or third trimester. In addition, transport of patients at 20 weeks gestation age or greater requires tilting of the back board to the left to avoid aortocaval collapse. Elevating the right hip approximately 4 to 6 inches with a wedge can provide a similar effect.

Management of blunt traumatic injury in pregnant patients largely follows the algorithms generated for nonpregnant patients [29]. Specifically, nonoperative management of solid organ injury is commonly successful. However, maternal hypotension is more commonly associated with fetal distress. Therefore, the threshold to intervene operatively should be lowered in the pregnant patient. In the second trimester, as the uterus becomes an abdominal organ, risk of direct trauma to the uterus rises dramatically despite natural tendencies of the uterine muscle and the amniotic sac to absorb energy. Hemorrhage from the traumatized gravid uterus can be extensive. Fortunately, even at later stages of pregnancy, the rate of uterine rupture remains extremely low (Table 4).

Treatment of penetrating trauma to the pregnant patient is also largely impacted by the gestational age of the fetus with the safety of the pelvis disappearing after week 12 (see Table 4) [30]. As in all cases of gunshot wounds, the type of firearm and the distance from the shooter dramatically impacts the outcome. Ultimately, if the bullet has entered or traversed the uterus and the fetus is viable, cesarean section should be performed. Hysterectomy is indicated if the uterus is beyond repair.

In the scenario of a lack of maternal pulses, cardiopulmonary resuscitation is initiated. Chest compressions become less effective as the gestational age enters the third trimester. Monitoring of fetal blood flow is judged not only by the generation of a carotid pulse and a return of end-tidal carbon dioxide in the mother but also by the presence of appropriate fetal heart tones. Suggestion of fetal distress during cardiopulmonary resuscitation potentially from inadequate chest compressions should raise considerations for open cardiac massage. If open cardiac massage proves ineffective in the setting of gestational age greater than 24 weeks, immediate cesarean section should be performed. Even in the setting of maternal death, a cesarean section performed within 5 to 10 minutes of cardiac arrest is believed to provide the fetus with a high probability of survival [25,27]. Trauma surgeons, likely unfamiliar with the technique, are urged to abandon the typical low transverse incision in the uterus in favor of a midline opening that facilitates delivery and avoids damage to the uterine vessels. An even more challenging ethical dilemma that fortunately remains rare is the scenario of maternal brain death with a viable fetus. In general, the fetus may remain in utero to mature. Maintaining the mother's body until after 28 weeks gestational age offers the fetus the greatest opportunity for survival, but making this decision requires the assistance of an ethics team along with the patient's family and treating surgeons.

Table 4
American Association for the Surgery of Trauma gravid uterus injury scale

Grade[a]	Injury description	ICD-9	AIS90
I	Contusion/hematoma (without placental abruption)	867.4/.5	2
II	Superficial laceration ($\leq$1 cm) or partial placental abruption <25%	867.4/.5	3
III	Deep laceration (>1 cm) occurring in second trimester or placental abruption >25% but <50%	867.4/.5	3
	Deep laceration (>1 cm) in third trimester	867.4/.5	4
IV	Laceration involving uterine artery	902.55	4
	Deep laceration (>1 cm) with >50% placental abruption	867.4/.5	4
V	Uterine rupture		
	Second trimester	867.4/.5	4
	Third trimester	867.4/.5	5
	Complete placental abruption	867.4/.5	4–5

[a]Advance one grade for multiple injuries up to grade III.

From Moore EE, Jurkovich GJ, Knudson MM, et al. Organ injury scaling. VI: Extrahepatic biliary, esophagus, stomach, vulva, vagina, uterus (nonpregnant), uterus (pregnant), fallopian tube, and ovary. *J Trauma* 1995;39(6):1069-1070; with permission.

LESS COMMON EMERGENCIES

Hepatic adenomas

Development of hepatic adenomas, generally solitary, is commonly associated with oral contraceptives and other hormone therapy. However, pregnancy is also associated with adenoma growth and risk of rupture [31]. Right upper quadrant pain should be evaluated with ultrasound. Although a cystic structure requires no immediate follow-up, a solid mass requires a noncontrasted MRI [32]. Although smaller adenomas benefit from frequent follow-up ultrasounds to assess their growth, surgeons should consider resecting adenomas greater than 5 cm in diameter because they are associated with high risk of rupture and bleeding [33].

Inflammatory bowel disease

Fortunately, the new diagnosis of Crohn disease is less common in pregnancy than in the general public. Symptoms are commonly vague and misinterpreted as other benign intestinal maladies leading to a delay in diagnosis [34]. Crohn disease flare ups are common during pregnancy and typically present in the first trimester, but the course of disease is commonly dictated by the state of disease at the time of conception [35]. Ultrasound is unlikely to provide definitive information with most practitioners relying more on MRI and/or CT imaging. Operative intervention should favor conservative dogma including a tendency toward fecal diversion rather than primary anastomosis [36]. Abscesses developing in the setting of Crohn disease are challenging to control during pregnancy [37]. Moreover, free perforation in the setting of Crohn disease occurs at an even higher incidence. Therefore, patients with peritoneal signs require immediate evaluation and likely surgical intervention. A three-stage surgical approach is common including initial resection, secondary reconstruction with proximal fecal diversion, and eventual reversal of the proximal diversion after delivery [38].

Renal colic

Urolithiasis is a common disease associated with severe abdominal/flank pain and ureteral obstruction. A history and physical commonly narrows the differential diagnosis. Laboratory tests including urinalysis and renal ultrasound are confirmatory. Pain control is affected by the safety of analgesics during pregnancy [39]. Fortunately, acetaminophen and antispasmodics are commonly successful because nonsteroidal anti-inflammatory medications are contraindicated in the later stages of pregnancy. Corticosteroids, considered when analgesics fail, are effective in postponing surgical intervention [40]. Persistent obstruction necessitates placement of a ureteral stent [41].

Splenic artery aneurysm

Splenic artery aneurysm is the most common splanchnic arterial aneurysm and the third most common abdominal aneurysm following aorta and iliac arteries [42]. Although splenic artery aneurysms generally are asymptomatic or generate vague symptoms, they may rupture during pregnancy (95% of cases present during pregnancy) presenting as sudden unexpected shock or even death [43]. Rupture is of greatest risk in mothers less than 45 year old and in the third trimester of pregnancy. Mortality risk is high for the mother and the fetus. Therefore, a timely diagnosis is key for a successful rescue, but rupture prevention is the preferred treatment strategy. The diagnosis may be raised with auscultation of a bruit in the abdominal left upper quadrant, observation of a calcified ring within the left upper quadrant, or with an ultrasound or CT. Treatment generally involves rupture avoidance through splenectomy with arterial resection or ligation of the artery with subsequent splenectomy [44].

Abdominal wall hernias

The incidence of primary abdominal wall hernias (ventral and groin) has been shown to be 0.002% in a cohort of 20,714 pregnant patients [45]. None of these patients required elective or emergent repair during their pregnancy and in some their groin hernias disappeared spontaneously after delivery. Watchful waiting is, therefore, the currently recommended approach for primary hernias in a pregnant patient. When an operation is required to address a strangulated hernia, timely surgical repair is advised.

CONSIDERATIONS DURING TREATMENT

Fetal monitoring

Any evaluation and treatment of a pregnant patient should include an assessment of the fetus and determination of fetal health. The most rudimentary assessment remains the physical examination from which estimated gestational age, auscultated fetal heart tones, and palpation of fetal movement are obtained. For patients in the earlier phases of pregnancy, ultrasound is a key component of this assessment. Formal ultrasonography helps assess the fetus in depth, but a Doppler probe or continuous fetal heart rate monitoring is an important adjunct to determining fetal health. The presence of a fetal heart rate between 120 and 160 beats per minute suggests good health, whereas decelerations suggest distress. The combination of tocographic monitoring with fetal cardiac monitoring provides a highly sensitive and specific assessment of fetal and maternal condition and identifies elements of preterm labor. In fact, the combination of cardio and tocographic monitoring for fetal distress is more effective than direct fetal ultrasonographic evaluation for identifying uterine catastrophic events including abruption or rupture.

Operative technique

On initial assessment of a pregnant patient who may require operative intervention, a surgeon should consult and maintain consistent communication with obstetric experts. Fetal monitoring before and after an operation is important but can present challenges when attempted intraoperatively; the value of the latter has not been conclusively shown and, therefore, is not routinely recommended [3]. Appropriate fluid resuscitation takes into consideration the increased plasma volume during pregnancy and supplemental oxygenation avoids maternal and fetal hypoxia. If operative intervention is necessary in patients in the second and third trimesters, a modified left lateral position is used to prevent uterine compression of primarily the inferior vena cava and less commonly the aorta. Abdominal surgery requires recognition of the changing uterine size and its impact on the placement of the initial port in laparoscopic surgery or the location of the incision in open procedures. Recognition of the changing uterine fundal height and adjustment of the location of initial port placement should allow surgeons to use the technique with which they are most comfortable and confident: open (Hasson), Veress needle, or optical trocar [3]. Insufflation pressures can initially be set at levels consistent with the general population. However, adjustment of the pressure should be considered if the patient's physiology does not support higher pressures (eg, persistent maternal hypotension) or limited visibility sacrifices safety in lower pressures. In addition to the risk of fetal hypoxia from maternal hypoxia or hypotension, fetal acidosis associated with maternal and fetal hypercarbia is equally detrimental. As a result, intraoperative monitoring of maternal capnography is strongly recommended [3].

Complications

Thromboembolic events represent the most common cause of maternal morbidity and mortality in a normal pregnancy. In addition to amniotic fluid embolism resulting from uterine trauma, this rings true for postoperative pregnant patients. In general, a hypercoagulable state exists during pregnancy with elevated levels of thrombotic factors and reduced levels of fibrinolysis. One of the most significant hematologic complications during pregnancy is disseminated intravascular coagulation.

Preventative measures should be used to limit the risk of thrombotic events. Placement of pneumatic compression devices on the lower extremities is strongly recommended [3]. Early mobilization, generally encouraged after all operative interventions today, is more easily attained after laparoscopic surgical procedures. Prophylactic use of chemoprophylaxis is less well researched. Surgeons should consider use of these agents during prolonged operative procedures. Unfractionated heparin is generally the preferred agent [3].

Signs of preterm labor, more common in the third trimester, should dictate the use of tocolytic therapy. Prophylactic use of tocolytics is not recommended [3].

SUMMARY

Emergencies in the general population that necessitate abdominal surgery can generate diagnostic and ethical dilemmas that challenge the surgeon and the health care team. Similar emergencies occurring in the pregnant patient create even more challenging clinical decision making. The most common surgical emergencies during pregnancy including appendicitis, cholecystitis, bowel obstruction, and trauma are still fairly infrequent and commonly extrapolate to only a couple of patients annually for most hospitals. A lack of familiarity with this clinical scenario is a setting for diagnostic missteps and delays in diagnosis that likely result from an overemphasis on protecting the fetus that ultimately negatively impacts the mother and the fetus.

Physiologic monitoring perioperatively with the assistance of tocographic equipment is an important component of assessing fetal condition. Predictable changes in maternal laboratory tests should be considered during the evaluation process. Radiology tests are commonly used to confirm the diagnosis. Of the commonly used modalities, ultrasound should be used preferentially followed by noncontrasted MRI and then x-ray techniques including radiographs, fluoroscopy, and CT imaging with or without iodinated contrast materials. Limiting radiation exposure to avoid teratogenic effects and risks of childhood cancer is key, but it should not compromise diagnostic accuracy to the detriment of the mother and the fetus.

Surgical intervention offers definitive therapy for common emergencies that present during pregnancy. If one takes into consideration the physiologic and anatomic changes that occur to the mother during pregnancy, operative intervention can be offered safely with appropriate monitoring, patient positioning, preventative prophylactic measures, and operative techniques. When appropriate, minimally invasive options including laparoscopy offer the benefits of the same quick recovery as that witnessed in the general population.

References

[1] Bouyou J, Gaujoux S, Marcellin L, et al. Abdominal emergencies during pregnancy. J Visc Surg 2015;152(6 Suppl):S105–15.

[2] Parangi S, Levine D, Henry A, et al. Surgical gastrointestinal disorders during pregnancy. Am J Surg 2007;193(2):223–32.
[3] Pearl JP, Price RR, Tonkin AE, et al. SAGES guidelines for the use of laparoscopy during pregnancy. Surg Endosc 2017;31(10):3767–82.
[4] Maternal Physiology. In: Cunningham F, Leveno KJ, Bloom SL, editors. Williams Obstetrics, 25e. New York: McGraw-Hill; 2018.
[5] McCollough CH, Schueler BA, Atwell TD, et al. Radiation exposure and pregnancy: when should we be concerned? Radiographics 2007;27(4):909–17 [discussion: 917–8].
[6] Sadro C, Bernstein MP, Kanal KM. Imaging of trauma: part 2, Abdominal trauma and pregnancy–a radiologist's guide to doing what is best for the mother and baby. AJR Am J Roentgenol 2012;199(6):1207–19.
[7] Duke E, Kalb B, Arif-Tiwari H, et al. A systematic review and meta-analysis of diagnostic performance of MRI for evaluation of acute appendicitis. AJR Am J Roentgenol 2016;206(3): 508–17.
[8] Elraiyah T, Hashim Y, Elamin M, et al. The effect of appendectomy in future tubal infertility and ectopic pregnancy: a systematic review and meta-analysis. J Surg Res 2014;192(2): 368–74.e1.
[9] Prodromidou A, Machairas N, Kostakis ID, et al. Outcomes after open and laparoscopic appendectomy during pregnancy: a meta-analysis. Eur J Obstet Gynecol Reprod Biol 2018;225:40–50.
[10] Maimaiti A, Aierkin A, Mahmood KM, et al. Laparoscopic appendectomy in pregnancy with acute appendicitis: single center experience with world review. Surg Laparosc Endosc Percutan Tech 2017;27(6):460–4.
[11] Wilasrusmee C, Sukrat B, McEvoy M, et al. Systematic review and meta-analysis of safety of laparoscopic versus open appendicectomy for suspected appendicitis in pregnancy. Br J Surg 2012;99(11):1470–8.
[12] Cox TC, Huntington CR, Blair LJ, et al. Laparoscopic appendectomy and cholecystectomy versus open: a study in 1999 pregnant patients. Surg Endosc 2016;30(2):593–602.
[13] Nasioudis D, Tsilimigras D, Economopoulos KP. Laparoscopic cholecystectomy during pregnancy: a systematic review of 590 patients. Int J Surg 2016;27:165–75.
[14] Sedaghat N, Cao AM, Eslick GD, et al. Laparoscopic versus open cholecystectomy in pregnancy: a systematic review and meta-analysis. Surg Endosc 2017;31(2):673–9.
[15] Sasaki KJ, Miller CE. Adnexal torsion: review of the literature. J Minim Invasive Gynecol 2014;21(2):196–202.
[16] Smorgick N, Pansky M, Feingold M, et al. The clinical characteristics and sonographic findings of maternal ovarian torsion in pregnancy. Fertil Steril 2009;92(6):1983–7.
[17] Morton MJ, Masterson M, Hoffmann B. Case report: ovarian torsion in pregnancy - diagnosis and management. J Emerg Med 2013;45(3):348–51.
[18] Sherer DM, Dalloul M, Schwartzman A, et al. Point-of-care sonographic diagnosis of maternal small bowel obstruction during pregnancy. Ultrasound Obstet Gynecol 2016;48(3):403–4.
[19] Ceresoli M, Coccolini F, Catena F, et al. Water-soluble contrast agent in adhesive small bowel obstruction: a systematic review and meta-analysis of diagnostic and therapeutic value. Am J Surg 2016;211(6):1114–25.
[20] Azagury D, Liu RC, Morgan A, et al. Small bowel obstruction: a practical step-by-step evidence-based approach to evaluation, decision making, and management. J Trauma Acute Care Surg 2015;79(4):661–8.
[21] Webster PJ, Bailey MA, Wilson J, et al. Small bowel obstruction in pregnancy is a complex surgical problem with a high risk of fetal loss. Ann R Coll Surg Engl 2015;97(5):339–44.
[22] Zachariah SK, Fenn MG. Acute intestinal obstruction complicating pregnancy: diagnosis and surgical management. BMJ Case Rep 2014;2014 [pii:bcr2013203235].
[23] Shah AJ, Kilcline BA. Trauma in pregnancy. Emerg Med Clin North Am 2003;21(3): 615–29.

[24] Barraco RD, Chiu WC, Clancy TV, et al. Practice management guidelines for the diagnosis and management of injury in the pregnant patient: the EAST Practice Management Guidelines Work Group. J Trauma 2010;69(1):211–4.
[25] Petrone P, Marini CP. Trauma in pregnant patients. Curr Probl Surg 2015;52(8):330–51.
[26] Thorp JM. Utilization of anti-RhD in the emergency department after blunt trauma. Obstet Gynecol Surv 2008;63(2):112–5.
[27] Lucia A, Dantoni SE. Trauma management of the pregnant patient. Crit Care Clin 2016;32(1):109–17.
[28] Raptis CA, Mellnick VM, Raptis DA, et al. Imaging of trauma in the pregnant patient. Radiographics 2014;34(3):748–63.
[29] Mirza FG, Devine PC, Gaddipati S. Trauma in pregnancy: a systematic approach. Am J Perinatol 2010;27(7):579–86.
[30] Moore EE, Jurkovich GJ, Knudson MM, et al. Organ injury scaling. VI: extrahepatic biliary, esophagus, stomach, vulva, vagina, uterus (nonpregnant), uterus (pregnant), fallopian tube, and ovary. J Trauma 1995;39(6):1069–70.
[31] Jabbour N, Brenner M, Gagandeep S, et al. Major hepatobiliary surgery during pregnancy: safety and timing. Am Surg 2005;71(4):354–8.
[32] Wilson CH, Manas DM, French JJ. Laparoscopic liver resection for hepatic adenoma in pregnancy. J Clin Gastroenterol 2011;45(9):828–33.
[33] van Aalten SM, Broker ME, Busschbach JJ, et al. Pregnancy and liver adenoma management: PALM-study. BMC Gastroenterol 2012;12:82.
[34] Mahadevan U, Matro R. Care of the pregnant patient with inflammatory bowel disease. Obstet Gynecol 2015;126(2):401–12.
[35] Bar-Gil Shitrit A, Grisaru-Granovsky S, Ben Ya'acov A, et al. Management of inflammatory bowel disease during pregnancy. Dig Dis Sci 2016;61(8):2194–204.
[36] Killeen S, Gunn J, Hartley J. Surgical management of complicated and medically refractory inflammatory bowel disease during pregnancy. Colorectal Dis 2017;19(2):123–38.
[37] McConnell RA, Mahadevan U. Pregnancy and the patient with inflammatory bowel disease: fertility, treatment, delivery, and complications. Gastroenterol Clin North Am 2016;45(2):285–301.
[38] Winter R, Norgard BM, Friedman S. Treatment of the pregnant patient with inflammatory bowel disease. Inflamm Bowel Dis 2016;22(3):733–44.
[39] Somani BK, Dellis A, Liatsikos E, et al. Review on diagnosis and management of urolithiasis in pregnancy: an ESUT practical guide for urologists. World J Urol 2017;35(11):1637–49.
[40] Semins MJ, Matlaga BR. Management of stone disease in pregnancy. Curr Opin Urol 2010;20(2):174–7.
[41] Pedro RN, Das K, Buchholz N. Urolithiasis in pregnancy. Int J Surg 2016;36(Pt D):688–92.
[42] Al-Habbal Y, Christophi C, Muralidharan V. Aneurysms of the splenic artery: a review. Surgeon 2010;8(4):223–31.
[43] Ha JF, Phillips M, Faulkner K. Splenic artery aneurysm rupture in pregnancy. Eur J Obstet Gynecol Reprod Biol 2009;146(2):133–7.
[44] Sadat U, Dar O, Walsh S, et al. Splenic artery aneurysms in pregnancy: a systematic review. Int J Surg 2008;6(3):261–5.
[45] Oma E, Bay-Nielsen M, Jensen KK, et al. Primary ventral or groin hernia in pregnancy: a cohort study of 20,714 women. Hernia 2017;21(3):335–9.

Advances in Surgery 53 (2019) 179–193

ADVANCES IN SURGERY

Transoral Endoscopic Thyroidectomy Vestibular Approach

Neeta J. Erinjeri, MD[a,*], Robert Udelsman, MD, MBA[a,b,c]

[a]Endocrine Neoplasia Institute, Miami Cancer Institute, 8900 North Kendall Drive, Miami, FL 33176, USA; [b]Florida International University, 11200 SW 8th St, Miami, FL 33199, USA; [c]Yale University School of Medicine, 333 Cedar St, New Haven, CT 06510, USA

Keywords

• Transoral thyroidectomy • Endoscopic thyroidectomy • Transoral neck surgery • Natural orifice thyroidectomy • NOTES • TOETVA

Key points

- Aesthetic concerns regarding anterior neck incisions have driven innovation to develop alternative access to the thyroid gland.
- Transoral endoscopic thyroidectomy vestibular approach (TOETVA) is a safe and effective alternative approach to thyroidectomy.
- TOETVA maximizes minimally invasive principles compared with other remote access approaches.
- Adoption of this method requires meticulous preparation and patient selection.

INTRODUCTION

Transcervical thyroidectomy, as refined by Theodor Kocher, has been the standard operative approach since his landmark work more than one hundred years ago. Although surgical and anesthetic techniques have evolved, the transcervical approach has endured. Mirroring other surgical procedures, the last 2 decades brought forth a debate regarding minimally invasive neck surgery to diminish or eliminate anterior cervical collar incisions. This cosmetic concern is most prominent in Asian countries where an anterior neck scar is considered a violation of aesthetics, especially among young female patients. The concern

Disclosure Statement: The authors have nothing to disclose.

*Corresponding author. *E-mail address:* NeetaE@BaptistHealth.net

https://doi.org/10.1016/j.yasu.2019.04.009

led to the development of multiple remote access approaches for thyroidectomy, including transaxillary, transbreast, and retroauricular routes. Each of these is associated with unique difficulties, risks, and complications, including the potential for significant nerve and vascular injuries. More recently, a technique was developed that eliminates external scarring, using a natural orifice transluminal endoscopic surgical (NOTES) approach.

EVOLUTION OF THYROID SURGERY

Thyroidectomy was first described more than 1000 years ago; however, until relatively recently, the high morbidity limited extensive application [1–3]. Morbidity was so profound that operative outcomes led to the imprisonment of a surgeon in 1646, and the French Academy of Medicine enacted a total ban of the operation in 1850 [2]. In 1866 in the United States, Samuel Gross, future president of the American Medical Association and one of the founders of the American Surgical Association, wrote regarding surgeons performing thyroidectomies, "every stroke of his knife will be followed by a torrent of blood and lucky it would be for him if his victim lives long enough to enable him to finish his horrid butchery" [4]. Multiple world renowned surgeons advanced and modified thyroid surgery, but it is Theodor Kocher, with his pioneering work in Berne during the late 1800s and early 1900s, who revolutionized the procedure [1,2]. His emphasis of meticulous technique using delicate instruments through a transverse transcervical approach, focused on careful dissection to reduce morbidity and mortality from bleeding, nerve injury, and hypoparathyroidism. This practice was improved upon and fine-tuned by other eminent surgeons, including William S. Halsted, Charles Mayo, and George Crile in the United States and has remained the standard of care [1,2]. Over the last 20 years, to limit or eliminate an anterior neck scar, a variety of endoscopic approaches were developed.

Endoscopic approaches to parathyroidectomy and thyroid lobectomy were published in 1996 and 1997, respectively [5,6]. These techniques used small anterior cervical incisions and video assistance with a laparoscope [7–12]. These methods evolved permitting remote access, eliminating all anterior neck incisions, as summarized in Table 1.

The transaxillary approach uses 3 axillary ports, allowing access to the ipsilateral neck [13,14]. The transbreast approach uses a trocar at the parasternal border of the breast and bilateral trocars at the superior areolar margin, enabling access to both thyroid lobes [15–17]. A combined axillary and breast approach improves triangulation but results in multiple incisions and significant flap dissection. The unilateral axillobreast approach allows for access to the ipsilateral thyroid lobe, and the axillobilateral breast and bilateral axillobreast approaches allow for visualization and resection of the entire thyroid gland [18–22]. To avoid breast involvement, the retroauricular approach was developed, involving 3 ports behind the ipsilateral ear [23].

Each of these approaches, although avoiding a cervical incision, impose incremental risks compared with conventional surgery. The large flaps and

Table 1
Remote access approaches to the thyroid gland

Transaxillary	Transbreast	Retroauricular
With or without robot assistance	Bilateral supra-areolar incisions with parasternal incision	With or without robot assistance
Three ports in axilla	Bilateral breast incisions with axillary incision	Three ports posterior to the ear
Option of single incision laparoscopic approach	Ipsilateral breast and axillary approach	Incision along the hairline
Access only to ipsilateral lobe	Bilateral axillary, bilateral breast approach	Can facilitate concomitant neck lift
	Access to entire thyroid gland	

extensive dissections are associated with increased bleeding and seroma formation. Specific peripheral nerves, including branches of the brachial plexus (transaxillary approach), the greater auricular nerve, and the spinal accessory nerve (retroauricular approach), are at increased risk. Furthermore, given the extent of dissection, these techniques are not minimally invasive. Ideally, minimally invasive thyroidectomy should follow the principles summarized in Box 1.

DEVELOPMENT OF TRANSORAL THYROIDECTOMY

With the dual goals of creating a minimally invasive approach and improving cosmetic results, transoral access to the thyroid gland developed. NOTES techniques were used, eliminating external incisions and visible scarring. Using the embryologic development and migration of the thyroid gland as a guide, the surgery was developed in a porcine model and in cadavers. Initially, an incision was made in the floor of the mouth and dissection carried down to the thyroid navigating and protecting the submandibular gland, esophagus, hypoglossal muscle, and the hypoglossal, superior laryngeal, and internal laryngeal nerves

Box 1: Principles of minimally invasive surgery

Minimal trauma from access
Close proximity to the operative field
Optimal operative visualization
Surgical resection equivalent to conventional approach
Morbidity profile similar to conventional approach
Equivalent specimen retrieval for histologic analysis
Improved cosmetic outcome

[24–26]. However, this technique caused significant tissue damage and had a high complication rate, most notably hypoglossal nerve injuries [24,27].

The vestibular technique was subsequently developed to improve the risk profile of this NOTES approach [28,29]. The transoral endoscopic thyroidectomy vestibular approach (TOETVA) allows for thyroidectomy using conventional laparoscopic instruments accessing the thyroid through the oral vestibule of the lower lip, traversing the premandibular space. This technique has been proven to be a safe and feasible approach, causing less tissue trauma compared with other remote access methods [29]. Specifically, the hypoglossal nerve is no longer in the operative field.

TOETVA has been refined by Anuwong and colleagues [29–32], who published their 60-patient series in 2016 and subsequently performed more than 500 cases at Police General Hospital, Bangkok, Thailand with minimal complications and excellent results. Having visited and observed Anuwong operating in Bangkok and then having him assist with the development of the first transoral thyroidectomy program in the United States, the authors can attest to his skills and continuous improvement of this technique [33]. Its use has been increasing, and it is now being performed in at least 14 countries: Thailand, Singapore, Indonesia, the Philippines, China, South Korea, Taiwan, Hong Kong, India, Italy, Mexico, Ecuador, Japan, and the United States [34]. In the United States, programs have been established in a few cities, including New Haven, Baltimore, Boston, San Francisco, New York, and Miami.

INDICATIONS AND PATIENT SELECTION

TOETVA can be used for a multitude of thyroid pathologic conditions. Although individual programs may limit cases in the initial phase of implementation, once adopted, these programs generally expand the applications. It can be used for unilateral or bilateral thyroid resection and central lymph node dissection. Indications include benign or indeterminate thyroid nodules, thyroid cysts, toxic adenomas, Graves disease, and many thyroid cancers. Table 2 summarizes the general indications and relative contraindications for TOETVA. Additional patient characteristics that must be considered include

Table 2
Indications and relative contraindications for transoral endoscopic thyroidectomy vestibular approach

Indications	Relative contraindications
Benign thyroid nodule(s)	Nodule size >10 cm
Indeterminate thyroid nodule(s)	Unable to tolerate general anesthesia/nasal intubation
Follicular neoplasm	Caution in patients with:
Hürthle cell neoplasm	Previous neck surgery
Thyroid cancer without lateral neck disease	Previous neck radiation
Well-controlled Graves disease	Compromised oral hygiene

body habitus, chin size, neck extension, previous cervical surgery, and oral hygiene.

SURGICAL TECHNIQUE

Preparation and positioning

Preoperative antibiotics are administered approximately 30 minutes before incision. General anesthesia is induced with nasotracheal intubation to keep the mouth free for surgical instrumentation. The patient is placed in the supine position, using a thyroid pillow behind the shoulders and a head ring under the occiput to obtain optimal neck extension. The skin is prepared from the upper lip to the upper chest and draped, permitting exposure from the mouth to the sternal notch, including the lateral aspects of the neck, as shown in Fig. 1. The wide skin preparation facilitates conversion to a conventional transcervical approach if necessary. The oral vestibule is prepared and rinsed with a chlorhexidine gluconate solution.

Access

A 10-mm transverse incision is made in the midline of the oral vestibule, just above the inferior labial frenulum, as depicted in Fig. 2. Electrocautery and blunt dissection are used to divide the submucosa and mentalis muscle to reach the edge of the mandible. Hydrodissection using a Varess needle and injecting an epinephrine/saline solution (1 mg epinephrine in 500 mL normal saline) initiates the creation of the subplatysmal flap to the level of the sternal notch. A blunt dissector, as exampled in Fig. 3, is passed into this space in a fan-shaped manner to create a working dome. A 10-mm trocar is inserted, and CO_2 insufflation is initiated and maintained at 6 mm Hg. Bilateral 5-mm incisions are made lateral to the canine teeth, perpendicular to and just inside the lower vermillion border to avoid the terminal branches of the mental nerves. Two 5-mm trocars are inserted parallel to the central port, as shown in Fig. 4.

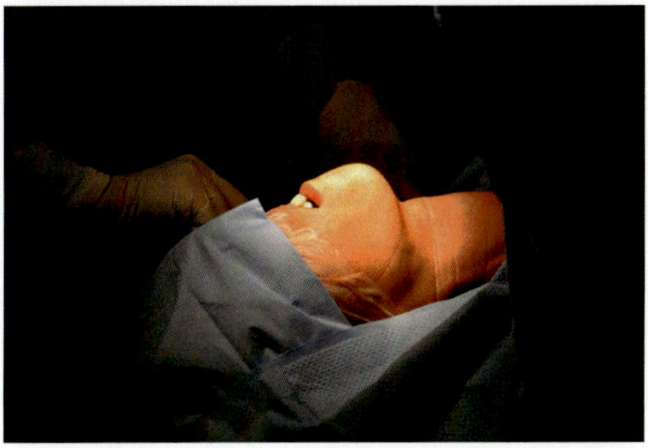

Fig. 1. Patient position after nasotracheal intubation. The head is hyperextended, and the patient is draped with exposure of the mouth and anterior neck.

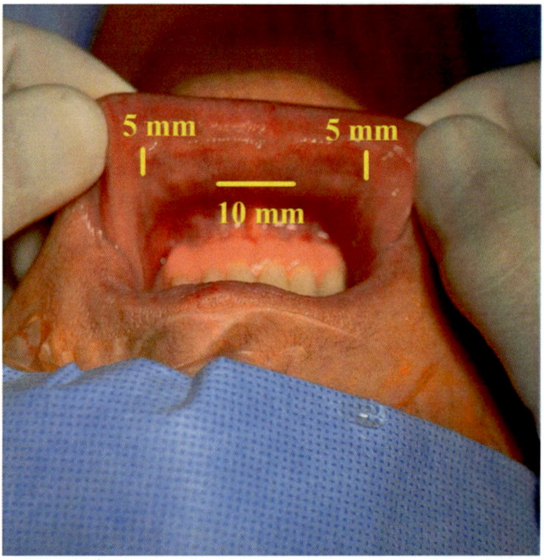

Fig. 2. Incision location in the oral vestibule of the lower lip. The 10-mm transverse incision is placed in the midline just anterior to the inferior labial frenulum. Bilateral 5-mm incisions are made internal to the lower vermillion border, lateral to the canine teeth.

Exposure

A 10-mm 30° laparoscope is placed in the central port. It is helpful to use a continuous airflow system to evacuate gas and smoke, which can compromise operative visualization while insufflating because the working space is relatively small. An external trapdoor suture is placed in the anterior midline of the neck to elevate the skin, subcutaneous tissue, and platysma, expanding the operative space. A combination of monopolar electrocautery and an ultrasonic or thermal energy device is used to complete dissection of the subplatysmal space inferiorly to the sternal notch, laterally to the edges of sternocleidomastoid muscles, and superiorly to the border of the thyroid cartilage. The strap

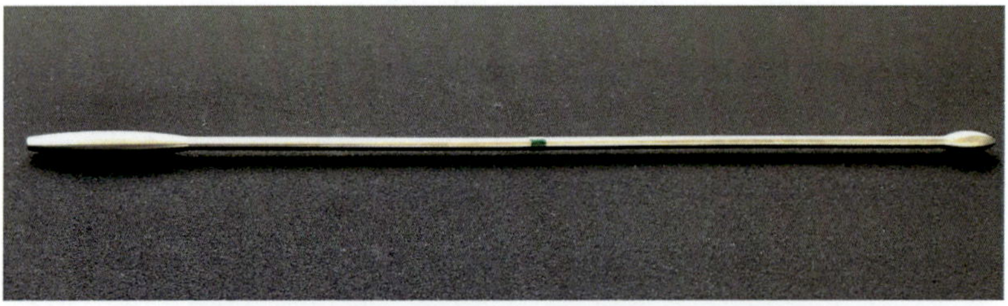

Fig. 3. Anuwong-Udelsman dual-head blunt transoral dissector. This instrument was custom made to fit through a 10-mm port for creation of the operative dome. This dilator was manufactured by DM Surgical LLC, Cheshire, Connecticut, USA.

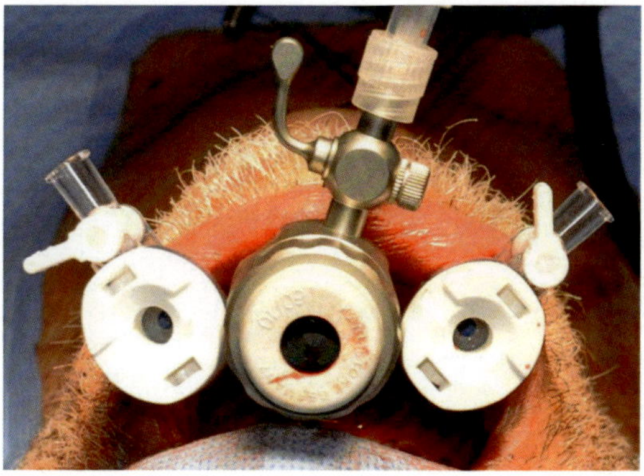

Fig. 4. Port placement in the lower lip. The central 10-mm port is used for insufflation with continuous air exchange and for use of a 10-mm 30° laparoscope. The two 5-mm ports are used for instrumentation.

muscles are mobilized by dividing the median raphe and dissecting them off the thyroid to expose the ipsilateral lobe. A second trap door suture can be used laterally through the skin to retract the strap muscles. If necessary, the sternothyroid muscle can be divided partially or completely at its superior insertion to facilitate visualization of the superior pole of the thyroid.

Dissecting the thyroid

Thyroid mobilization is initiated at the pyramidal lobe, extended along the trachea, transecting the gland through the isthmus along the border of the contralateral lobe. The avascular plane between the thyroid and cricothyroid muscle is opened, exposing the superior pole vessels. These vessels are ligated directly on the thyroid capsule to protect the external branch of the superior laryngeal nerve and the superior parathyroid gland. The gland is rotated medially to expose the tracheoesophageal groove and the recurrent laryngeal nerve (RLN). The RLN is traced proximally as the thyroid is mobilized and retracted medially, as shown in Fig. 5. Inferiorly, dissection of the thyroid gland stays on the capsule to preserve the lower parathyroid gland. The ligament of Berry is divided, protecting the RLN and trachea as the remaining pretracheal fascia is transected. For a total thyroidectomy, the procedure is replicated on the contralateral side. When indicated, a central neck lymph node dissection can easily be performed with this approach. Fig. 6 shows an extracted thyroid lobe with the ipsilateral central neck lymph node dissection.

Specimen retrieval and closure

A specimen retrieval pouch is placed through the center port. The specimen is placed into the pouch and delivered through the central incision after removal of the trocar. If necessary with large specimens, the thyroid capsule may be cut within the retrieval pouch to facilitate specimen compression and extraction. To preserve the specimen for histopathologic analysis, thyroid nodules are

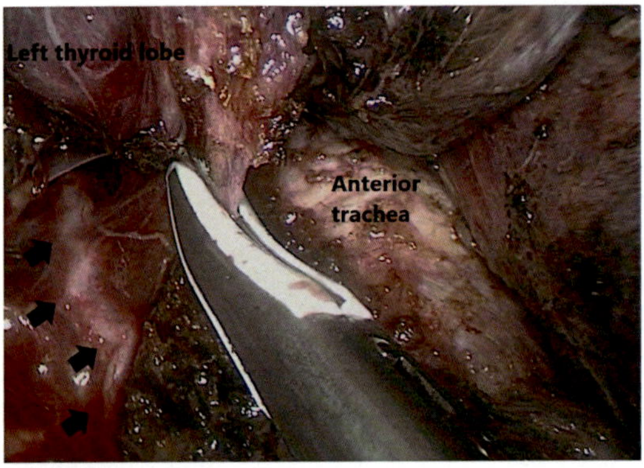

Fig. 5. Intraoperative dissection of the thyroid gland. The left thyroid lobe has been mobilized and rotated medially, and the thermal energy device is transecting the ligament of Berry. The left RLN is demarcated with black arrows.

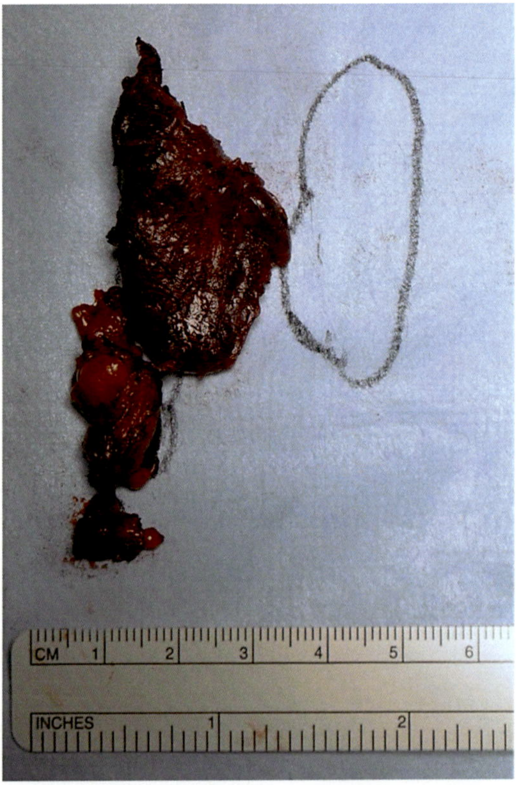

Fig. 6. Right thyroid lobe with the associated central lymph nodes after extraction on a patient with papillary thyroid cancer.

not compromised. After ensuring hemostasis, the strap muscles are reapproximated with a running suture. Residual CO_2 is evacuated, and the trocars are removed. The mentalis muscle is reapproximated, and the lip mucosa is closed with absorbable sutures.

Postoperative management

A facelift compression wrap is placed over an anterior cervical gauze pressure dressing. The patient is admitted to the hospital, and prophylactic antibiotics are continued for 24 hours. Patients are restricted to a liquid diet for the night of surgery, and an oral mouthwash is used 4 times a day. These patients are closely monitored for signs of bleeding, vocal cord paresis, or difficulty breathing. If they have undergone a total thyroidectomy, serum calcium levels are measured. On postoperative day 1, patients are offered a solid diet and generally discharged home.

SURGICAL RESULTS

Surgical procedures include thyroid lobectomy, isthmusectomy, subtotal or near-total thyroidectomy, and total thyroidectomy with or without a central neck dissection. The results following these procedures are favorable, and complication rates are low. The largest published experience shows complication rates at or less than 5% for major complications, and reported infections are rare. Overall, the morbidity profile is comparable to that of a conventional approach. A review of the published worldwide data for TOETVA is summarized in Table 3 [28–33,35–52].

SURGICAL COMPLICATIONS

In addition to the complications associated with conventional thyroidectomy, including bleeding, RLN injury, injury to the external branch of the superior laryngeal nerve, and hypoparathyroidism, TOETVA carries added risk. Although infection after conventional thyroidectomy is rare, the infection risk with TOETVA is theoretically increased. Using the oral cavity for access changes the case categorization from a clean to a clean-contaminated field. Consequently, perioperative antibiotic prophylaxis is standard for TOETVA, while unnecessary for a conventional approach [29–32]. Although reported infection rates vary, the largest single-institution case series showed a 0% infection rate [32]. Careful oral preparation, prophylactic antibiotics, and meticulous technique minimizing tissue trauma and eliminating dead space contribute to this success [26,29,30,32]. Seroma formation and subcutaneous emphysema are more common, occurring 3.5% to 5% of the time, but rarely require intervention. Subcutaneous emphysema is not in itself a complication and should be expected in most patients because of insufflation. It is almost always self-limiting and resolves spontaneously within 3 to 5 days.

Mental nerve palsy or injury causing sensory disorders of the lower lip and chin is a complication unique to this approach because the lateral ports traverse close to terminal branches of the mental nerve. The transposition of the lateral

Table 3
Worldwide transoral endoscopic thyroidectomy vestibular approach experience

Author, y	Cases	Indications	Procedures	Complications
Nakajo et al [35], 2013	8	3 PTC 4 Follicular adenoma 1 Goiter	5 Lobectomy 3 Subtotal, CND	1 RLN injury
Wang et al [28], 2014	12	12 Goiter	8 Lobectomy 4 TT	None
Yang et al [36], 2015	41	34 Goiter 3 Hyperthyroidism 4 PTC	19 Lobectomy 18 Subtotal/near-TT 4 TT, CND	2 Jaw ecchymosis 1 Skin puncture 1 Skin burn 1 Transient RLN palsy
Pai et al [37], 2015	1	1 Indeterminate	1 Lobectomy	None
Anuwong [29], 2016	60	42 Single nodule 2 Graves 2 PTC	42 Lobectomy 2 TT or near-TT 2 TT, CND	2 Transient hoarseness 1 Delayed hematoma 1 Transient hypoparathyroidism
Udelsman et al [33], 2016	5	1 Toxic adenoma 2 Goiter 1 Indeterminate 1 PTC	3 Lobectomy 1 TT 1 TT, CND	None
Inabnet et al [38], 2017	1	1 Toxic adenoma	1 Lobectomy	
Park et al [39], 2016	1	1 Indeterminate	1 Lobectomy	None
Jitpratoom et al [40], 2016	45	45 Graves	45 TT or near-TT	1 Conversion to open 10 Transient hypoparathyroidism
Yang et al [41], 2016	6	6 Solitary nodule	5 Partial thyroidectomy 1 Unilateral subtotal	1 Wound infection
Zeng et al [42], 2016	4	4 Goiter	4 TT	None
Dionigi et al [43], 2017	15	7 Single nodule 5 Goiter 2 Toxic adenoma 1 PTC	10 Lobectomy 5 TT	1 Transient hypocalcemia
Park & Sun [44], 2017	18[a]	6 Single nodule 11 PTC 1 Follicular carcinoma	15 Lobectomy 1 Completion 2 TT	1 Transient hypocalcemia 2 Seroma

(*continued on next page*)

Table 3
continued

Author, y	Cases	Indications	Procedures	Complications
Chai et al [45], 2017	10	10 PTC	7 Lobectomy 3 Isthmusectomy	2 Transient RLN palsy
Russell et al [46], 2017	6	6 Single nodule	6 Lobectomy	1 Temporary RLN palsy
Anuwong et al [32], 2018	200	110 Single nodule/cyst 66 Goiter 13 Graves 11 PTC	111 Lobectomy 89 TT or near-TT	8 Transient RLN palsy 35 Transient hypoparathyroidism 3 Transient mental nerve palsy 10 Seroma formation 1 Postoperative hematoma
Bakkar et al [47], 2018	5	5 Single nodule	5 Lobectomy	1 Conversion to open 1 Flap perforation
Anuwong et al [30], 2018	425	245 Single nodule/cyst 118 Goiter 33 Graves 26 PTC	245 Lobectomy 177 TT or near-TT	3 Conversion to open 25 Transient RLN palsy 46 Transient hypoparathyroidism 3 Transient mental nerve palsy 20 Seroma formation 1 Postoperative hematoma
Razavi et al [48], 2018	2[a]	1 Single nodule 1 Hürthle cell carcinoma	1 Lobectomy 1 Completion thyroidectomy	None
Yi et al [49], 2018	20	19 PTC 1 Follicular neoplasm	12 Lobectomy 1 Isthmusectomy 7 TT	1 Transient RLN palsy 1 Seroma 3 Transient hypocalcemia
Zhang et al [50], 2018	1	1 Indeterminate	1 TT	1 Transient hypocalcemia, extensive subcutaneous emphysema
Sivakumar and Amizhthu [51], 2018	11	11 Goiter	11 TT	None
Fu et al [52], 2018	81	65 Unilateral nodule 5 Goiter 6 Isthmus nodule 5 PTC	65 Lobectomy 6 Isthmusectomy 5 Subtotal 5 TT	2 Converted to open 2 Transient perioral numbness

Abbreviations: CND, central neck dissection; PTC, papillary thyroid cancer; TT, total thyroidectomy.
[a]Greater than 1 case in same patient.
Data from Refs [28–33,35–52].

working ports from anterior to the canines to the inferior vermillion border lateral to the canines appears to have reduced this risk; however, transient paresthesia from terminal branch mental nerve palsy is seen in 1% to 2% of these patients.

IMPLEMENTATION

Developing a successful transoral thyroidectomy program is a complex process that requires a multidisciplinary effort. After obtaining approval from institutional review committees, there must be an organized approach with anesthesia, pathology, operating room staff, surgical nursing, the postoperative surgical team, and hospital leadership. Specifically, a dedicated operating room team, including anesthesia, nursing, and scrub staff, greatly improves adoption, and more importantly, patient safety. Pathology needs to be involved, in case there is disruption or distortion of the specimen from extraction through the oral vestibule. Hospital credentialing will vary among institutions but must be obtained preemptively.

To succeed in implementation of the TOETVA program, a surgeon's preparation is extensive. Although the concept of dissecting the thyroid remains the same, this technique is more difficult to learn and perform. It is advantageous to practice using laparoscopic trainers and to visit centers already performing the procedure to observe. Ideally, a mentor who is actively performing the procedure will assist in training and implementation.

PARATHYROID APPLICATION

The transoral endoscopic vestibular approach has also been used for parathyroidectomy in patients with a well-localized adenoma and primary hyperparathyroidism. Although feasible, it is not an ideal alternative to the traditional approach for multiple reasons. Primarily, it is not clear preoperatively when a planned minimally invasive resection of a presumed single adenoma will require bilateral exploration for occult multigland disease and a subtotal parathyroid resection to achieve cure. Although bilateral exploration via the transoral approach is possible, it is more complicated than with the conventional approach. In addition, multiple ectopic parathyroid gland locations are best approached by a traditional transcervical incision, such as accessing a parathyroid gland within the carotid sheath or low within the mediastinal thymus.

DISCUSSION

The development of alternative and remote approaches to the thyroid is driven by cosmetic concerns. There are significant social differences and aesthetic concerns around the world that push this to the forefront. In Asia, an anterior neck scar is often considered disfiguring. In every population, however, there are subgroups whereby aesthetics and cosmetic surgical results are prioritized. For these patients, TOETVA offers an excellent alternative to the conventional cervical incision. Compared with other remote access approaches, TOETVA is particularly attractive. It has a similar morbidity profile to conventional thyroid surgery with low complication rates and is truly a minimally invasive approach. Although implemented in many institutions, the other remote access techniques have frequently been abandoned.

In the western world, TOETVA is not likely a method that will become the standard of care in all centers. Rather, it is a specialized approach, likely to be offered in select institutions for appropriate patients, performed by surgeons committed to learning and implementing this technique. Although current results are favorable, those with the most experience continue to adjust and fine tune the procedure to improve outcomes. Although it is applicable for multiple indications, the case numbers required to become and remain proficient necessitate a large referral base because a fraction of those patients will be willing and appropriate to proceed. During the initial implementation, operative times are longer. With increased experience, however, operative times approach conventional thyroid surgery.

SUMMARY

Kocher's transverse cervical incision has been the standard surgical approach for thyroidectomy for more than 100 years. Now, for those patients with aesthetic concerns who wish to avoid an anterior neck scar, remote access surgical techniques have been developed. TOETVA offers a minimally invasive NOTES approach without visible scarring and a low complication rate. Although it is increasingly performed in Asian countries, the western experience is limited. TOETVA shows great potential to become an accepted alternative approach for select surgeons in institutions committed to establishing programs.

References

[1] Welbourn RB, Friesen SR, Johnston IDA, et al. The history of endocrine surgery. New York: Praeger Publishers; 1990.
[2] Giddings AEB. The history of thyroidectomy. J R Soc Med 1998;91(33_Supplemental):3–6.
[3] Sarkar S, Banerjee S, Sarkar R, et al. A review on the history of 'thyroid surgery'. Indian J Surg 2016;78(1):32–6.
[4] Gross SD. 4th edition. A system of surgery: pathologic, diagnostic, therapeutic, and operative, vol. ii. Philadelphia: Henry C Lea; 1866.
[5] Gagner M. Endoscopic subtotal parathyroidectomy in patients with primary hyperparathyroidism. Br J Surg 1996;83(6):875.
[6] Huscher CS, Chiodini S, Napolitano C, et al. Endoscopic right thyroid lobectomy. Surg Endosc 1997;11(8):877.
[7] Miccoli P, Berti P, Raffaelli M, et al. Comparison between minimally invasive video-assisted thyroidectomy and conventional thyroidectomy: a prospective randomized study. Surgery 2001;130(6):1039–43.
[8] El-Labban GM. Minimally invasive video-assisted thyroidectomy versus conventional thyroidectomy: a single-blinded, randomized controlled clinical trial. J Minim Access Surg 2009;5(4):97–102.
[9] Miccoli P, Bellantone R, Mourad M, et al. Minimally invasive video-assisted thyroidectomy: multiinstitutional experience. World J Surg 2002;26(8):972–5.

[10] Terris DJ, Gourin CG, Chin E. Minimally invasive thyroidectomy: basic and advanced techniques. Laryngoscope 2006;116(3):350–6.
[11] Bellantone R, Lombardi CP, Raffaelli M, et al. Minimally invasive, totally gasless video-assisted thyroid lobectomy. Am J Surg 1999;177(4):342–3.
[12] Shimizu K, Akira S, Jasmi AY, et al. Video-assisted neck surgery: endoscopic resection of thyroid tumors with a very minimal neck wound. J Am Coll Surg 1999;188(6):697–703.
[13] Ikeda Y, Takami H, Niimi M, et al. Endoscopic thyroidectomy and parathyroidectomy by the axillary approach. A preliminary report. Surg Endosc 2002;16(1):92–5.
[14] Ikeda Y, Takami H, Sasaki Y, et al. Endoscopic neck surgery by the axillary approach. J Am Coll Surg 2000;191(3):336–40.
[15] Ohgami M, Ishii S, Arisawa Y, et al. Scarless endoscopic thyroidectomy: breast approach for better cosmesis. Surg Laparosc Endosc Percutan Tech 2000;10(1):1–4.
[16] Sasaki A, Nakajima J, Ikeda K, et al. Endoscopic thyroidectomy by the breast approach: a single institution's 9-year experience. World J Surg 2008;32(3):381–5.
[17] Kim YS, Joo KH, Park SC, et al. Endoscopic thyroid surgery via a breast approach: a single institution's experiences. BMC Surg 2014;14:49.
[18] Shimazu K, Shiba E, Tamaki Y, et al. Endoscopic thyroid surgery through the axillo-bilateral-breast approach. Surg Laparosc Endosc Percutan Tech 2003;13(3):196–201.
[19] Choe JH, Kim SW, Chung KW, et al. Endoscopic thyroidectomy using a new bilateral axillo-breast approach. World J Surg 2007;31(3):601–6.
[20] Choi JY, Lee KE, Chung K-W, et al. Endoscopic thyroidectomy via bilateral axillo-breast approach (BABA): review of 512 cases in a single institute. Surg Endosc 2012;26(4):948–55.
[21] Koh YW, Kim JW, Lee SW, et al. Endoscopic thyroidectomy via a unilateral axillo-breast approach without gas insufflation for unilateral benign thyroid lesions. Surg Endosc 2009;23(9):2053–60.
[22] Bodade RM, Dhoran AP, Dhurve AS, et al. Endoscopic thyroidectomy-axilla breast approach: the experience of 26 cases. International Surgery Journal 2018;5(2):593–7.
[23] Lee KE, Kim HY, Park WS, et al. Postauricular and axillary approach endoscopic neck surgery: a new technique. World J Surg 2009;33(4):767–72.
[24] Karakas E, Steinfeldt T, Gockel A, et al. Transoral thyroid and parathyroid surgery. Surg Endosc 2010;24(6):1261–7.
[25] Karakas E, Steinfeldt T, Gockel A, et al. Transoral thyroid and parathyroid surgery–development of a new transoral technique. Surgery 2011;150(1):108–15.
[26] Karakas E, Anuwong A, Ketwong K, et al. [Transoral thyroid and parathyroid surgery: implementation and evaluation of the transoral endoscopic technique via the vestibular approach (TOETVA)]. Chirurg 2018;89(7):537–44.
[27] Wilhelm T, Metzig A. Endoscopic minimally invasive thyroidectomy (eMIT): a prospective proof-of-concept study in humans. World J Surg 2011;35(3):543–51.
[28] Wang C, Zhai H, Liu W, et al. Thyroidectomy: a novel endoscopic oral vestibular approach. Surgery 2014;155(1):33–8.
[29] Anuwong A. Transoral endoscopic thyroidectomy vestibular approach: a series of the first 60 human cases. World J Surg 2016;40(3):491–7.
[30] Anuwong A, Ketwong K, Jitpratoom P, et al. Safety and outcomes of the transoral endoscopic thyroidectomy vestibular approach. JAMA Surg 2018;153(1):21–7.
[31] Anuwong A, Kim HY, Dionigi G. Transoral endoscopic thyroidectomy using vestibular approach: updates and evidences. Gland Surg 2017;6(3):277–84.
[32] Anuwong A, Sasanakietkul T, Jitpratoom P, et al. Transoral endoscopic thyroidectomy vestibular approach (TOETVA): indications, techniques and results. Surg Endosc 2018;32(1):456–65.
[33] Udelsman R, Anuwong A, Oprea AD, et al. Trans-oral vestibular endocrine surgery: a new technique in the United States. Ann Surg 2016;264(6):e13–6.

[34] Dionigi G, Chai YJ, Tufano RP, et al. Transoral endoscopic thyroidectomy via a vestibular approach: why and how? Endocrine 2018;59(2):275–9.
[35] Nakajo A, Arima H, Hirata M, et al. Trans-oral video-assisted neck surgery (TOVANS). A new transoral technique of endoscopic thyroidectomy with gasless premandible approach. Surg Endosc 2013;27(4):1105–10.
[36] Yang J, Wang C, Li J, et al. Complete endoscopic thyroidectomy via oral vestibular approach versus areola approach for treatment of thyroid diseases. J Laparoendosc Adv Surg Tech A 2015;25(6):470–6.
[37] Pai VM, Muthukumar P, Prathap A, et al. Transoral endoscopic thyroidectomy: a case report. Int J Surg Case Rep 2015;12:99–101.
[38] Inabnet WB 3rd, Suh H, Fernandez-Ranvier G. Transoral endoscopic thyroidectomy vestibular approach with intraoperative nerve monitoring. Surg Endosc 2017;31(7):3030.
[39] Park JO, Kim MR, Kim DH, et al. Transoral endoscopic thyroidectomy via the trivestibular route. Ann Surg Treat Res 2016;91(5):269–72.
[40] Jitpratoom P, Ketwong K, Sasanakietkul T, et al. Transoral endoscopic thyroidectomy vestibular approach (TOETVA) for Graves' disease: a comparison of surgical results with open thyroidectomy. Gland Surg 2016;5(6):546–52.
[41] Yang K, Ding B, Lin C, et al. The novel transvestibule approach for endoscopic thyroidectomy: a case series. Surg Laparosc Endosc Percutan Tech 2016;26(1):e25–8.
[42] Zeng YK, Li ZY, Xuan WL, et al. Trans-oral glasses-free three-dimensional endoscopic thyroidectomy-preliminary single center experiences. Gland Surg 2016;5(6):628–32.
[43] Dionigi G, Bacuzzi A, Lavazza M, et al. Transoral endoscopic thyroidectomy: preliminary experience in Italy. Updates Surg 2017;69(2):225–34.
[44] Park JO, Sun DI. Transoral endoscopic thyroidectomy: our initial experience using a new endoscopic technique. Surg Endosc 2017;31(12):5436–43.
[45] Chai YJ, Chung JK, Anuwong A, et al. Transoral endoscopic thyroidectomy for papillary thyroid microcarcinoma: initial experience of a single surgeon. Ann Surg Treat Res 2017;93(2):70–5.
[46] Russell JO, Clark J, Noureldine SI, et al. Transoral thyroidectomy and parathyroidectomy—a North American series of robotic and endoscopic transoral approaches to the central neck. Oral Oncol 2017;71:75–80.
[47] Bakkar S, Al Hyari M, Naghawi M, et al. Transoral thyroidectomy: a viable surgical option with unprecedented complications-a case series. J Endocrinol Invest 2018;41(7):809–13.
[48] Razavi CR, Tufano RP, Russell JO. Completion thyroidectomy via the transoral endoscopic vestibular approach. Gland Surg 2018;7(Suppl 1):S77–9.
[49] Yi JW, Yoon SG, Kim HS, et al. Transoral endoscopic surgery for papillary thyroid carcinoma: initial experiences of a single surgeon in South Korea. Ann Surg Treat Res 2018;95(2):73–9.
[50] Zhang D, Wu CW, Inversini D, et al. Lessons learned from a faulty transoral endoscopic thyroidectomy vestibular approach. Surg Laparosc Endosc Percutan Tech 2018;28(5):e94–9.
[51] Sivakumar T, Amizhthu RA. Transoral endoscopic total thyroidectomy vestibular approach: a case series and literature review. J Minim Access Surg 2018;14(2):118–23.
[52] Fu J, Luo Y, Chen Q, et al. Transoral endoscopic thyroidectomy: review of 81 cases in a single institute. J Laparoendosc Adv Surg Tech A 2018;28(3):286–91.

Advances in Surgery 53 (2019) 195–208

ADVANCES IN SURGERY

Firearm Violence in America

Is There a Solution?

Rachel L. Choron, MD[a], Sarabeth Spitzer[b], Joseph V. Sakran, MPH, MD, MPA[c,*]

[a]Division of Acute Care Surgery, Department of Surgery, The Johns Hopkins Hospital, 1800 Orleans Street, Sheikh Zayed Tower, Suite 6107, Baltimore, MD 21287, USA; [b]Stanford University School of Medicine, 291 Campus Drive, Stanford, CA 94305, USA; [c]Department of Surgery, The Johns Hopkins University School of Medicine, Emergency General Surgery, The Johns Hopkins Hospital, 1800 Orleans Street, Sheikh Zayed Tower, Suite 6107, Baltimore, MD 21287, USA

Keywords

• Gun violence • Firearms • Injury • Death • Trauma • Public health • Suicide

Key points

- Firearm-related violence is a public health crisis that results in nearly 40,000 deaths per year.
- This is a uniquely American problem; the United States has the highest firearm-related mortality worldwide among industrialized countries.
- Suicide and homicide account for 60% and 40% of firearm-related deaths, seen primarily in older white communities and younger black communities, respectively.
- Although there is a perceived national divide regarding gun legislation reform, literature shows that Americans have more commonalities than often thought regarding firearm injury prevention.
- A multipronged approach is needed to bolster firearm injury–prevention programs and reduce firearm-related injury and death. Some of the important steps forward include increasing federal funding for research, expanding universal background checks, uniting professional organizations to promote and create change, and improving mental health access.

Disclosure Statement: The authors do not have any relationships with commercial companies with direct financial interest in the subject matter or materials discussed in this article or with any company making competing products.

*Corresponding author. *E-mail address:* Jsakran1@jhmi.edu

https://doi.org/10.1016/j.yasu.2019.04.019
0065-3411/19/

INTRODUCTION

Firearm injury is a public health crisis in the United States. Every day, an average of 109 individuals are killed, and more than 240 people suffer injuries secondary to firearm violence [1,2]. Although the United States is a world leader in many arenas, we are failing when it comes to firearm injury prevention. Firearm-related injury and death is a public health problem creating a vast burden of disease across the spectrum of ages and socioeconomic groups in this country. In addition, firearm-related violence has a substantial economic burden of more than 229 billion dollars per year to the United States health care system [3,4]. Most concerning, despite advances in trauma systems and health care capabilities, the fatality rate secondary to firearms has not significantly changed or improved [5,6].

EPIDEMIOLOGY OF FIREARM VIOLENCE

In 2017, the Centers for Disease Control and Prevention (CDC) reported 39,773 deaths from firearm injury. This figure accounts for 58% of all intentional injuries in the United States. Of these firearm-related deaths, 23,854 (60%) were suicides and 15,919 (40%) were homicides [1,6]. These numbers are the highest that have been seen in the past 40 years. Since 1999, there has been a 17% increase in firearm-related intentional injury mortalities, with 7000 more suicide deaths secondary to firearms in 2017 compared with 1999 [1,7].

In the United States, we have nearly the same number of deaths from firearms as compared with motor vehicle collisions (MVC). MVCs account for 10.6 deaths/100,000, whereas firearms account for 10.5 deaths/100,000, followed by falls at 10.4 deaths/100,000 [8]. Interestingly, although there is nearly the same number of deaths from MVCs as firearms, only 5% of patients cared for by trauma centers are from firearm-related injuries; this emphasizes the high severity of injury and associated firearm mortality [8].

Firearm violence: a uniquely American problem

Although we have so much to be proud of in America, it is clear that one of the areas where we have fallen short compared with our peer nations is preventing firearm-related injury and death. The rate of firearm-related violence, suicides, and unintentional injuries in the United States is the highest among industrialized countries. Specifically, the US firearm homicide rate is 25.2 times higher and the suicide rate is 8 times higher than other developed nations [9,10]. This problem is an American problem for our children as well. The mortality of American children is 11 times the rate seen in other high-income countries [9].

Estimates based on self-reporting projections indicate there are nearly 400 million firearms owned privately by civilians in the United States, putting the United States first among all nations when comparing the number of privately owned firearms across different countries [11,12]. There is now substantial literature confirming that the presence of firearms in the home increases the likelihood of homicide, suicide, and unintentional injury for the firearm owner and those with access [5,11,13,14].

Not only does America continue to face an extraordinary mortality nationwide secondary to firearm-related violence, but also the intensity of violence appears to be increasing. Patients are experiencing higher-caliber wounds and multiple gunshot wounds opposed to one; overall, the proportion of nonsurvivable traumatic injuries has increased [15]. The fatality rate secondary to firearm-related violence in 1 urban trauma center showed a significant increase from 9.5% during 2000 to 2003 to 18.3% during 2004 to 2005, and this trend is continuing to increase [6,15].

Firearm-related homicide

The greatest burden of homicide is seen most prominently in young men, specifically in black and Hispanic communities. The overall firearm mortality between the ages of 20 to 29 is 5 times higher in the black community than in the Hispanic community, and 17 times higher than the white community in the same age distribution [1]. In addition, firearm-related mortality among black women in the United States is higher than all other races in each age bracket [1].

Overall, a disproportionate burden of firearm-related death falls on our minorities. In addition, these rates have not been affected by previous legislation with the goal for reform. Previous firearm legislation aimed at decreasing pediatric, unintentional, self-harm, and overall firearm-related fatality rates has shown no effect on the overall homicide rate nor the mortality among the black community [16].

Firearm-related suicide

Firearm-related suicide is seen primarily in older, white communities. Although 85% of firearm-related injury and death among the black population is related to homicide, 75% of injury and death in the white population is related to suicide. The highest rate of mortality due to suicide by firearms is among white men older than 70 years of age [1]. Availability of firearms has been shown to be associated with increased risk of suicide in the home among both adolescents and adults [13,14]. Although mental illness has been shown not to be a significant contributor to homicide-related deaths, access to firearms among patients with preexisting mental illness results in a significantly increased rate of suicide [17,18].

High-risk populations: children and adolescents

Children and adolescents are especially at risk for injury and mortality attributed to firearms. Among children and teenagers less than 20 years of age, 8 children are killed by firearms every day [1]. Unfortunately, children account for 45% of fatalities in domestic mass shootings and 10% of fatalities in mass shootings [19]. Not only are children direct victims of injury and death secondary to firearms but also 1 in every 5 teenagers (aged 14–17 years) have also witnessed shootings [18].

Mass shootings

Although mass shootings are only responsible for less than 2% of all firearm-related deaths, mass shootings in the United States have been increasing in frequency since at least 2011. Although the term "mass shooting" has different definitions among organizations, it is defined here as any firearm-related incident resulting in injury or death of 4 or more people. In 2000, the Federal Bureau of Investigation (FBI) identified only 7 deaths secondary to active shooter incidents [20]. In comparison, the Gun Violence Archives reported 376 mass shootings in 2017 alone [21]. Other sources report the number of mass shootings in 2017 to be even higher, with deaths totaling 590 persons [21]. Most importantly, semiautomatic weapons are commonly used in active shooter incidents, resulting in more people being injured or killed [22].

CHALLENGES TO FIREARM-RELATED INJURY PREVENTION

Despite the massive toll firearm violence takes on the United States, our nation continues to struggle with tackling this public health crisis. One of the barriers to moving the needle forward has been that the manner in which this process has been approached. Similar to how the health care community has addressed other public health problems, firearm-related injury should follow a similar approach. For example, when MVC fatalities were rising, the nation moved toward safer roads, developing seatbelts and ensuring compliance, and improving vehicle safety. With high mortalities seen secondary to cigarette smoking and lung cancer, an effective antismoking campaign was developed. Public health advances regarding firearm-related violence must be a priority in this country as well.

Two conflicting narratives

One important obstacle to improving firearm injury prevention is the assumption that there are 2 conflicting viewpoints in the United States related to firearms. The leaders of the American College of Surgeons Committee on Trauma (ACS COT) described these 2 "conflicting narratives" [7].

One narrative sees firearms as a fundamental American right, necessary in society for protection. This viewpoint links "gun control" to "freedom control." People who share this viewpoint see firearm regulations as a reduction in personal liberty. The second narrative sees firearms as harmful and unnecessary. Those who hold this viewpoint believe guns represent violence and therefore link "gun control" to "violence control." They believe firearms put their personal safety and their families at risk [7].

It is thought that these vastly different viewpoints have brought our nation to a standstill and prevented improvement in violence and injury prevention. However, the reality is that we, as Americans, have more in common than we have that divides us; research has demonstrated that we are not nearly as different as is often portrayed.

In 2015, a public opinion survey from the Johns Hopkins Center for Gun Policy and Research was conducted among gun owners and nonowners. Both 84% of gun owners and 84% of nonowners favored background checks for all gun sales. In addition, 78% of gun owners and 80% of nonowners favored preventing sales to people with temporary domestic violence restraining orders. Most of both owners and nonowners also supported the release of data on which gun dealers sell the most guns used in crimes, requiring a license before buying a gun to verify identify, and temporarily removing guns from individuals who pose immediate threat of harm to self or others [23].

Limitations to research funding

In 1996, Congress passed the Dickey Amendment in the omnibus spending bill mandating that none of the funds made available for injury prevention and control at the CDC could be used to "advocate or promote gun control" [24]. In addition, in that same spending bill, Congress stripped the CDC of 2.6 million dollars, which happened to be the exact amount allocated in the prior year to firearm research. These actions severely limited research funding dedicated to firearm-related violence over the past 2 decades [25]. In 2011, this was extended to include all federal agencies, including the National Institutes of Health (NIH) [26]. More recently, in 2013, President Obama signed an executive order permitting the CDC to study or sponsor research dedicated to firearm injury prevention [27]. Although this executive order created opportunities for funding injury prevention secondary to firearm-related injury and death, Congress has failed to appropriate the necessary funds to allow for research in this arena.

This funding limitation has substantially impacted firearm-related violence research. Violent injury secondary to firearms is the most poorly addressed public health problem in the United States and is drastically underfunded given its substantial burden of disease [7]. One study compared the mortality and research funding of different disease states. The number of deaths from firearm violence and sepsis were nearly the same in 2014. However, when comparing funding, the aid dedicated to gun violence research was 0.7% that of sepsis, and the publication volume was only 4% [28]. Of all diseases compared in this study, firearm violence was the least researched cause of death [28].

SOLUTIONS TO DECREASING FIREARM-RELATED INJURIES

Expand universal background checks

The Brady Handgun Violence Prevention Act, or "The Brady Bill," was signed into law in 1993 by President Clinton and instituted background checks at federally licensed gun dealerships; it was designed to prevent high-risk individuals from purchasing firearms. This bill instituted the FBI to run each firearm purchaser through the National Instant Criminal Background Check System. Prohibited users include felons, fugitives, domestic abusers, and dangerously mentally ill individuals. Since the success of the Brady Bill and Brady Campaign, more than 3 million attempts to purchase firearms have been prevented; about half of these blocked attempts were attempted purchases by felons [29].

Background checks are a strongly evidence-based method to reduce firearm violence and mortality. In addition, this process is critical to ensuring appropriate individuals have access to obtaining firearms, and avoiding sales or transfer of firearms to criminals or others who should not have access to these weapons.

Although the Brady Bill has been successful in limiting gun sales in federally licensed gun dealerships, 40% of firearms are sold through nonlicensed dealers who are not mandated to perform background checks [30,31]. Currently, background checks are not required for guns sold at gun shows, online, or through private transfers. In total, these sales account for an estimated 6.6 million firearms [31,32]. Another way to think about it is 1 in 5 gun sales take places with "no questions asked," resulting in thousands of guns going into the hands of people that should not have them.

Many health care organizations, along with firearm research experts, believe universal background checks would decrease firearm violence [33]. Some of the pending legislation that has not yet been passed has attempted to expand Brady background checks to all gun sales, including those sold at gun shows and over the Internet. It would prohibit the transfer of firearms between private parties unless a licensed importer, manufacturer, or dealer has first taken possession of the firearm to submit a background check. In addition, it calls for gun owners to report lost or stolen firearms to the US Department of Justice and local law enforcement within 48 hours of discovery. Although this legislation is pending, nothing has been passed to move these initiatives forward.

Expansion of extreme risk protective orders

Extreme risk protective orders currently are state-level firearm-prevention measures that allow police or family members to petition state courts to have firearms temporarily removed from an individual who may be at risk to themselves or others. These laws are referred to differently in different states, such as "Gun Violence Restraining Orders" or "Extreme Risk Protection Orders" [34]. Connecticut was the first state to enact such a regulation in 1999 [35]. By the end of 2018, a total of 13 states had enacted such laws.

Although specifics of these provisions differ by state, each allows for a period of court-ordered temporary removal of a firearm from a high-risk individual on the order of weeks to months. Experts believe that expanding such laws to all states would significantly improve firearm safety, allowing for action to be taken to prevent high-risk individuals from harming themselves or others once a weapon is already in their possession [36]. In addition, the National Rifle Association (NRA) has voiced limited support for such laws [37].

Bolster funding for firearm-related research

As discussed, firearm-related research is drastically underfunded and does not match the national burden of disease. Improving funding is absolutely critical to produce high-quality, rigorous academic analysis of firearm injury in the United States and is the best way to prevent it. The CDC, the NIH, and the National Institute of Justice need to increase funding allocation toward firearm injury–prevention research.

Recently, private organizations and a select group of local and state governments have worked to improve funding irrespective of the federal funding for this research. However, funding does not match the burden of death and injury attributed to gun violence in comparison to other mechanisms in this country. As funding improves and more research is completed, this research must be made available so legislators, policy makers, and health care providers alike can enact evidence-based policy changes to decrease firearm-related injury and mortality.

Physician's role in prevention

Physicians and health care providers have a unique role in preventing firearm-related injury. As trusted sources of health information, physicians are able to counsel patients regarding firearm ownership and safety and identify individuals who might be particularly high risk for firearm injury [38]. Motivational interviewing and physician counseling have been shown to be effective in improving safe storage of firearms in the home [39]. Safe storage is especially important in homes in which there are children present or in those persons who have increased risk of suicide or self-harm. Training for medical students, resident physicians, and practicing physicians regarding important firearm safety assessment tools and knowledge is crucial to improve the physician's role in preventing firearm violence. It is especially important this occurs across specialties and includes a spectrum of physicians, including surgeons, pediatricians, emergency physicians, family medicine practitioners, intensivists, and internists.

Physician involvement in firearm violence prevention was questioned by the NRA with a strong response from both the physician and the nonmedical community alike [37,40]. Encouraging and training providers to discuss firearms with patients is a crucial way physicians can begin to reduce the firearm epidemic in the United States.

Organizations working toward a mutual goal

Medical and surgical professional organizations and societies have historically supported a public health approach to major issues resulting in mortality. For example, tobacco use, MVC, and unintentional poisonings were all managed from a public health standpoint to reduce fatalities by professional organizations. Throughout the United States, physicians have first-hand experience with firearm-related violence and the resulting impact on their patients' lives. In turn, many professional organizations have developed consensus statements and recommendations regarding firearm violence that use a public health approach to tackle this difficult issue.

The ACS COT is strongly pursuing prevention efforts and has published a clear position statement promoting injury prevention [41]. This strategy supports approaching firearm violence from a public health standpoint, evaluating evidence regarding trauma center networks' violence-prevention programs and committing to a collegial and professional dialogue to work toward reducing mortality (Box 1) [8,41,42]. The ACS COT is pursuing these commitments

Box 1: American College of Surgeons Committee on Trauma's position statement on firearm injury–prevention strategy

1. Commitment to approach firearm violence as a public health problem
2. Evaluation of evidence for violence-prevention programs, particularly those implemented through trauma center networks
3. Commitment to create a forum for civil, collegial, and professional dialogue on reducing deaths

Data from Jenkins DH, Winchell RJ, Coimbra R, et al. Position statement of the American College of Surgeons Committee on Trauma on the National Academies of Sciences, Engineering and Medicine Report: A national trauma care system: integrating military and civilian trauma systems to achieve zero preventable deaths after injury. J Trauma Acute Care Surg. 2016; 81:819-823.

by holding town hall meetings, conferencing with stakeholders to create policy development for firearm injury prevention, and supporting a research agenda. The ACS COT has also proposed how to engage movement toward this solution (Box 2) [8]. They have also proposed solutions to reduce firearm violence that include restricting firearm ownership for anyone who is a danger to themselves or others, encouraging responsible ownership regarding safety and educations, and improving mental health access and understanding of the proximate causes of violence (Box 3) [7].

The American Association for the Surgery of Trauma has also identified firearm-related injury and mortality as an unacceptable public health problem. In a 2018 publication in the *Trauma Surgery Acute Care Open Access Journal*, they challenged branches of government and professional organizations to address firearm violence and proposed more detailed solutions to the problem

Box 2: American College of Surgeons Committee on Trauma's proposed engagement to solution on firearm injury–prevention strategy

1. Bridge the chasm of the 2 narratives' sides with professionalism, respect, and tolerance
2. Center on what is the right thing to do for our patients
3. Recognize and respect philosophic differences
4. Acknowledge opposing views and respect them
5. Appeal to the middle
6. Commit to not move forward with legislative initiatives until there is consensus that involves elements of both narratives
7. Focus on making guns safer rather than eliminating guns
8. Articulating not just freedom, but freedom with responsibility

Data from Stewart RM, Kuhls DA. Firearm injury prevention: a consensus approach to reducing preventable deaths. J Trauma Acute Care Surg. 2016; 80:850-852.

Box 3: American College of Surgeons Committee on Trauma's proposed solution to firearm injury prevention

1. Anyone who is a danger to themselves or others should not have a firearm
2. Responsible ownership includes safe storage, education, training, and a commitment to keep firearms out of the hands of family members at high risk of self-harm, unlawful purchasers, and violent offenders
3. Improvement of mental health access, hygiene, and treatment
4. Identification, understanding, and addressing proximate causes of violence

Data from Stewart RM, Kuhls DA, Rotondo MF, et al. Freedom with responsibility: A consensus strategy for preventing injury, death, and disability from firearm violence. J Am Coll Surg. 2018; 227:281-283.

(Box 4) [43]. Similarly, a consensus statement with recommendations regarding decreasing firearm-related injuries was developed by the leaders of the following organizations: American Academy of Family Physicians, American Academy of Pediatrics, American College of Emergency Physicians, American

Box 4: American Association for the Surgery of Trauma's statement on firearm injury solution

1. Strengthen National Instant Criminal Background Check System and require background check on all firearm sales
2. Standardize a waiting period for firearm sales
3. Promote responsible firearm ownership, including training of new owners, safe storage, and application of practical technologic safety strategies
4. Strictly regulate the sale of high-capacity magazine-fed semiautomatic rifles
5. Strictly regulate the sale of bump stocks and trigger actuators
6. Strictly regulate high-volume ammunition sales
7. Require reporting of all firearm sales: both public and private
8. Require firearm owners to report lost or stolen weapons to law enforcement
9. Remove firearms from accused perpetrators of intimate partner violence and those threatening violence to others until their case is adjudicated
10. Encourage and train physicians to counsel their patients about firearm safety and health risks associated with firearm ownership
11. Improve access to quality of medical care, including behavioral health services to reduce suicide and gun-related violence
12. Mandate new federal funding from the NIH and CDC for research on firearm injuries and injury-prevention strategies commensurate with the burden of disease
13. Support bleeding control training for the public and public access to bleeding control kits
14. Create a National Trauma Care System

Data from Croce MA. AAST statement on firearm injury. Trauma Surg Acute Care Open. 2018;3:e000204. https://doi.org/10.1136/tsaco-2108-000204.

Congress of Obstetricians and Gynecologists, American College of Physicians, American College of Surgeons, American Psychiatric Association, American Public Health Association, and American Bar Association [33].

The Eastern Association for the Surgery of Trauma (EAST) recently released a Firearm Injury Prevention Statement in January 2019 underscoring their commitment to the health and safety of patients and their communities along with the recognition that current efforts are insufficient to reduce firearm-related injuries. The EAST consensus statement appropriately describes firearm violence as a public health crisis and supports evidence-based strategies to reduce firearm injuries; this statement emphasizes federal funding, programs to prevent violence and teach conflict resolution, firearm safety related to storage and usage, universal background checks with waiting periods, and limited access to highly lethal firearms and accessories (Box 5) [44].

Although these organizations continue to work toward common goals, there is still more that can be accomplished. The medical and surgical organizations need to work together in a cohesive manner to improve funding, publish firearm-related research, and use their collective power to influence regulatory decisions that reduce the number of injuries and deaths attributable to firearm violence. Overall, a united approach is required to move toward solving this complex health problem.

Box 5: Eastern Association for the Surgery of Trauma's consensus statement on firearm injury prevention

1. Federal funding of firearm-related research to inform solutions
2. Violence and injury–prevention programs that address conflict resolution
3. Programs that teach nonviolent conflict resolution, coping strategies, and anger management
4. Improved access and quality of mental health services
5. Recognition of other factors (structural violence, domestic violence, mental health)
6. Limited access to firearms through mandatory safe storage, gun locks, trigger locks, and so forth
7. Expanded universal background checks to include all firearms sales in any venue
8. Mandatory waiting periods and universal background checks for firearm acquisition
9. Limited civilian access to highly lethal firearms and firearm accessories (high-velocity rifles, high-capacity magazines, trigger cranks, and bump stocks)
10. Limited dissemination of technology to enhance lethality or bypass standard safety and/or screening (eg, 3D printing firearms)

Data from EAST Board of Directors. Eastern Association for the Surgery of Trauma Firearm Injury Prevention Statement. J trauma Acute Care Surg. 2019; 86(1):168-170.

Campaigns to raise public awareness and change legislation

One of the most important aspects of any public health crisis is creating public awareness that a problem exists and how to resolve it. Currently, multiple campaigns exist to help improve firearm violence and injury prevention. For example, The Brady Campaign to Prevent Gun Violence is a mission of the Brady organization and its Million Mom March to create a safer America. Their goal is to decrease firearm-related deaths in the United States by half by 2025 by impact-driven, engaging campaigns (Box 6) [45].

A second well-known campaign in the United States is the End Family Fire campaign. Brady and The Ad Council have led the End Family Fire campaign by dedicating resources to improve safe gun storage and responsible gun ownership. Through television commercials and public service announcements, education and encouragement are provided to the public to learn more about proper gun safety, storage, and responsible ownership [46]. These efforts must be expanded and ideally funded by federal and state funds similar to the public health campaigns that have existed in the past.

Better access and availability to mental health resources

Overall, the percentage of violent injury committed by people affected by mental health illnesses and substance abuse disorders is relatively low. One study revealed less than 5% of patients with firearm-related injuries from 2006 to 2014 at a level 1 trauma center had mental health disorders [2]. However, although mental health accounted for a low percentage of overall injuries, the mortality of this subgroup was 38.5%, indicating the severity of injury and the association with suicide [2].

Although mental health is only a small overall contributing factor to firearm-related homicide in our society, there is a strong relationship between mental health disorders and suicide. Therefore, improving access to mental health treatment and resources is an important aspect of any public policy aimed at reducing injury.

There needs to be an open discussion surrounding mental health to foster an environment of support rather than social stigma. Although there is a low percentage of violent acts committed by people with mental health disorders, studies have shown patients who receive adequate treatment from health

Box 6: Brady Campaign to Prevent Gun Violence's proposed solutions to decrease firearm-related deaths

1. Policy focus for Brady background checks to be applied to all gun sales
2. Stop the 5% of gun dealers who supply 90% of all crime guns
3. Lead a new conversation, change social norms regarding the real dangers of guns in the home to prevent homicides, suicides, and unintentional shootings

From Brady: United Against Gun Violence. Available at: https://www.bradyunited.org/the-brady-plan; with permission.

professionals are less likely to commit violence [47]. Enhanced mental healthcare has been proposed by policy makers as a way to improve firearm violence, and data reveal this would likely decrease deaths associated with mental health disorders, specifically those secondary to suicide [48,49]. Resources and support are also needed to help coordinate mental health and substance use disorders among state, local, and community-based behavioral health systems.

SUMMARY

Firearm-related injury and death is a public health crisis in this country with mortality nearly equivalent to MVC. Despite the massive burden of disease that exists, the funding dedicated to research is grossly deficient. This complex health problem requires a multidisciplinary, interprofessional approach to create the multimodal solution to develop data-driven policies to reduce firearm injury and death in this country. Understanding that most Americans are united in the approach to dealing with firearm-related violence, a commitment is needed to approach this in a nonpartisan manner that mitigates the spread of false narratives and allows us to work across disciplines with stakeholders in the pursuit for common sense legislation that allows us to reduce firearm-related injuries and death.

References

[1] Centers for Disease Control and Prevention, National Center for Health Statistics. Underlying Cause of Death. 1999-2017 on CDC WONDER Online Database, released December, 2018. Data are from the Multiple Cause of Death Files, 1999-2017, as compiled from data provided by the 57 vital statistics jurisdictions through the Vital Statistics Cooperative Program. Available at: http://wonder.cdc.gov/ucd-icd10.html. Accessed February 15, 2019.

[2] Gani F, Sakran JV, Canner JK. Emergency Department visits for firearm-related injuries in the United States, 2006-14. Health Aff (Millwood) 2017;36(10):1729–38.

[3] Tasigiorgos S, Economopoulos KP, Winfield R, et al. Firearm injury in the United States: an overview of an evolving public health problem. J Am Coll Surg 2015;221(6): 1005–14.

[4] Follman M, Lurie J, Lee J, et al. The true cost of gun violence in America 2015. Available at: http://www.motherjones.com/politics/2015/04/true-cost-of-gun-violence-in-america. Accessed February 15, 2019.

[5] Gross BW, Cook AD, Rinehart CD, et al. An epidemiologic overview of 13 years of firearm hospitalizations in Pennsylvania. J Surg Res 2017;210:188–95.

[6] Tessler RA, Arbabi S, Bulger EM, et al. Trends in firearm injury and motor vehicle crash case fatality by age group, 2003-2013. JAMA Surg 2018; https://doi.org/10.1001/jamasurg.2018.4685.

[7] Stewart RM, Kuhls DA, Rotondo MF, et al. Freedom with responsibility: a consensus strategy for preventing injury, death, and disability from firearm violence. J Am Coll Surg 2018;227: 281–3.

[8] Stewart RM, Kuhls DA. Firearm injury prevention: a consensus approach to reducing preventable deaths. J Trauma Acute Care Surg 2016;80:850–2.

[9] Richardson EG, Hemenway D. Homicide, suicide, and unintentional firearm fatality: comparing the United States with other high-income countries. J Trauma 2011;70(1):238–43.

[10] Grinshteyn E, Hemenway D. Violent death rates: the US compared to other high-income OECD Countries, 2010. Am J Med 2016;129(3):266–73.

[11] Alpers P, Rossetti A, Salinas D, et al. Rate of civilian firearm possession per 100 population. United States—gun facts, figures and the law. Sydney (Australia): Sydney School of Public

Health, The University of Sidney; 2015. Available at: www.gunpolicy.org/firearms/region/unite-states.
[12] Ingraham C. There are more guns than people in the United States, according to a new study of global firearm ownership 2018. Available at: https://www.washingtonpost.com/news/wonk/wp/2018/06/19/there-are-more-guns-than-people-in-the-united-states-according-to-a-new-study-of-global-firearm-ownership/?noredirect=on&utm_term=.ab2d056491a6. Accessed February 15, 2019.
[13] Kellermann AL, Rivara FP, Somes G, et al. Suicide in the home relation to gun ownership. N Engl J Med 1992;327:467–72.
[14] Anglemyer A, Horvath T, Rutherford G. The accessibility of firearms and risk for suicide and homicide victimization among household members: a systematic review and meta-analysis. Ann Intern Med 2014;160:101–10.
[15] Efron DT, Haider A, Change D, et al. Alarming surge in nonsurvivable urban trauma and the case for violence prevention. Arch Surg 2006;141:800–5.
[16] Resnick S, Smith RN, Beard JH, et al. Firearm deaths in America: can we learn from 462,000 lives lost? Ann Surg 2017;266(3):432–40.
[17] Briggs JT, Tabarrok A. Firearms and suicides in the US states. Int Rev Law Econ 2014;37: 180–8.
[18] Finkelhor D, Turner H, Ormrod R, et al. Children's exposure to violence: a comprehensive national survey. Washington, DC: U.S. Department of Justice, Office of Juvenile Justice and Delinquency Prevention; 2009. p. P6.
[19] Every town for Gun Safety. Mass shootings in the United States: 2009-2016. Available at: https://everytownresearch.org/reports/mass-shootings-analysis/. Accessed February 15, 2019.
[20] Federal Bureau of Investigation. Quick Look: 250 active shooter incidents in the United States from 2000 to 2017. Available at: https://www.fbi.gov/about/partnerships/office-of-partner-engagement/active-shooter-incidents-graphics. Accessed February 15, 2019.
[21] Gun Violence Archives. Available at: http://www.gunviolencearchive.org. Accessed February 15, 2019.
[22] De Jager E, McCarty JC, Hashmi ZG, et al. Lethality of civilian active shooter incidents with and without semiautomatic rifles in the United States. JAMA 2018;320(10):1–2.
[23] Barry CL, McGinty EE, Vernick JS, et al. Two years after Newton—public opinion on gun policy revisited. Prev Med 2015;79:55–8.
[24] Kellerman AL, Rivara FP. Silencing the science on gun research. JAMA 2013;309(6): 549–50.
[25] He K, Sakran JV. Elimination of the moratorium on gun research is not enough. The need for the CDC to set a budgetary agenda. JAMA Surg 2018; https://doi.org/10.1001/jamasurg.2018.4211.
[26] Consolidated appropriations act 2023; PublNo.112-74. Available at: http://www.gpo.-gov/fdsys/pkg/PLAW-112publ74/pdf/PLAW-112publ74.pdf. Accessed February 15, 2019.
[27] Presidential Memorandum—engaging in public health research on the causes and prevention of gun violence. Available at: https://www.whitehouse.gov/the-press-office/2013/01/16/presdiential-memorandum-engagin -public-health-research-causes-and-pre-0. Accessed February 15, 2019.
[28] Stark DE, Shah NH. Funding and publication of research on gun violence and other leading causes of death. JAMA 2017;317(1):84–6.
[29] Frandsen RJ, Naglich D, Lauver GA, et al. Background checks for firearm transfers, 2010—statistical tables. Washington, DC: Department of Justice. Bureau of Justice Statistics; 2013.
[30] Miller M, Hepburn L, Azrael D. Firearm acquisition without background checks: results of a national survey. Ann Intern Med 2017;166(4):233–9.

[31] Cook PJ, Ludwig J. Guns in America: national survey on private ownership and use of firearms. Washington, DC: US Department of Justice, National Institute of Justice Research in Brief; 1997. Available at: www.ncjrs.gov/pdffiles/165476.pdf.
[32] Wintemute GJ, Braga AA, Kennedy DM. Private-party gun sales, regulation, and public safety. N Engl J Med 2010;363(6):508–11.
[33] Weinberger SE, Hoyt DB, Lawrence HC III, et al. Firearm-related injury and death in the United States: a call to action from 8 health professional organizations and the American Bar Association. Ann Intern Med 2015;162(7):513–6.
[34] Data behind extreme risk protective order policies: a look at Connecticut's risk-warrant law. Educational Fund to Stop Gun Violence. May 2018. Available at: http://efsgv.org/wp-content/uploads/2018/05/Data-behind-Extreme-Risk-Laws-FINAL-2.pdf. Accessed May 14, 2019.
[35] Hanna J, Ly L. After the Parkland massacre, more states considered "Red Flag" gun bills. CNN 2018.
[36] Wintemute GJ. How to stop mass shootings. N Engl J Med 2018;379(13):1193–6.
[37] Gaudiano N. Under pressure, NRA voices support for gun violence restraining orders 2018. Available at: https://www.usatoday.com/story/news/politics/2018/03/19/under-pressure-nra-voices-support-gun-violence-restraining-orders/433716002/. Accessed February 15, 2019.
[38] Wintemute GJ, Garen J, Betz ME, et al. Yes, you can: physicians, patients, and firearms. Ann Intern Med 2016;165(3):205–13.
[39] Barkin SL, Finch SA, Ip EH, et al. Is office-based counseling about media use, timeouts, and firearm storage effective? Results from a cluster-randomized, controlled trial. Pediatrics 2008;122:e15–25.
[40] Mueller KL, Ranney ML. Our lane needs all of us. Acad Emerg Med 2018; https://doi.org/10.1111/acem.13675.
[41] Jenkins DH, Winchell RJ, Coimbra R, et al. Position statement of the American College of Surgeons Committee on Trauma on the National Academies of Sciences, Engineering and Medicine Report: a national trauma care system: integrating military and civilian trauma systems to achieve zero preventable deaths after injury. J Trauma Acute Care Surg 2016;81:819–23.
[42] Kuhls DA, Campbell BT, Burke PA, et al. Survey of American College of Surgeons Committee on Trauma members on firearm injury: consensus and opportunities. J Trauma Acute Care Surg 2016;82:877–86.
[43] Croce MA. AAST statement on firearm injury. Trauma Surg Acute Care Open 2018;3: e000204.
[44] EAST Board of Directors. Eastern Association for the Surgery of Trauma Firearm Injury Prevention Statement. J Trauma Acute Care Surg 2019;86(1):168–70.
[45] Brady Campaign to Prevent Gun Violence. Available at: https://www.bradyunited.org/the-brady-plan. Accessed February 15, 2019.
[46] Ad Council. Gun safety: end family fire. https://www.adcouncil.org/Our-Campaigns/Safety/Gun-Safety-End-Family-Fire. Accessed February 15, 2019.
[47] Friedman RA. Violence and mental illness—how strong is the link? N Engl J Med 2006;355: 2064–6.
[48] Rubin R. Mental health reform will not reduce US gun violence, experts say. JAMA 2016;315(2):119–21.
[49] McGinty EE, Frattaroli S, Appelbaum PS, et al. Using research evidence to reframe the policy debate around mental illness and guns: process and recommendations. Am J Public Health 2014;104(11):e22–6.

Advances in Surgery 53 (2019) 209–220

ADVANCES IN SURGERY

Musculoskeletal Disorders in Minimally Invasive Surgery

H. Reza Zahiri, DO[a], Alex Addo, MD, MPH[a], Adrian E. Park, MD, FRCSC, FCS(ECSA)[a,b,*]

[a]Department of Surgery, Anne Arundel Medical Center, 2000 Medical Parkway, Annapolis, MD 21401, USA; [b]Johns Hopkins University School of Medicine, Baltimore, MD, USA

Keywords

• Ergonomics • Ergonomic challenges • Musculoskeletal disorders • Musculoskeletal strain • Minimally invasive surgery • Laparoscopic surgery • Robotic surgery • Endoscopic surgery

Key points

- Laparoscopic surgery has led to profound patient benefit since its introduction, but this has come at a great cost to the surgeon.
- Several studies have established that the association between musculoskeletal disorders and minimally invasive surgery are mainly attributed to ergonomic violations by the operative team.
- The solution to improving the ergonomic challenges among surgeons performing MIS will involve both high-tech and low-tech approaches.

BACKGROUND

The physical and mental demands of surgery have exacted their toll on surgeons over the centuries as they have performed their craft. Before the advent of general anesthesia, the hallmark of a successful surgeon, apart from expert knowledge and clinical judgment, was speed and accuracy in the conduct of operations. As the field has blossomed in the subsequent 170-odd years, the call upon surgeons to master an ever-expanding knowledge domain and the judgment that must keep pace has been joined by new physical demands of the profession. Surgeons have been able to develop longer more complex surgical

Disclosure statement: No conflicts of interest to declare. No financial support was received for this study.

*Corresponding author. Department of Surgery, Anne Arundel Medical Center, 2000 Medical Parkway, Belcher Pavilion, Suite 106, Annapolis, MD 21401, USA *E-mail address:* apark@aahs.org

https://doi.org/10.1016/j.yasu.2019.04.020

solutions to patients' disease and in the process have to assume prolonged, static, and often unhealthy postures in the operating room. As new imaging modalities, "energy sources," and aids to dissection/tissue manipulation entered routine use in the operating room, patient options, outcomes, and experiences improved tremendously. Not so the surgeon's experience during the course of bringing these advances in care to their patients.

Although our understanding of pathology, patient safety and outcomes, operative flow, and implementation of technology has almost arithmetically advanced, the essence of the surgeon-patient interface in the operating room (OR) has advanced not one whit. We still stand for extended periods at the patient's bedside (operating table) stretching, bending, and twisting ourselves while maintaining laser-like focus on the surgical task at hand. In this regard, the surgeon's workspace has changed little over the past several centuries.

Few examples better underscore this reality than the far more recent (25–30 years) advent of minimally invasive surgery (MIS). As Cushieri observed in MIS' infancy, "laparoscopic surgery represents a rare instance in surgical history where an advance has been so profound in patient benefit in so short a period of time." [1] These advantages enjoyed by the patient–which are profound in terms of decreased perioperative pain, enhanced return to function, and reduced surgical morbidity–come at great cost to the surgeon [2]. Surgeons' visualization of the target anatomy is no longer direct and is often at odds with their "working axes." We assume even more unhealthy and prolonged, static postures than in "open surgery." Furthermore, we contort ourselves to get our "end effectors" to anatomic destinations made immeasurably more difficult by the degrees of movement we have lost with laparoscopic instruments, all of which has given rise to the long overdue interest in and study of surgical ergonomics and surgeons' physical well-being.

As defined by the International Ergonomics Association, ergonomics comprehensively addresses the intellectual, physical, and organizational dimensions of human activity through assessment of safety, comfort, ease of use, productivity, performance, and aesthetics parameters [3]. Physical ergonomics regards how the body relates to its surrounding environment and accounts for resultant bodily consequences derived from posture, motion repetition, workplace design, material handling, and musculoskeletal strain. Mental ergonomics centers around the workings of cognitive operations, encompassing perceptual memory, sensory, and motor functions. Organizational ergonomics focuses on the influences of surroundings, workflow processes, and even employed guidelines.

In this article the authors review the most current studies of the risks of work-related injuries and symptoms faced by surgeons and some suggested strategies to mitigate the assaults on physical well-being that surgeons encounter by simply going to work every day.

LAPAROSCOPIC MINIMALLY INVASIVE SURGERY

As laparoscopy has become established as a predominant technical approach for a variety of surgeries across nearly all specialties, it has progressively replaced many open approaches [4,5].

Despite its many benefits for patients and the health care system as a whole, MIS has presented ergonomic challenges to surgeons, increasing their physical and psychological stress and compounding work-related injuries and burnout [6–10].

These challenges begin with the restricted degrees of freedom that constrain surgeons and for which they often compensate with suboptimal surgical postures and movement. They also have had to adjust to working from a two-dimensional image while working in a three-dimensional space [11,12]. Laparoscopic instrument designs have not meaningfully progressed over time with regard to facility of use [11,13]. Finally, the OR setup has failed to advance appropriately with time to optimize its interactions with surgeons and other staff.

A comparison of axial skeletal motions of surgeons during MIS versus open surgery show that although surgeons maintain more erect posture with respect to their head, neck, and axial spine during MIS, they are limited in motion [14]. In addition, their center of gravity favors a forward shift. Therefore, surgeons are more prone to short-term musculoskeletal strain with the risk of injuries over a prolonged period of MIS practice.

Electromyography (EMG) studies have been conducted to gain a more in-depth understanding of the ergonomic impact of MIS on specific muscles. One study analyzed the activation patterns of deltoid, trapezius, bicep, pronator teres, flexor carpi ulnaris, and extensor digitorum superficialis muscles of surgeons performing simulated laparoscopic tasks [15]. The emphasis was on the duration rather than the intensity of muscle activation. The results showed that muscle activation patterns were influenced most by the complexity of the task, followed by the design of instruments used and the physical adjustments of the operator to the task. Overall, proximal arm and shoulder muscle activations were greatest for all tasks, irrespective of complexity or instrument design, whereas forearm muscle activation became more prominent during complicated exercises.

The challenges of MIS extend beyond physical demands to also encumber surgeons with an increased mental workload. To quantify this mental workload, one study analyzed 28 surgeons performing simulation tasks using open versus video-endoscopic approaches. Measurements of mental stress were accomplished objectively with validated skin conductance and electrooculogram evaluations and subjectively with a survey query. There was congruence between subjective and objective measures showing that the endoscopic approach required greater concentration than the open approach. These findings are consistent with early experience that MIS demands greater focus and may amplify mental stress for surgeons [10].

Although investigations into ergonomic risk factors have been limited in the clinical domain of surgical practice, numerous studies have supported findings that show consistent ergonomic risk factor violations by nursing and surgeons in the OR during laparoscopic surgery [16–18]. Studies have also shown that simply performing MIS cases on a regular basis will subject practitioners to its perils, irrespective of age, experience, gender, height, or handedness [4]. An online survey study of 317 MIS surgeons found high rates of fatigue/strain/injury with frequent laparoscopic surgery (87%). Most implicated poor design of instruments as the primary factor and identified postural adjustments as the most employed counterstrategy to their physical symptoms. Finally, the majority reported lack of education/awareness about proper ergonomic practices during MIS.

Other studies have supported these findings. A systematic review by Alleblas and colleagues [19] showed that the weighted average prevalence of physical complaints among laparoscopic surgeons was 74%. Another recent study showed a strong association between musculoskeletal disorders and MIS among a group of 14 pediatric surgeons [13]. These musculoskeletal disorders have involved the cervical spine, thoracic spine, upper limbs, lower limbs, and lumbar spine [20]. Their clinical manifestations include pain, muscle stiffness, numbness, and fatigue. These symptoms have a significant impact on surgical performance, indirectly affect patient safety, and may shorten surgeons' career longevity [13,19,21,22].

Overall, such studies are important in highlighting the current deficits in sound ergonomic practices among surgeons [23]. They also advocate task-specific positions, postures, and movements that promote excellent ergonomics and maximally counter fatigue and strain during MIS. The potential for these findings is significant in optimizing current surgeon/OR interactions. They also set the foundation for training future surgeons to acquire the proper ergonomic knowledge and skills to enhance their function and longevity while improving patient safety.

ROBOTIC MINIMALLY INVASIVE SURGERY

Robotic surgery has gained tremendous momentum across the world since its introduction in 2000. Nearly 450,000 cases were performed using robotic systems in 2012, a number 29% higher than the previous year [24]. This rate of growth has stemmed from novel MIS technologies affording 3-dimensional perception, enhanced degrees of freedom, motion scaling, and tremor reduction. Furthermore, this technology has allowed surgeons without prior MIS training to more easily adopt MIS techniques to deliver less-invasive care to their patients.

Studies have sought to determine whether robotic surgery improves on the ergonomic challenges posed by traditional laparoscopy. Several have shown improved ergonomics with reduced physical strain and mental stress for surgeons on robotic systems in comparison with those performing laparoscopy [25–28]. Some studies have used EMG and the National Aeronautics and Space Administration Task Load Index (NASA-TLX) to measure physical and mental workload, respectively [8,29]. Targeted anatomic regions for motion analysis with EMG included the:

- Elbow (biceps and triceps)
- Shoulders (deltoid and trapezius)

- Wrists (flexor carpi ulnaris and extensor digitorum)
- Thumbs (thenar compartment)
- Back (erector spinae)

A global performance score was also tabulated with respect to the partial or total task completion and performance errors. The results showed that robotic techniques were slower and less precise, but less stressful than laparoscopic techniques.

These studies found lesser mental and physical ergonomic demands of robotic surgery in comparison with laparoscopy. In addition, surgeons derived greater benefit from these ergonomic advantages by using better posture on the robot with lower shoulder position and reduced application of pressure to the armrest.

Nevertheless, the studies also indicated that while surgeons may be less negatively affected physically and mentally during robotic surgery, they derive the most benefit when they employ sound ergonomic principles during surgery [8,9]. Thus, even such sophisticated technology may lead to strain and injury if ergonomic considerations are not implemented during utilization.

Giberti and colleagues [20] evaluated a group of robotic surgeons who reported (41.2%) musculoskeletal disorders mostly in the cervical spine and upper limbs. These results were attributed to posture discomfort secondary to lack of an ergonomic seat and static position of the console operator, resulting in poor spine posture. A study by Zihni and colleagues [30] found no differences in activation of bilateral trapezius muscle groups between traditional laparoscopic surgery (TLS) and robotic-assisted laparoscopic surgery (RALS) using surface EMG measurement. These findings likely reflect the ergonomic strain placed on this muscle group secondary to cervical spine posture during TLS and RALS.

Thus, although the robotic console has been "purpose designed" to mitigate the ergonomic risk factor violations so rampant in MIS, whereby the patient-surgeon interface has seen no improvement over the years, the evidence to date suggests that the benefits to the surgeon are far from those anticipated. In fact, surgeons who spend regular operative time at the "robotic console" describe injury and symptom patterns consistent with those who regularly work at microscopes [31].

One would hope that as robotic surgery evolves and competition grows, surgeon console design will also evolve and improve ergonomically.

SURGICAL ENDOSCOPY

Surgeons commonly use endoscopic techniques via the upper or lower gastrointestinal tract to treat patients. When applicable, endoscopy that allows access to target anatomy and pathologic conditions by means of a natural orifice is considered the most minimally invasive of surgical techniques and offers patients the opportunity to avoid abdominal wall incisions altogether.

Flexible endoscopy still poses unique and major challenges to surgeons beyond laparoscopy [32]. The challenges revolve around the main tool, the flexible endoscope, with a comparatively condensed field of vision, diminished lighting, less focal length, and reduced depth projection than the laparoscope. The endoscope's small diameter results in a restricted working domain, limiting the manipulation of operative instruments. Moreover, an accurate bimanual control of instruments is compromised secondary to the inability to triangulate when needed. Finally, lengthier procedures potentiate the physical and mental hazards of these techniques for those who may use them in their practice.

These travails have been echoed by surgeons and gastroenterologists who participate in high-volume endoscopic practices. Most report regular pain in their neck, upper back, shoulders, wrists, and thumbs [33,34]. Unfortunately, there remains a paucity of research to describe and characterize ergonomic risk factors associated with surgical endoscopy to improve equipment design and corresponding human factors and ergonomic issues.

INTERVENTIONS TO MITIGATE THE EFFECTS OF MUSCULOSKELETAL DISORDERS IN MINIMALLY INVASIVE SURGERY

Surgeon-directed efforts

Nearly 50% of doctors in the United States have experienced burnout [35]. Fortunately, in recent years there has been progress in shedding light on physician injuries, burnout, and the prospect of shortened career longevity [36–39]. The surgical culture of self-forfeit and sacrifice in the pursuit of patient care has come into question [40]. Today, physician and health care professional well-being programs are being established across health care facilities and institutions and are highly supported. These efforts are in recognition of not only a prevalent problem among health care professionals but also the critical importance of maintaining a precious workforce.

Targeted factors have included physician work hours, physical fitness, nutrition, and the use of mental coaching to address burnout [36,40,41]. Specific to surgeons, one evidence-based strategy has been the use of breaks during surgery. Its objective is to ensure that surgeons take a break from prolonged and static postures during MIS while at the same time allowing them to improve mental focus and physical function. The implementation of breaks to counter fatigue, reduce errors, and ensure safety has been a valuable strategy employed in many demanding and "high-stakes" work environments, including the air traffic control, translation, computer science, and even professional mountain climbing [42–44].

The impact of breaks during surgery has previously been investigated as a viable countermeasure to surgeon stress [45,46]. Engelmann and colleagues [46] randomized surgeons to perform surgery with and without taking 5-min breaks every half-hour during surgery. Their results showed that with regular breaks, there were gains in quality of technical execution while fatigue, strain, pain, hormone levels associated with stress (cortisol and testosterone), intraoperative "events," and error rates were reduced without adding significant operative time. Recently, a multicenter prospective study was conducted to determine the impact of intraoperative targeted stretching micro breaks

(TSMB) on surgeon pain, function, and focus. Surgeons and OR staff rated pain/fatigue, and physical and mental performance using validated scales during 2 operative days, one with and the other without intraoperative TSMB [47]. TSMB included standardized (90 s) guided TSMB at appropriate 30- to 40-min intervals throughout each case. Case type and duration were recorded as were surgeon pain data before and after each procedure and at the end of the surgical day. Sixty-eight participants (69% men, 31% women; mean 47 years) completed 193 "non-TSMB" and 146 "TSMB" procedures; 47% of surgeons were concerned that musculoskeletal pain may shorten their career. The most common approaches used to deal with musculoskeletal pain were changing position (60%), taking a break (34%), adjusting some aspect of the surgical field (29%), adjusting height (26%), and ignoring the pain (26%) (Fig. 1). TSMB improved surgeon postprocedural pain scores in the neck, lower back, shoulders, upper back, wrists/hands, knees, and ankles (Fig. 2). Operative duration did not differ ($P>.05$). Improved pain scores with TSMB were statistically equivalent ($P>.05$) for laparoscopic and open procedures. Surgeons perceived improvements in physical performance (57%) and mental focus (38%); 87% of respondents planned to continue TSMB beyond study completion. Overall, Park and colleagues [47] concluded intraoperative TSMB represents a practical and effective means to reduce surgeon pain, enhance performance, and increase mental focus without extending operative time. Other related studies have reported similar findings [48].

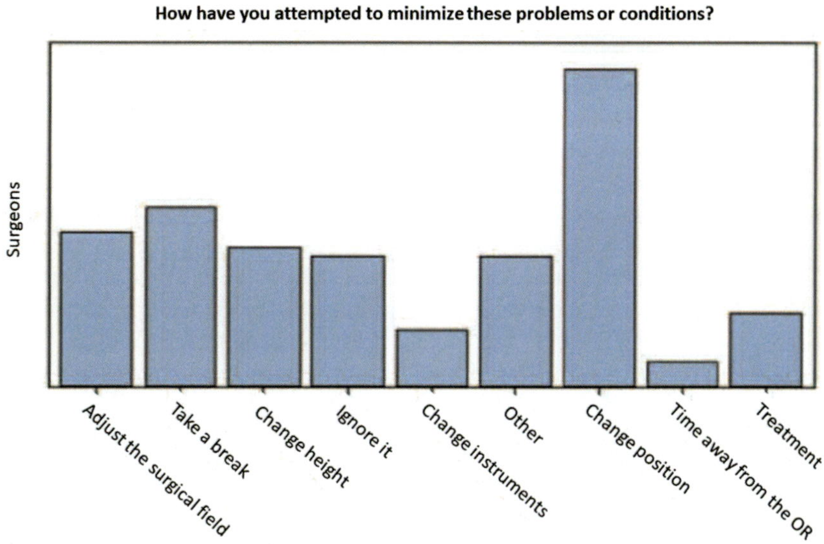

Fig. 1. Most popular counterstrategies by surgeons against pain and fatigue. (*From* Park A, Zahiri H, Hallbeck S, et al. Intraoperative "Micro Breaks" with targeted stretching enhance surgeon physical function and mental focus: a multicenter cohort study. Ann Surg 2017;265;340–6; with permission.)

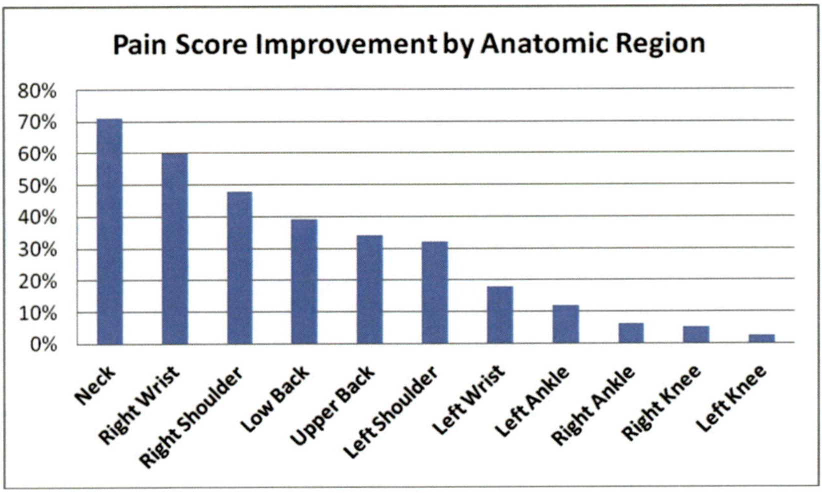

Fig. 2. Impact of TSMB on pain scores by anatomic site. (*From* Park A, Zahiri H, Hallbeck S, et al. Intraoperative "Micro Breaks" with targeted stretching enhance surgeon physical function and mental focus: a multicenter cohort study. Ann Surg 2017;265;340–6; with permission.)

Postural balance training is another tool that can help alleviate the ergonomic stress associated with laparoscopic and endoscopic procedures. Reddy and colleagues [49] evaluated the effect of improving posture and surgical ergonomics by teaching subjects completing laparoscopic skill assessment, a posture balance technique known as the Alexander technique. This technique improves postural balance and coordination while at the same time minimizing strain and maximizing comfort. Results from this study showed that subjects reported decreased discomfort, and posture assessment data revealed significant improvement in scores after adopting the Alexander technique. These findings demonstrate that postural training can aid in reducing ergonomic strain and stress during MIS.

Although these strategies are evidence-based and promising, their implementation, regular use, and effectiveness remain to be established among the surgical community. Without a concerted effort by health care leaders and, foremost, physicians, these strategies will continue largely as abstractions.

Operating room design

The need to optimize the OR environment to improve safety, efficiency, and workflow well predates the advent of MIS although its widespread adoption has overly magnified the inadequacies of the current state [50]. No longer are traditional ORs set up (geared toward open surgery) with bulky laparoscopic equipment crammed into a limited space adequate to accommodate the minimally invasive surgeon, patient, and OR staff. Unfortunately, these outdated designs, which can amplify risks of workflow disruptions, fatigue, strain, and injury to the entire operative team, continue to persist in most ORs in use today. Multidisciplinary collaboration including physicians, registered nurses and associated health professional, biomedical engineers, and administration as well as the requisite funding need to be corralled to focus on significant new OR design. As new technologies constantly enter into use in the OR, both the surgeon-technology interface and the surgeon-patient interface need to be completely revisited, informed by our latest understanding of optimal ergonomic and human factor considerations in workspace design.

Laparoscopic instrument design

Another major challenge to overcome, geared toward the MIS industry, is updating the interaction of the surgeon with his or her instruments. Although laparoscopy has now been in existence for nearly 30 years, many of the instruments used by surgeons today have retained their original design without any innovation to accommodate MIS practitioners [51]. This is largely secondary to an inexplicable acceptance of the status quo and the lack of demand for better instruments by the surgical community! However, to ensure career longevity of surgeons it is essential to adopt a clinically driven approach whereby engineers work with surgeons to design the next generation of MIS instruments, centered around comfort and sound ergonomic principles. The time of a "one size fits all" surgical instrument handle is well past. At the least, they must now be designed and tailored to surgeon gloves/hands.

SUMMARY

A comprehensive approach to enhance ergonomics, prevent strain/injury, elevate performance, and ensure safety for surgeons will require more than isolated and disjointed surgeon-directed efforts. Rather, the environment surrounding and involving the surgeon and operating room staff must be ergonomically sophisticated to facilitate workflow while optimizing the patient and the entire OR team. As awareness has risen in recent years regarding the critical need to preserve our health care workforce, there is room for optimism that the culture of the health care industry will more rapidly change among all key stakeholders including doctors, nurses, executive leaders, and industry to demand protection, with the goal always of improving patients' outcomes and experiences.

References

[1] Cuschieri A. The spectrum of laparoscopic surgery. World J Surg 1992;16:1089–97.
[2] Park A, Lee G, Seagull FJ, et al. Patients benefit while surgeons suffer: an impending epidemic. J Am Coll Surg 2010;210(3):306–13.
[3] Int Ergon Assoc (IEA): what is ergonomics?. Available at: https://www.iea.cc/whats/index.html. Accessed October 10, 2018.
[4] Cuschieri A. Whither minimal access surgery: tribulations and expectations. Am J Surg 1995;169:9–19.
[5] Klein M, Anderson LPH, Alamili M, et al. Psychological and physical stress in surgeons operating in a standard or modern operating room. Surg Laparosc Endosc Percutan Tech 2010;20(4):237–42.

[6] Bohm B, Rotting N, Schwenk W, et al. A prospective randomized trial on heart rate variability of the surgical team during laparoscopic and conventional sigmoid resection. Arch Surg 2001;136:305–10.
[7] Vereczkei A, Feussner H, Negele T, et al. Ergonomic assessment of the static stress confronted by surgeons during laparoscopic cholecystectomy. Surg Endosc 2004;18: 1118–22.
[8] Berguer R, Smith W. An ergonomic comparison of robotic and laparoscopic technique: the influence of surgeon experience and task complexity. J Surg Res 2006;134:87–92.
[9] Matern U, Faist M, Kehl K, et al. Monitor position in laparoscopic surgery. Surg Endosc 2005;19:436–40.
[10] Berguer R, Smith WD, Chung YH. Performing laparoscopic surgery is significantly more stressful for the surgeon than open surgery. Surg Endosc 2001;15:1204–7.
[11] Seagull F. Disparities between industrial and surgical ergonomics. Work 2012;41: 4669–72.
[12] Kenngott H, Fischer L, Nickel F, et al. Status of robotic assistance—a less traumatic and more accurate minimally invasive surgery? Langenbecks Arch Surg 2012;397:333–41.
[13] Esposito C, Najmaldin A, Schier F, et al. Work-related upper limb musculoskeletal disorders in pediatric minimally invasive surgery: a multicentric survey comparing laparoscopic and SILS ergonomy. Pediatr Surg Int 2014;30:395–9.
[14] Berguer R, Rab GT, Abu-Ghaida H, et al. A comparison of surgeons' posture during laparoscopic and open surgical procedures. Surg Endosc 1997;11:139–42.
[15] Quick NE, Gillette JC, Shapiro R, et al. The effect of using laparoscopic instruments on muscle activation patterns during minimally invasive surgical training procedures. Surg Endosc 2003;17:462–5.
[16] Lee YH, Chiou WK. Ergonomic analysis of working posture in nursing personnel: example of modified Ovako Working Analysis System application. Res Nurs Health 1995;18: 67–75.
[17] Kant IJ, de Jong LC, van Rijssen-Moll M, et al. A survey of static and dynamic work postures of operating room staff. Int Arch Occup Environ Health 1992;63:423–8.
[18] Rademacher K, Pichler KV, Erbse S, et al. Using human factor analysis and VR simulation techniques for the optimization of the surgical worksystem. Stud Health Technol Inform 1996;29:532–41.
[19] Alleblas CC, de Man AM, van den Haak L, et al. Prevalence of musculoskeletal disorders among surgeons performing minimally invasive surgery. Ann Surg 2017;266(6):905–20.
[20] Giberti C, Gallo F, Francini L, et al. Musculoskeletal disorders among robotic surgeons: a questionnaire analysis. Arch Ital Urol Androl 2014;86:96–8.
[21] Huysmans M, Hoozemans M. Fatigue effects on tracking performance and muscle activity. J Electromyogr Kinesiol 2008;18:410–9.
[22] Huysmans M, Hoozemans M. Position sense acuity of the upper extremity and tracking performance in subjects with non-specific neck and upper extremity pain and healthy controls. J Rehabil Med 2010;42:876–83.
[23] Lee G, Lee T, Dexter D, et al. Methodological infrastructure in surgical ergonomics: a review of tasks, models, and measurement systems. Surg Innov 2007;14(3):153–67.
[24] Lee GI, Lee MR, Clanton T, et al. Comparative assessment of physical and cognitive ergonomics associated with robotic and traditional laparoscopic surgeries. Surg Endosc 2014;28:456–65.
[25] Lee EC, Rafiq A, Merrell R, et al. Ergonomics and human factors in endoscopic surgery: a comparison of manual vs. telerobotic simulation systems. Surg Endosc 2005;19: 1064–70.
[26] Stefanidis D, Wang F, Korndorffer JR, et al. Robotic assistance improves intracorporeal suturing performance and safety in the operating room while decreasing operator workload. Surg Endosc 2010;24:377–82.

[27] Stefanidis D, Hope WW, Scott DJ. Robotic suturing on the FLS model possesses construct validity, is less physically demanding, and is favored by more surgeons compared with laparoscopy. Surg Endosc 2011;25(7):2141–6.
[28] Klein MI, Warm JS, Riley MA, et al. Mental workload and stress perceived by novice operators in the laparoscopic and robotic minimally invasive surgical interfaces. J Endourol 2012;26(8):1089–94.
[29] Marecik SJ, Prasad LM, Park JJ, et al. Evaluation of midlevel and upper-level residents performing their first robotic-sutured intestinal anastomosis. Am J Surg 2008;195(3): 333–7.
[30] Zihni A, Ohu I, Cavallo J, et al. Ergonomic analysis of robot-assisted and traditional laparoscopic procedures. Surg Endosc 2014;28:3379–84.
[31] Park A. "Physician heal thyself" isn't working. Ann Surg 2017;266(6):921–2.
[32] Lee G, Sutton E, Clanton T, et al. Higher physical workload risks with NOTES versus laparoscopy: a quantitative ergonomic assessment. Surg Endosc 2011;25:1585–93.
[33] Shergill AK, McQuaid KR, Rempel D. Ergonomics and GI endoscopy. Gastrointest Endosc 2009;70:145–53.
[34] Liberman AS, Shrier I, Gordon PH. Injuries sustained by colorectal surgeons performing colonoscopy. Surg Endosc 2005;19:1606–9.
[35] West CP. Physician well-being: expanding the triple aim. J Gen Intern Med 2016;31(5): 458–9.
[36] Hamidi MS, Boqqild MK, Cheung AM. Running on empty: a review of nutrition and physicians' well-being. Postgrad Med J 2016;92(1090):478–81.
[37] Rothenberger DA. Physician burnout and well-being: a systematic review and framework for action. Dis Colon Rectum 2017;60(6):567–76.
[38] Arora M, Asha S, Chinnappa J, et al. Review article: burnout in emergency medicine physicians. Emerg Med Australas 2013;25(6):491–5.
[39] Arora M, Diwan AD, Harris IA. Burnout in orthopaedic surgeons: a review. ANZ J Surg 2013;83(7–8):512–5.
[40] Schneider S, Kingsolver K, Rosdahl J. Physician coaching to enhance well-being: a qualitative analysis of a pilot intervention. Explore (NY) 2014;10960:372–9.
[41] Blum AB, Shea S, Czeisler CA, et al. Implementing the 2009 Institute of Medicine recommendations on resident physician work hours, supervision and safety. Nat Sci Sleep 2011;3:47–85.
[42] Farmer E, Brownson A. Review of workload measurement, analysis and interpretation methods (CARE-Integra-RES-130-02-WP2). Technical report prepared for the European Organisation for the Safety of Air Navigation. Brussels, Belgium: Eurocontrol.
[43] McLean L, Tingley M, Scott RN, et al. Computer terminal work and the benefit of microbreaks. Appl Ergon 2001;32(3):225–37.
[44] Caceres-Munoz VS, Magallances-Meneses A, Torres-Coronel D, et al. Effect of rest pauses combined with information leaflets on the decrease in musculoskeletal pain in administrative workers. Rev Peru Med Exp Salud Publica 2017;34(4):611–8.
[45] Mukhopadhyay BK. Strategic rest break in laparoscopic surgery: a need. World J Laparosc Surg 2012;5(2):85–8.
[46] Englemann C, Schneider M, Kirschbaum C, et al. Effects of intraoperative breaks on mental and somatic operator fatigue: a randomized clinical trial. Surg Endosc 2011;25:1245–50.
[47] Park AE, Zahiri HR, Hallbeck MS, et al. Intraoperative "Micro Breaks" with targeted stretching enhance surgeon physical function and mental focus: a multicenter cohort study. Ann Surg 2017;265(2):340–6.
[48] Schrempf M, Anthuber M. Intraoperative microbreaks reduce pain and improve concentration. Chirurg 2017;88(3):256.

[49] Reddy P, Reddy T, Roig-Francoli J, et al. The impact of the Alexander technique on improving posture and surgical ergonomics during minimally invasive surgery: pilot study. J Urol 2011;186:1658–62.
[50] Herron DM, Gagner M, Kenyon TL, et al. The minimally invasive surgical suite enters the 21st century. Surg Endosc 2001;15:415–22.
[51] Sancibrian R, Gutierrez-Diez MC, Torre-Ferrero C, et al. Design and evaluation of a new ergonomic handle for instruments in minimally invasive surgery. J Surg Res 2014;188: 88–99.

Advances in Surgery 53 (2019) 221–233

ADVANCES IN SURGERY

What's New in Trauma Resuscitation?

Elizabeth Dauer, MD*, Amy Goldberg, MD

Department of Surgery, Lewis Katz School of Medicine at Temple University, 3401 North Broad Street, Zone C, 4th Floor, Philadelphia, PA 19140, USA

Keywords

• Trauma resuscitation • Damage control resuscitation • Permissive hypotension • Permissive hypoventilation • Whole blood

Key points

- Trauma resuscitation continues to evolve over time as the understanding of the physiology of hemorrhagic shock changes.
- Existing literature supports rapid transport of traumatically injured patients to a trauma center for definitive care.
- Trauma-induced coagulopathy should be addressed early in resuscitation to improve outcomes.
- Further studies are needed to define the optimal prehospital care.
- Trauma team training and video review improve patient care quality.

INTRODUCTION

Traumatic injury is the leading cause of death for individuals up to the age of 45 and the fourth leading cause of death among all ages in the United States [1]. Outside of preventive actions, little can be done for those who suffer immediate loss of life, but for the remainder of patients, the care provided in the very early stages after their injury can have profound impact on their eventual outcome. A better understanding of the physiology of hemorrhagic shock, trauma-induced coagulopathy, and goal-directed therapy has led to changes in the delivery of care early after injury. The objective of this article was to summarize approaches to the resuscitation of the critically injured patient that have recently come to the forefront. This article focuses on the role of the prehospital care

Disclosure Statement: The authors have no disclosures.

*corresponding author. *E-mail address:* Elizabeth.dauer@tuhs.temple.edu

https://doi.org/10.1016/j.yasu.2019.04.010
0065-3411/19/

providers, damage control resuscitation (DCR) strategies, and the team approach to trauma care.

SIGNIFICANCE

Since 1978, the fundamental principles of Advanced Trauma Life Support (ATLS) have given trauma care providers a standardized framework for the rapid assessment and resuscitation of the injured patient. The structure is based on the concept that injuries kill patients in a reproducible pattern and allows for the prompt identification of those that are potentially fatal [2]. This paradigm was created largely from physician experience, not clinical study, as a comprehensive, reproducible way to provide trauma care that could be applied in any setting.

During the time that ATLS was being adopted, prehospital care was evolving. The development of sophisticated trauma systems and the implementation of prehospital emergency medical services (EMS) have contributed to an overall decrease in morbidity and mortality of traumatically injured patients; however, the addition of advanced life support (ALS) techniques in the 1980s has led to considerable discussion regarding the role of prehospital interventions, such as intravenous fluids (IVF) and endotracheal intubation (ETI). The use of IVF for hypotensive trauma patients was largely based on animal models in the 1960s that showed that end organ perfusion was restored with volume expansion and survival was increased [3,4]. In 1994, Bickell and colleagues [5,6] performed a landmark study in which patients with hypotensive penetrating trauma were assigned to receive immediate continuous IVF versus delayed fluid administration until operative intervention of their injuries. A significant survival advantage was seen in those patients with penetrating injuries not receiving IVFs. He and others theorized that IVF could accentuate blood loss, disrupt clot formation, and dilute coagulation factors [7].

In addition to circulatory support, prehospital providers are trained to prioritize management of the airway. In certain instances, the decision to perform ETI is clear, but at other times it requires significant expertise and clinical judgment. Traditionally, a Glasgow Coma Score (GCS) of 8 or less has been used to indicate a need for intubation, but this does not take into consideration assessment of potential injuries, hemodynamic status, or environmental factors.

There is mounting evidence against the use of prehospital ETI for patients with penetrating trauma who are in hemorrhagic shock. The positive pressure ventilation and changes in intrathoracic pressure with ETI lead to decreased venous return and cardiac output, and end organ perfusion. Drugs used in medication-assisted ETI potentiate these effects and may result in complete cardiovascular collapse in patients in hemorrhagic shock. At our institution, we compared ETI and mask ventilation in a rat and swine hemorrhagic shock model. There was no difference in the time to death [8,9]. When compared with swine receiving only supplemental oxygen via face mask (FM), the FM group had higher body temperatures, higher cardiac output, and lower lactate levels, but worse respiratory acidosis; however, the resultant hypercapnia did not result in worse survival. We concluded that "permissive hypoventilation" might allow for improved perfusion and oxygen delivery with decreased physiologic compromise [10].

In a clinical study, Stockinger and McSwain [11] showed there was no survival advantage to ETI in the penetrating population, whereas Rhee and colleagues [12] suggested that Bag-Valve-Mask is often adequate ventilatory support for the obtunded patient. Furthermore, ETI has a negative impact on survival in those patients requiring resuscitative thoracotomy [13], while not decreasing the rate of in-hospital complications [14]. EMS providers should have a clear airway algorithm that takes into account injury patterns, mechanisms, transport time to a trauma center, and physiologic consequences of ETI in order to reserve ETI situations where there is a benefit.

Although instituting the ATLS algorithm improved standardization and introduction of ALS changed practice, over time there has been a growing understanding of the physiologic burden of hemorrhagic shock. The development of the lethal triad of coagulopathy, acidosis, and hypothermia related to blood loss can be a precursor to mortality. The introduction of damage control surgery to control hemorrhage and contamination, minimize operative time, and allow for ongoing resuscitation to occur in the intensive care unit changed the way trauma surgeons managed those in profound shock [15]. Similarly, DCR aims to recognize coagulopathy early and address all elements of the lethal triad concurrently [16]. With this idea, the rigid adherence to the ATLS sequence of airway, breathing, circulation has come into question, with many advocating a circulation first method of trauma care resuscitation [17–19].

PRESENT RELEVANCE AND FUTURE AVENUES

Prehospital care

In 1996, Demetriades and colleagues [20] performed the first large-scale comparison of patients transported via paramedics versus private vehicle and showed that those patients with an Injury Severity Score greater than 15 transported by EMS had a mortality rate that was double that of the non-EMS patients. The investigators contended that the improved survival was likely due to decreased transport times and fewer therapeutic interventions being performed in the field. Since that time, there has been a continued attempt to define what components of ALS care should be provided that would be of benefit to the care of the trauma patient. Most of these studies are limited by study design, limited data availability, and reliance on bystander observations in the case of private and police transport. Even with these limitations, the data support foregoing procedural interventions prehospital and rapid transport to a trauma center where patients can receive definitive management of their injuries improves outcomes [21–25] (Table 1).

Damage control resuscitation and its adjuncts

Permissive hypotension

Permissive hypotension is the practice of keeping blood pressure low enough to avoid exsanguination, but still allow for end organ perfusion. In permissive

Table 1
Summary of studies comparing transport type

Author	Transport type	Study design	Outcome
Demetriades et al [20], 1996	Paramedic vs private	Retrospective	ISS >15 with EMS mortality 29% vs 14% in private transport
Liberman et al [22], 2003	ALS vs BLS	Retrospective	ALS mortality 29% vs BLS 18% ALS mortality 30% vs BLS mortality 26% in patients with survivable injuries
Seamon et al [13], 2007	EMS vs police/ private vehicle	Retrospective	Prehospital procedures have a negative effect on mortality in patients requiring resuscitative thoracotomy
Steill et al [23], 2008	ALS vs BLS	Before—after controlled trial	GCS <9 with decreased survival with ALS Overall survival not significantly different
Band et al [24,25], 2010 and 2011	EMS vs police	Retrospective	Increased survival in GSW/stab when brought via police
Seamon et al. [26], 2013	ALS vs BLS	Prospective observational	Prehospital interventions do not benefit rapidly transported penetrating trauma patients
Rappold et al [21], 2015	ALS vs BLS vs police	Retrospective	ISS <30 with increased odds of death with ALS ISS >30 no survival advantage with ALS
Evans et al [27], 2016	ALS	Retrospective	No prehospital procedures associated with survival benefit Airway insertion portends worse odds for survival

Abbreviations: ALS, advanced life support; BLS, basic life support; EMS, emergency medical services; GCS, glasgow coma score; ISS, injury severity score

Data from Refs [20,21,23–27].

hypotension, systolic blood pressure is targeted to 80 to 90 mm Hg to help avoid clot disruption and minimize the sequela of hemorrhagic shock. Dutton and colleagues [28] and Schreiber and colleagues [29] performed randomized controlled trials of patients in hemorrhagic shock comparing outcomes after fluid administration targeted to a goal systolic blood pressure. The investigators of both studies determined that hypotensive resuscitation was safe, but were unable to show an overall mortality difference; however Schreiber and colleagues [29] did show a trend toward improved 24-hour and in-hospital mortality in the hypotensive group. When applied in the operating theater, permissive hypotension may lessen postoperative coagulopathy and nonsurgical bleeding [30]. The combination of demonstrated safety of permissive hypotension and the increasing evidence to support minimizing crystalloid fluid administration led to a change in the ATLS content. The new recommendations advocate for permissive hypotension and limiting crystalloid to 1 to 2 L before consideration of blood products [2]. Careful consideration of this approach should be taken in patients with traumatic brain injury in which hypotension may result in secondary brain injury.

Hemostatic resuscitation

The coagulopathy of trauma represents a significant challenge in DCR with an incidence of more than 50% in the most critically ill patients [31]. The development of coagulopathy is the result of tissue injury and hypoperfusion that is perpetuated by hemodilution, acidosis, hypothermia, and inflammation [32]. As platelet and coagulation factors are consumed, pH drops and body temperature decreases, and the body's ability to form clot is impaired. Many of these changes occur very early after injury, necessitating early recognition and prevention or correction. Hemostatic resuscitation attempts to address these issues using a strategy of limited crystalloid and early transfusion of blood products with high fresh frozen plasma (FFP) to packed red blood cell (PRBC) ratios.

The use of massive transfusion protocols (MTPs) has allowed for more uniformity in achieving these ratios. The Pragmatic Randomized Optimal Platelet and Plasma Ratios trial randomized patients to a 1:1:1 versus a 1:1:2 platelet:-plasma:PRBC transfusion strategies and attempted to define the ideal ratio. Although they were not able to show a 30-day all-cause mortality benefit, the 1:1:1 group did have more patients achieve hemostasis and fewer patients die from bleeding within the first 24 hours [33]. Most MTPs aim to deliver close to a 1:1 ratio of FFP:PRBC, as it confers a survival advantage to lower ratios and historical transfusion strategies [34,35]. The implementation of MTP practices have resulted in earlier blood administration, decreased cost, and lower total blood use over the course of a patient's hospital stay [36]. MTPs correlate with a decrease in the incidence of death from exsanguinating hemorrhage and an increase survival to discharge in the patients requiring the highest number of transfusions [37,38]. The rate-limiting step in supplying blood at these ratios is the need for FFP to be thawed before release from the blood bank. The process for thawing plasma takes approximately 20 to 30 minutes, which can lead to lag times to the start of the first plasma transfusion in comparison with the first PRBC. Several large studies, including the Prospective Observational Multicenter Major Trauma Transfusion study, have shown the advantages of early plasma administration [39]. Initiation of thawed plasma (TP) protocols, whereby TP is available in either the blood bank or the emergency department at all times, significantly decreases mortality, blood product utilization, and massive transfusion rates [40,41].

Platelet transfusion is also a crucial element in DCR; however, the exact timing and ratio of platelets to FFP and PRBC remains an area of debate. Higher platelet to PRBC and platelet to FFP ratios result in increased 24-hour and 30-day survival [42], but studies to date have examined only intraoperative platelet transfusion. The effect of immediate platelet administration is yet to be elucidated. Difficulties with storage, availability, risk of contamination, and immunologic sensitization poses a significant challenge to incorporation of platelets in the very early stages of resuscitation [43] (Box 1).

Whole blood transfusion

Although component therapy is commonplace, the use of whole blood (WB) has made a resurgence. WB provides higher platelet counts and increased coagulation factors while containing less preservative and anticoagulants, leading to greater hemostatic potential than 1:1:1 component therapy [44]. During the wars in Iraq and Afghanistan, warm fresh WB (WFWB) became a logistical necessity because of scarce supply and difficulty with transporting and maintaining blood products in the remote environment [45]; however, in retrospective studies from military practice, the use of WB has been associated with mixed effects on mortality and total transfusion needs [46,47]. In civilian practice, there has been resistance to use of WB due to misconceptions regarding safety of non-ABO group specific WB, loss of platelet presence with leukoreduction, and loss of platelet function in cold storage. The risk of significant hemolytic reactions with low-titer anti-A and anti-B group O WB is minimal and the recent production of platelet sparing leukoreduction filters will allow for platelet containing WB products to be available. In 2015, the Food and Drug Administration approved the storage of apheresis platelets at temperatures of 1 to 6° Celsius to be used in the resuscitation of actively bleeding patients [44].

Clinical application of WB in the civilian arena has shown promising results. In a randomized controlled pilot trial, Cotton and colleagues [48] compared modified WB and component therapy in patients predicted to require massive transfusion. When excluding patients with traumatic brain injury, the WB group received significantly less PRBC, FFP, platelets, and total transfusions. WB products have also been shown to improve platelet function and decrease the acute coagulopathy after trauma, while not impacting clinical outcomes [49–51]. The encouraging results of WB use in trauma centers and the prehospital care of military casualties has led to the development and implementation of prehospital WB transfusion protocols in 3 areas of Texas beginning in 2017.

Viscoelastic hemostatic assays

With approximately one-third of patients presenting to the hospital with coagulopathy, it is essential to be able to have early monitoring of coagulation.

Box 1: Key elements of damage control resuscitation

- Control of hemorrhage
- Permissive hypotension
- Hemostatic resuscitation
- Prevention/Correction of acidosis
- Normothermia
- Correction of hypocalcemia

Conventional plasma-based coagulation test, such as prothrombin time, activated partial thromboplastin time, and international normalized ratio serve mainly to measure clot initiation time and do not assess the interplay of platelets and coagulation factors in forming clot. Viscoelastic hemostatic assay (VHA), thrombelastography (TEG), or rotational thromboelastometry measure clot formation and dissolution in WB and can identify the etiology of coagulopathy (Fig. 1). On admission to a trauma center, TEG has been shown to be a more accurate predictor of need for blood product transfusion than conventional coagulation assays, and if reduced clot strength is present, there is associated increased 30-day mortality [52,53]. Also, VHAs provide clinically pertinent information in a short time frame, making it relevant for clinical decision-making regarding transfusion. Patients receiving TEG-guided MTP have better survival, less use of FFP and platelets, and better characterization of their unique coagulation profile [54]. Identification of factor depletion or fibrinolysis as the underlying cause of coagulopathy can steer resuscitation efforts and inform decisions regarding administration of antifibrinolytic agents.

VHA has benefits in resuscitation of the severely injured patient, but it has several obstacles to widespread adaption. Performance of the VHA test requires trained personnel and readily available equipment. Many hospitals house their equipment in a central laboratory and the times to results are influenced by limitations of laboratory resources. Point of care testing is appealing for trauma resuscitation, as it eliminates the need for involvement of a central laboratory, but those performing the test must be trained to ensure quality of results and the equipment requires frequent calibration and upkeep. As the technology of VHA evolves to become less labor intensive, it will be incorporated into more resuscitation algorithms due to its clinical advantages.

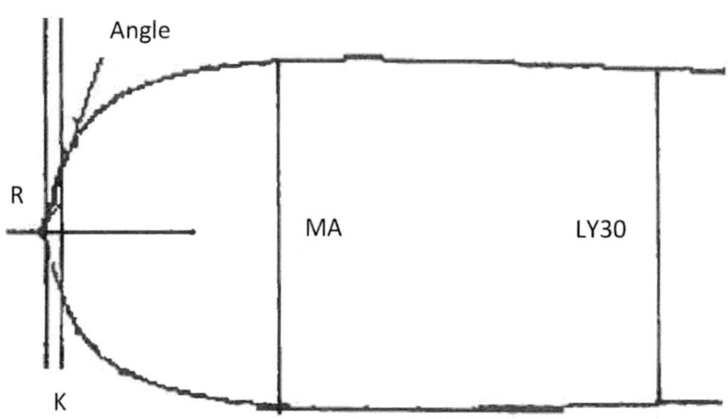

Fig. 1. Sample TEG tracing. K, clot amplification; LY30, % decrease of amplitude at 30 minutes; MA, maximum clot strength; R, clot initiation; α, speed of fibrin buildup and crosslinking.

Tourniquet placement

Hemorrhage control is a crucial component of DCR. Previously, tourniquet use for exsanguinating extremity injuries fell out of favor because of the concern for compounding the ischemic insult by restricting collateral circulation. The military conflicts in Iraq and Afghanistan saw many casualties from isolated limb injuries that were potentially preventable. This changed the military's stance on tourniquet use and availability in the field [55]. This has been extrapolated to the civilian trauma by EMS providers and through the Stop the Bleed campaign, which supplies citizens with tourniquets and education on their application.

Resuscitative endovascular balloon occlusion of the aorta

In recent years, the use of resuscitative endovascular balloon occlusion of the aorta (REBOA) has been gaining momentum as an endovascular approach to control noncompressible torso hemorrhage. White and colleagues [56,57] published a series of animal studies looking at the use of REBOA in a swine hemorrhagic shock model and showed that balloon aortic occlusion resulted in similar increases in central aortic pressure and carotid blood flow with less acidosis and less fluid and pressor requirements compared with open occlusion. Small clinical case series from various institutions showed that REBOA is a feasible option for control of noncompressible torso bleeding, but mortality rates are equivocal and safety concerns exist regarding access site complications [58–62]. Currently, the American Association for the Surgery of Trauma Aortic Occlusion for Resuscitation in Trauma and Acute Care Surgery study group is evaluating indications and outcomes for REBOA use. Early data from the registry suggested that there is no significant difference in mortality between open and endovascular occlusion of the aorta; however, this group and others have shown there may be a benefit in specific subsets of patients, including those with significant pelvic fractures [58,63].

The ultimate role of REBOA in the clinical setting remains in question. In the Joint Statement from the American College of Surgeons Committee on Trauma and the American College of Emergency Physicians regarding the clinical use of REBOA, it was recommended that practitioners undergo formal procedural training, have proficiency in ultrasound-guided and open access to the common femoral artery and participate in ongoing competency programs related to use of REBOA [64]. This statement received criticism in both the civilian and military community because it was overly restrictive and because of its lack of acknowledgment of the Joint Trauma System Clinical Practice Guideline for the use of REBOA published in 2017, which established clear indications for considering the use of REBOA in the combat setting, performing quality improvement, and system reporting [65,66].

The ultimate role of REBOA in the clinical setting remains in question. As the evidence continues to evolve regarding its use, practitioners will hopefully see clarification surrounding its indications, pitfalls, training, and outcomes.

TEAM TRAINING AND VIDEO REVIEW

A systematic and team-based approach to trauma bay resuscitation is a critical component of an injured patient's care. Medical errors most frequently occur as a result of ineffective leadership, poor communication, and lack of situational awareness [67,68]. Training of health care professionals in nontechnical skills, such as teamwork, stress management, decision-making, and communication, has long been recommended to improve patient care quality and patient safety. Following modeling approaches seen in the aviation industry and the military over many decades, trauma centers have begun to incorporate simulation-based team training into their performance improvement initiatives. Although still in its relative infancy, human patient simulator training has shown promising results in improving trauma bay efficiency, teamwork, and interpersonal and closed loop communication skills [69,70].

In concert with simulation training, the use of trauma video review (TVR) has become an invaluable tool for appraising trauma team performance. Hoyt and colleagues [71] first introduced this concept in the literature in 1988 and found that the use of TVR improved adherence to assigned responsibilities and a decrease in time to definitive care for the patients. Since that time, TVR has been used to identify and monitor system issues, to develop leadership skills, to ensure adherence to protocols, and more recently for procedural training [72].

FUTURE ADVANCES

The current available literature in trauma resuscitation has notable limitations from study design, selection bias, unmeasured confounders, and availability of resources, making widespread application of their results problematic. Future research efforts should be planned to minimize these issues to provide concrete evidence of best practices in early-phase trauma care.

There is a large volume of literature to support immediate transport of penetrating trauma victims to a trauma center for definitive care; however, EMS providers are still performing prehospital interventions that potentially delay transport and surgical intervention. At the same time, the early administration of blood components and/or WB decreases trauma-induced coagulopathy and many EMS systems are beginning prehospital transfusion protocols. These 2 statements seem to be contradictory and evoke many questions that are yet to be answered. When does the benefit of rapid transport no longer outweigh the benefit of prehospital blood product administration? In Philadelphia, most penetrating trauma victims are transported via police to the nearest trauma center for definitive care. Should other urban areas look to their other public service workers, such as police, to transport patients in order to get them to the hospital more quickly? A prospective randomized controlled trial designed to investigate the role of prehospital interventions is needed to definitively answer these questions.

SUMMARY

Trauma resuscitation continues to change over time. The role of prehospital care providers remains to be fully defined and the optimal resuscitation strategies are in evolution. The initial management of the trauma patient will continue to improve as the understanding of the physiology and coagulopathy of trauma is better refined.

References

[1] Heron M. Deaths: leading causes for 2016. Natl Vital Stat Rep 2018;67(6):1–77.
[2] Committee on Trauma, American College of Surgeons. Advanced trauma life support for doctors. 9th edition. Chicago: American College of Surgeons; 2012.
[3] Shires T, Coln D, Carrico J, et al. Fluid therapy in hemorrhagic shock. Arch Surg 1964;88(4):688–93.
[4] Dillon J, Lynch L, Myers R, et al. A bioassay of treatment of hemorrhagic shock. I. The roles of blood Ringer's solution with lactate and macromolecules (dextran and hydroxyethyl starch) in the treatment of hemorrhagic shock in the anesthetized dog. Arch Surg 1966;93(4): 537–55.
[5] Bickell W, Wall M, Pepe P, et al. Immediate versus delayed fluid resuscitation for hypotensive patients with penetrating torso injuries. N Engl J Med 1995;332:681–3.
[6] Bickell W, Bruttig S, Millnamow G, et al. The detrimental effects on intravenous crystalloid after aortotomy in swine. Surgery 1991;110(3):529–36.
[7] Kowalenko T, Stern S, Dronen S, et al. Improved outcome with hypotensive resuscitation of uncontrolled shock in a swine model. J Trauma 1992;33(3):349–53.
[8] Taghavi D, Durna J, Jayarajan S, et al. Still making the case against prehospital intubation: a rat hemorrhagic shock model. J Trauma Acute Care Surg 2012;73(2):332–7.
[9] Taghavi S, Jayarajan S, Koche S, et al. Examining prehospital intubation for penetrating trauma in swine hemorrhagic shock model. J Trauma Acute Care Surg 2013;74(5): 1246–51.
[10] Taghavi S, Jayarajan S, Ferrer L, et al. "Permissive hypoventilation" in a swine model of hemorrhagic shock. J Trauma Acute Care Surg 2014;77(1):14–9.
[11] Stockinger Z, McSwain N. Prehospital endotracheal intubation for trauma does not improve survival over bag-valve-mask ventilation. J Trauma 2004;56(3):531–6.
[12] Rhee K, O'Malley R, Turner J, et al. Field airway management of the trauma patient: the efficacy of bag mask ventilation. Am J Emerg Med 1988;6(4):333–6.
[13] Seamon M, Fisher C, Gaughan J, et al. Prehosptial procedures before emergency department thoracotomy: "scoop and run" saves lives. J Trauma 2007;63:113–20.
[14] Taghavi S, Vora H, Jayarajan S, et al. Prehospital intubation does not decrease complications in the penetrating trauma patient. Am Surg 2014;80(1):9–14.
[15] Rotondo M, Schwab C, McGonigal M, et al. 'Damage Control': an approach for improved survival in exsanguinating penetrating abdominal injury. J Trauma 1993;35:375–82.
[16] Holcomb J, Jenkins D, Rhee P, et al. Damage control resuscitation: directly addressing the early coagulopathy of trauma. J Trauma 2007;62(2):307–10.
[17] Petrosoniak A, Hicks C. Resuscitation resequenced: a rational approach to patients with trauma in shock. Emerg Med Clin North Am 2018;36(1):41–60.
[18] Seamon M, Feather C, Smith B, et al. Just one drop: the significance of a single hypotensive blood pressure reading during trauma resuscitations. J Trauma 2010;68(6):1289–94.
[19] Ferrada P, Callcut R, Skarupa D, et al. Circulation first—the time has come to question the sequencing in the ABCs of trauma; an American Association for the Surgery of Trauma multicenter study. World J Emerg Surg 2018;13:8.
[20] Demetriades D, Chan L, Cornwell E, et al. Paramedic vs private transportation of trauma patients: effects on outcome. Arch Surg 1996;131(2):133–8.

[21] Rappold J, Hollenbach K, Santora T, et al. The evil of good is better: making the care for basic life support transport for penetrating trauma victims in an urban environment. J Trauma Acute Care Surg 2015;79(3):343–8.
[22] Liberman M, Mulder D, Lavoie A, et al. Multicenter Canadian study of prehospital trauma care. Ann Surg 2003;237(2):153–60.
[23] Stiell I, Nesbitt L, Pickett W, et al. The OPALS Major Trauma Study: impact of advanced life-support on survival and morbidity. CMAJ 2008;178(9):1141–52.
[24] Band R, Pryor J, Gaiesji D, et al. Injury-adjusted mortality of patients transported by police following penetrating trauma. Acad Emerg Med 2011;18(1):32–7.
[25] Band R, Salhi R, Holena D, et al. Severity-adjusted mortality in trauma patients transported by police. Ann Emerg Med 2014;63(5):608–14.
[26] Seamon M, Doane S, Gaughan J, et al. Prehospital interventions for penetrating trauma victims: a prospective comparison between advanced life support and basic life support. Injury 2013;44(5):634–8.
[27] Evans C, Petersen A, Meier E, et al. Prehospital traumatic cardiac arrest: management and outcomes from the resuscitation outcomes consortium epistry-trauma and PROPHET registry. J Trauma Acute Care Surg 2016;81(2):285–93.
[28] Dutton R, Mackenzie C, Scalea T. Hypotensive resuscitation during active hemorrhage: impact on in-hospital mortality. J Trauma 2002;52(6):1141–6.
[29] Schreiber M, Meier E, Tisherman S, et al. A controlled resuscitation strategy is feasible and safe in hypotensive trauma patients: results of a prospective randomized pilot trial. J Trauma Acute Care Surg 2015;78(4):6887–95.
[30] Carrick M, Morrison C, Tapia N, et al. Intraoperative hypotensive resuscitation for patients undergoing laparotomy or thoracotomy for trauma: early termination of a randomized prospective clinical trial. J Trauma Acute Care Surg 2016;80(6):886–96.
[31] May A, Young J, Butler K, et al. Coagulopathy in severe closed head injury: is empiric therapy warranted? Am Surg 1997;63(3):233–6.
[32] Hess J, Brohi K, Dutton R, et al. The coagulopathy of trauma: a review of mechanisms. J Trauma 2008;65(4):748–54.
[33] Holcomb J, Tilley B, Baraniuk S, et al. Transfusion of plasma, platelets, and red blood cells in a 1:1:1 vs a 1:1:2 ratio and mortality in patients with severe trauma: the PROPPR randomized controlled trial. JAMA 2015;313:471–82.
[34] Borgman M, Spinella P, Perkins J, et al. The ratio of blood products transfused affects mortality in patients receiving massive transfusions at a combat support hospital. J Trauma 2007;63(4):805–13.
[35] Hirshberg A, Dugas M, Banez E, et al. Minimizing dilutional coagulopathy in exsanguinating hemorrhage: a computer simulation. J Trauma 2003;54(3):454–63.
[36] O'Keefe T, Refaai M, Tchorz K, et al. A massive transfusion protocol to decrease blood component use and costs. Arch Surg 2008;143(7):686–90.
[37] Biffl W, Smith W, Moore E, et al. Evolution of a multidisciplinary clinical pathway for the management of unstable pelvic fractures. Ann Surg 2001;233(6):843–50.
[38] Vaslef S, Knudsen N, Neligan P, et al. Massive transfusion exceeding 50 units of blood products in trauma patients. J Trauma 2002;53(2):291–5.
[39] Del Junco D, Holcomb J, Fox E, et al. Resuscitate early with plasma and platelets or balance blood products gradually: findings from the PROMMTT study. J Trauma Acute Care Surg 2013;75(1 Suppl 1):S24–30.
[40] Cotton B, Au B, Nunez T, et al. Predefined massive transfusion protocols are associated with a reduction in organ failure and post injury complications. J Trauma 2009;66(1):41–8.
[41] Radwan Z, Bai Y, Matijevic, et al. An emergency department thawed plasma protocol for severely injured patients. JAMA Surg 2013;148(2):170–5.
[42] Holcomb J, Wade C, Michalek J, et al. Increased plasma and platelet to red blood cell ratios improves outcome in 466 massively transfused civilian trauma patients. Ann Surg 2008;248(3):447–58.

[43] Pohlman T, Fecher A, Arreola-Garcia C. Optimizing transfusion strategies in damage control resuscitation: current insights. J Blood Med 2018;20(9):117–33.
[44] Spinella P, Pidcoke H, Strandenes G, et al. Whole blood for hemostatic resuscitation of major bleeding. Transfusion 2016;56(Supple 2):S190–202.
[45] Repine T, Perkins J, Kauver D, et al. The use of fresh whole blood in massive transfusion. J Trauma 2006;60(6 supple):S59–69.
[46] Spinella P, Perkins J, Grathwohl K, et al. Warm fresh whole blood is independently associated with improved survival for patients with combat related traumatic injuries. J Trauma 2009;66(4 Suppple):S69–76.
[47] Perkins J, Cap A, Spinella P, et al. Comparison of platelet transfusion as fresh whole versus apheresis platelets for massively transfused combat trauma patients. Transfusion 2011;51(2):242–52.
[48] Cotton B, Podbielski J, Camp E, et al. A randomized controlled pilot trial of modified whole blood versus component therapy in severely injured patients requiring large volume transfusions. Ann Surg 2013;258(4):527–32.
[49] Rahbar E, Cardenas J, Matijevic, et al. Trauma, time and transfusions: a longitudinal analysis of coagulation markers in severely injured trauma patients receiving whole blood or component blood products. Shock 2015;44(5):417–25.
[50] Sheppard F, Schaub L, Cap A, et al. Whole blood mitigates the acute coagulopathy of trauma and avoids the coagulopathy of crystalloid resuscitation. J Trauma Acute Care Surg 2018; https://doi.org/10.1097/TA.0000000000002046.
[51] Seheult J, Anto V, Alarcon L, et al. Clinical outcomes among low-titer group O whole blood recipients compared to recipients of conventional; components in civilian trauma resuscitation. Transfusion 2018;58:1838–45.
[52] Holcomb J, Minei K, Scerbo M, et al. Admission rapid thrombelastography can replace conventional coagulation tests in the emergency department. Ann Surg 2012;256:476–86.
[53] Nystrup k, Windelov N, Thomsen A, et al. Reduced clot strength upon admission, evaluated by thrombelastography (TEG), in trauma patients is independently associated with increased 30-day mortality. Scand J Trauma Resusc Emerg Med 2011;19:52.
[54] Gonazalez E, Moore E, Moore H. Management of trauma-induced coagulopathy with thrombelastography. Crit Care Clin 2017;33:119–34.
[55] Blackbourne L, Baer D, Eastridge B, et al. Military medical revolution: prehospital combat casualty care. J Trauma Acute Care Surg 2012;73(6 suppl 5):S372–7.
[56] White J, Cannon J, Stannard A, et al. A porcine model for evaluation the management of noncompressible torso hemorrhage. J Trauma 2011;71(1 Suppl):S131–8.
[57] White J, Cannon J, Stannard A, et al. Endovascular balloon occlusion of the aorta is superior to resuscitative thoracotomy with aortic clamping in a porcine model of hemorrhagic shock. Surgery 2011;150(3):400–9.
[58] Saito N, Matsumoto H, Yagi T, et al. Evaluation of the safety and feasibility of resuscitative endovascular balloon occlusion of the aorta. J Trauma Acute Care Surg 2015;78(5):897–903.
[59] Ogura T, Lefor A, Nakano M, et al. Nonoperative management of hemodynamically unstable abdominal trauma patients with angioembolization and resuscitative endovascular balloon occlusion of the aorta. J Trauma Acute Care Surg 2015;78(1):132–5.
[60] Moore L, Brenner M, Kozar R, et al. Implementation of resuscitative endovascular balloon occlusion of the aorta as an alternative to resuscitative thoracotomy for noncompressible truncal hemorrhage. J Trauma Acute Care Surg 2015;79(4):523–30.
[61] Abe t, uchida M, Nagata I, et al. Resuscitative endovascular balloon occlusion of the aorta versus aortic cross clamping among patients with critical trauma; a nationwide cohort study in Japan. Crit Care 2016;20(1):400.
[62] Inoue J, Shiraichi A, Yoshiyuki, et al. Resuscitative endovascular balloon occlusion of the aorta might be dangerous in patients with severe torso trauma: a propensity score analysis. J Trauma Acute Care Surg 2016;80(4):559–66.

[63] Brenner M, Inaba K, Aiolfi A, et al. Resuscitative endovascular balloon occlusion of the aorta and resuscitative thoracotomy in select patients with hemorrhagic shock: early results from the American Association for the Surgery of Trauma's aortic occlusion for the resuscitation in trauma and acute care surgery registry. J Am Coll Surg 2018;226(5):730–40.
[64] Brenner M, Bulger E, Perina D, et al. Joint statement from the American College of Surgeons Committee on Trauma (ACS COT) and the American College of Emergency Physicians (ACEP) regarding the clinical use of resuscitative balloon occlusion of the aorta. Trauma Surg Acute Care Open 2018;3(1):e000154.
[65] Qasim Z, Dubise J, Rasmussen T, et al. Breaking down silos: the joint statement about the clinical use of resuscitative endovascular balloon occlusion of the aorta (REBOA) warrants revision. Ann Emerg Med 2018;72(2):225–6.
[66] Allen B, Callaway D, Gibbs M, et al. Regarding the 'Joint statement from the American College of Surgeons Committee on Trauma (ACS COT) and the American College of Emergency Physicians (ACEP) regarding the clinical use of resuscitative endovascular balloon occlusion of the aorta (REBOA). Trauma Acute Care Open 2018;3(1):e000168.
[67] Doumouras A, Keshet I, Nathens A, et al. Trauma non-technical training (TNT-2): the development, piloting and multilevel assessment of a simulation-based, interprofessional curriculum for team-based trauma resuscitation. Can J Surg 2014;57(5):354–5.
[68] Sutcliffe K, Lewton E, Rosenthal M. Communication failures: an insidious contributor to medical mishaps. Acad Med 2004;79(2):186–94.
[69] Steinemann S, berg B, Skinner A, et al. In-situ, multidisciplinary, simulation-based teamwork training improves early trauma care. J Surg Educ 2011;68(6):472–7.
[70] Severson M, Maxson P, Wrobleski D, et al. Simulation-based team training and debriefing to enhance nursing and physician collaboration. J Contin Educ Nurs 2014;45(7): 297–303.
[71] Hoyt D, Shackford S, Firdland P, et al. Video recording trauma resuscitations: an effective teaching technique. J Trauma 1988;28(4):435–40.
[72] Dumas R, Chreiman K, Seamon M, et al. Benchmarking emergency department thoracotomy: using trauma video review to generate procedural norms. Injury 2018;49(9): 1687–92.

Advances in Surgery 53 (2019) 235–251

ADVANCES IN SURGERY

Anticoagulants and Surgery

So Many Agents, So Many Taking Them

Ronak B. Patel, MD, Apostolos K. Tassiopoulos, MD*

Division of Vascular and Endovascular Surgery, Department of Surgery, Stony Brook University Hospital, Stony Brook, NY 11794, USA

Keywords

• Anticoagulation • Anticoagulation bridging • Perioperative anticoagulation • Anticoagulation reversal • Direct oral anticoagulant (DOAC) • Idarucizumab (Praxbind) • Novel oral anticoagulant (NOAC) • Andexxa

Key points

- The increasing number of direct oral anticoagulants available and the increasing frequency of their use makes perioperative anticoagulation management a great challenge.
- Strategies to determine the appropriate perioperative anticoagulation management rely on estimated thromboembolic risk versus bleeding risk using risk calculators, clinical experience, and basic understanding of the pharmacokinetics of the oral anticoagulant.
- Food and Drug Administration-approved reversal agents are available for dabigatran, rivaroxaban, and apixaban; however, there are few data to evaluate their efficacy and appropriate use, and they remain costly and of limited availability.
- There is a need for further studies to help standardize perioperative anticoagulation management that can still be tailored to meet individual patients' needs.

INTRODUCTION

The perioperative management of anticoagulation among patients undergoing surgical procedures has always been a challenge; surgeons need to balance the benefit of protection from thromboembolic events to the risk of bleeding during

Disclosure Statement: No potential conflict of interest relevant to this article to report.

*Corresponding author. Division of Vascular and Endovascular Surgery, Health Sciences Center T19-090, Stony Brook Medicine, Stony Brook, NY 11794, USA. *E-mail address:* Apostolos.Tassiopoulos@stonybrookmedicine.edu

https://doi.org/10.1016/j.yasu.2019.04.011
0065-3411/19/

the perioperative period. This decision is not always easy and the increasing number of anticoagulation agents further complicates the perioperative decision if and when to interrupt therapy. Although vitamin K antagonists (VKA) have been the mainstay of anticoagulation therapy for decades, the relatively recent Food and Drug Administration (FDA) approval of several new direct oral anticoagulant (DOAC) agents has changed the landscape of anticoagulation therapy. DOACs are often preferred owing to their fixed dosing, decreased drug and food interactions, and lack of monitoring requirements. The 2014 American Heart Association/American College of Cardiology guidelines for the management of nonvalvular atrial fibrillation recommend DOACs as an alternative to warfarin, with several studies showing a reduced risk of intracranial hemorrhage with DOACs when compared with warfarin [1]. The 2016 American College of Chest Physicians guidelines favor DOACs over VKAs as a first-line therapy for venous thromboembolism (VTE) management in patients who do not have cancer [2]. This recommendation has resulted in a rapid increase in clinical use of DOACs, making encounter of these patients by surgeons increasingly more common. To further complicate the matter, newly FDA-approved reversal agents also exist for several of the DOACs, without sufficient data to evaluate their use in the perioperative setting. This article summarizes the FDA-approved DOACs and their reversal agents, and discusses strategies to determine the appropriate management of anticoagulation in the perioperative period to minimize both the thromboembolic and bleeding risks for patients undergoing surgical interventions.

PERIOPERATIVE ANTICOAGULATION MANAGEMENT

The management of anticoagulation in the perioperative setting requires an evaluation of the thromboembolic risk associated with interrupting anticoagulation therapy, the relative risk of bleeding associated with continuation of anticoagulation, the need for bridging therapy, and the specific anticoagulant agent itself.

Evaluation of thromboembolic risk

The most common indications for anticoagulation therapy include

- Atrial fibrillation,
- Recent VTE, and
- Prosthetic heart valves.

The CHA_2DS_2-VASc score is a validated risk stratification tool used to predict the risk of stroke and thromboembolism (TE) in a nonanticoagulated patient with nonvalvular atrial fibrillation (Table 1). Individuals can be stratified into low, moderate, or high thrombotic risk (Table 2) [3]. The degree of thrombotic risk can then be used to help determine the need for continuation of anticoagulation in the acute perioperative setting and whether or not the patient needs to be bridged with an unfractionated heparin (UFH) infusion preoperatively or postoperatively. A score of 0 is considered to be low risk for TE, a score of 1 is intermediate risk (0.6% at 1 year), and greater than 1 is high

Table 1
Thromboembolic risk stratification during anticoagulation interruption

Risk level	Atrial fibrillation	VTE	Mechanical heart valve
High	CHA_2DS_2-VASc score ≥2 Recent ischemic stroke or transient ischemic attack within 3 mo Rheumatic valvular heart disease	Recent VTE within 3 mo Severe thrombophilia (protein C/S deficiency, antiphospholipid antibodies, etc)	Any mitral valve prosthesis Recent stroke or TIA within 6 mo
Moderate	CHA_2DS_2-VASc Score of 1	VTE within 3–12 mo Nonsevere thrombophilia (eg, heterozygous Factor V Leiden) Recurrent VTE Active malignancy (treated within 6 mo or palliative)	Bileaflet aortic valve prosthesis with one or more: Atrial fibrillation, prior stroke or TIA, hypertension, diabetes, CHF, or age >75
Low	CHA_2DS_2-VASc score of 0	VTE ≥12 mo ago with no other risk factors	Bileaflet aortic valve prosthesis without atrial fibrillation or other risk factors

Abbreviations: CHF, congestive heart failure; TIA, transient ischemic attack.
Adapted from Douketis, J.D., Spyropoulos, A.C., Spencer, F.A., et al. Perioperative management of antithrombotic therapy. CHEST 2012;141(2):p. e326S–e350S; with permission.

risk (3% at 1 year) [4]. It is important to note that the CHA_2DS_2-VASc score has not been prospectively validated in the perioperative setting.

Up to 25% of patients undergoing abdominal surgery will develop deep vein thrombosis within 6 weeks of discharge [5]. Patients with a VTE within the

Table 2
CHA_2DS_2-VASc score calculator

Criterion	Value	Points
CHF	Yes	+1
Hypertension therapy	Yes	+1
Age	<65 years old	+0
	65–74 years old	+1
	≥75 years old	+2
Diabetes history	Yes	+1
Stroke/TIA/VTE history	Yes	+2
Vascular disease history	Yes	+1
Sex	Male	+0
	Female	+1

Abbreviations: CHF, congestive heart failure; TIA, transient ischemic attack.
Data from Lip, G.Y., Vieuwlaat, R., Pisters, R., et al. Refining clinical risk stratification for predicting stroke and thromboembolism in atrial fibrillation using a novel risk factor-based approach: the euro heart survey on atrial fibrillation. Chest 2010;137(2):p. 263–72.

preceding 3 months or with a history of VTE owing to a severe inherited thrombophilia are at high risk of a recurrent thromboembolic event in the perioperative setting if taken off therapeutic anticoagulation. Patients with a VTE within 3 to 12 months before surgery or who have an active malignancy are at moderate risk of VTE, and those with a history of VTE more than 12 months before surgery are at low risk of VTE perioperatively [3].

Patients with prosthetic valves are considered high risk for TE events. In general, bioprosthetic valves carry a lower TE risk compared with mechanical valves. It is not uncommon for patients with a bioprosthetic aortic valve to be on antiplatelet agents only, particularly those without atrial fibrillation. The TE risk is higher with mitral valve prostheses than with aortic valve prostheses; thus, patients with mechanical mitral valves should discontinue anticoagulation only for brief intervals during the perioperative period [3].

Estimating bleeding risk

The International Society on Thrombosis and Hemostasis for surgical studies defines major bleeding as bleeding that is fatal, involves a critical organ, requires surgery to correct, has a decrease in hemoglobin of 2 g/dL or more, or requires a transfusion of 2 or more units of packed red blood cells [5]. The consequences of bleeding complications depend on the nature of the surgical intervention being performed, as well as individual patient factors that may contribute to an increased volume of blood loss. Patients scheduled for eye procedures, neurosurgical or spine interventions, and those requiring neuraxial anesthesia are considered to be at high bleeding risk and should have all types of anticoagulation agents wear off completely before the planned procedure. In these situations, anticoagulants are restarted when the bleeding risk is minimal, usually several days after surgery. In addition, procedures that have a 2-day risk of major bleeding of 2% to 4%, such as vascular surgery, general surgery, prostatic resections, and polypectomies, are also considered high risk. Low risk of bleeding procedures have an estimated 2-day risk of major bleeding of 0% to 2%, such as abdominal hernia repair, axillary node dissection, and cholecystectomy, endoscopy [6].

In general, patients with a high surgical risk of bleeding should have their anticoagulant discontinued before surgical intervention. If they confer a high thromboembolic risk, elective surgery should be delayed until the thromboembolic risk is lower. If surgical intervention must be performed, the time period without anticoagulation should be as limited as possible, using a bridging agent such as low-molecular-weight heparin (LMWH) or UFH infusion if necessary. If the surgical risk of bleeding is low, patients can often continue their anticoagulant if at high risk of thromboembolic event without anticoagulation.

There are several patient factors that confer an increased risk of bleeding, regardless of the procedure being performed. These factors vary greatly and several attempts to quantify these risks have been made in both prospective and retrospective studies.

For patients with atrial fibrillation, a number of studies have attempted to predict bleeding complications based on patient-specific factors. The HAS-BLED score allows one to estimate the 1-year risk for major bleeding for patients with atrial fibrillation on oral anticoagulation. This score was developed based on a multivariate analysis of nearly 4000 real-world patients with atrial fibrillation on an oral anticoagulant in the Euro Heart Survey on Atrial Fibrillation (Table 3) [7]. HEMORR$_2$HAGES is a bleeding risk scheme used to help quantify the risk of hemorrhage in elderly patients with atrial fibrillation on warfarin, based on a multivariate analysis of various patient factors of nearly 4000 patients in the National Registry of Atrial Fibrillation [8]. Last, the ATRIA study used a Cox regression model of more than 9000 patients with atrial fibrillation on warfarin to develop a simple 5-variable hemorrhage risk stratification score that was effective in quantifying the risk of warfarin-associated hemorrhage in this patient population [9].

The predictive performance of the HAS-BLED, HEMORR$_2$HAGES, and ATRIA bleeding risk scores were compared in the AMADEUS trial, which demonstrated that the HAS-BLED score more accurately predicted clinically relevant bleeding in patients with atrial fibrillation on oral anticoagulation, and was the only score to significantly improve the rate of intracranial hemorrhage in this population [10]. In the BNK Online Bridging Registry (BORDER), an observational registry of perioperative outcomes in patients undergoing invasive cardiac procedures, a HAS-BLED score of 3 or greater was the most predictive variable for bleeding [11]. The majority of these patients were receiving VKAs, which were bridged with a LMWH before the

Table 3
HAS-BLED score

Criterion	Points
Uncontrolled hypertension	+1
Systolic blood pressure >160 mm Hg	
Renal disease	+1
Dialysis, renal transplant, or creatinine >2.26 mg/dL	
Liver disease	+1
Cirrhosis or bilirubin >2× normal and AST/ALT/ALP >3× normal	
Stroke history	+1
Prior major bleeding or predisposition to bleeding	+1
Labile INR	+1
Unstable/high INRs, time in therapeutic range <60%	
Age >65	+1
Medication usage predisposing to bleeding	+1
Aspirin, clopidogrel, NSAIDs	
Alcohol use ≥8 drinks/wk	+1

Abbreviations: ALP, alkaline phosphatase; ALT, alanine aminotransferase; AST, aspartate aminotransferase; NSAIDs, nonsteroidal anti-inflammatory drugs.

Data from Pisters, R., Lane, D.A., Nieuwlaat, R., et al. A novel user-friendly score (HAS-BLED) to assess 1-year risk of major bleeding in patients with atrial fibrillation: The Euro Heart Survey. Chest 2010;138(5):p. 1093–1100.

procedure. A small retrospective case-control study was recently investigated in patients receiving DOAC (specifically rivaroxaban), in which the HAS-BLED score demonstrated a modest ability to predict major bleeding events; however, this did not reach statistical significance [12].

For patients with VTE, only the International Medical Prevention Registry on Venous Thromboembolism (IMPROVE) bleeding risk score has been shown to consistently predict major and clinically relevant bleeding at 14 days, with a score of 7 or greater indicating an increased risk of bleeding [13]. The IMPROVE bleeding risk score is a multinational observational study of more than 15,000 patients for whom a multiple regression model analysis was performed to identify risk factors at admission associated with in-hospital bleeding for patients not on therapeutic anticoagulation [14]. However, the cohort studied was limited to medical inpatients not undergoing any surgical intervention [14].

As with surgical risk of bleeding, the discontinuation of anticoagulation based on a patient's propensity for major or clinically relevant bleeding is strongly recommended, with the duration of discontinuation determined by the patient's risk of thromboembolic event while not anticoagulated.

Bridging

For patients with a high to very high thromboembolic risk (recent ischemic stroke, CHA_2DS_2-VASc score of $\geq$7, mechanical heart valve, etc) for whom anticoagulation must be discontinued for surgery with a high risk of bleeding, it may be appropriate to bridge the patient with another form of anticoagulation both preoperatively and/or postoperatively. This is especially true for patients on VKAs, who are typically instructed to hold their warfarin dose 4 to 5 days before surgery and resume it postoperatively, resulting in several days of subtherapeutic anticoagulation. Postoperative bridging may also be considered for patients who are expected to remain without oral intake owing to postoperative ileus, ventilator dependence, and so on.

If a patient with a recent VTE (ie, within 3 months) requires urgent surgical intervention and cannot be anticoagulated perioperatively, a retrievable inferior vena cava filter may be placed preoperatively, with the caveat that, once anticoagulation can be safely resumed, the inferior vena cava filter should be removed. It is important to note that the American College of Chest Physicians does not support the use of inferior vena cava filters as a means of pulmonary embolism prophylaxis in high-risk populations, such as patients with multitrauma or spinal cord injury, without evidence of deep vein thrombosis [15].

In patients with a lower risk of TE, bridging is not recommended. The Bridging Anticoagulation in Patients who Require Temporary Interruption of Warfarin Therapy for an Elective Invasive Procedure or Surgery (BRIDGE) trial randomly assigned patients with a low TE risk who required interruption of warfarin for an invasive procedure to bridging with LMWH (dalteparin) versus bridging with placebo. Within 30 days, the incidence of arterial thromboembolic events were similar in the 2 cohorts, although the incidence of major bleeding was greater in those bridged with LMWH [16]. High-risk TE patients (those with mechanical heart valves, a recent VTE, or ischemic stroke/transient ischemic attack) were excluded from this trial. Similar results were reported in a metaanalysis of 34 observational studies of patients undergoing elective surgery or procedures. The authors found that there was no significant difference in the rate of TE in patients who received bridging when compared with those that did not. However, bridging was associated with a significantly increased risk of major bleeding [17].

In the Dresden NOAC registry of 8000 patients receiving a DOAC for any indication who underwent an invasive procedure, there were similar rates of cardiovascular events regardless of whether the patient was bridged, not bridged, or oral anticoagulation was continued perioperatively. However, bridging was not found to be an independent risk factor of major bleeding in this registry [18].

The PERIOP-2 trial is a randomized, controlled trial currently investigating postoperative bridging with LMWH in patients with a mechanical heart valve, all of whom received preoperative bridging, with a primary outcome of major TE within 90 days of randomization (ClinicalTrials.gov, NCT00432796).

In general, anticoagulation bridging should be reserved for those patients who are at high or very high risk of thromboembolic events during the time of anticoagulation interruption, because bridging with LWMH or UFH does seem to confer an increased risk of major bleeding without a documented decrease in the thromboembolic events in patients with a low to moderate TE risk.

ORAL ANTICOAGULANT AGENTS

Since the FDA approval of DOACs in 2010, there has been an approximate 10-fold increase in the number of prescription of DOACs, with a concurrent 4.5-fold decrease in the number of warfarin prescriptions, for adults with nonvalvular atrial fibrillation who filled a new prescription for an anticoagulant between 2010 and 2017 [19]. Among the DOACs, the predominant anticoagulant of choice varies with time as additional prospective studies are performed comparing the DOACs not only with VKAs, but also with other DOACs. Given the prescribing patterns favoring DOACs over VKAs, it is imperative that surgeons understand the properties of the most commonly used DOACs and how these agents affect the perioperative management of anticoagulation in the current era (see Table 3).

Warfarin

Warfarin inhibits a vitamin K-dependent enzyme, preventing the production of factors II, VII, IX, and X. It has a half-life of 36 to 42 hours, and thus is generally held for 4 to 5 days before elective surgery to allow the prothrombin time/international normalized ratio (INR) to normalize [20]. If the INR is still elevated before surgery, low doses of oral vitamin K (1–2 mg) can be administered to quicken the normalization of the INR. Just as it takes several days for the reversal of warfarin's anticlotting effect, it takes several days to achieve therapeutic anticoagulation. Postoperatively, warfarin can typically be resumed within 12 to 24 hours after surgery at the preoperative dose, assuming hemostasis was achieved intraoperatively. This step allows for therapeutic anticoagulation within a few days postoperatively. For patients at particularly high risk of TE, a bridging agent such as UFH or LMWH may be necessary in the interim, until the INR reaches the desired therapeutic goal.

In the event of minor bleeding, a dose of warfarin may be held, or low-dose vitamin K can be administered if there is a high risk of bleeding or if the INR is supratherapeutic [21]. Clinical trials involving phytonadione, a vitamin K derived from plants, showed that oral administration in conjunction with temporary interruption of warfarin can decrease an INR of 6 to 10 to less than 4 in approximately 1.4 days, assuming normal hepatic function [22]. For intravenous (IV) administration of phytonadione, this time frame is reduced to approximately 24 hours, and the decrease in the INR begins within 2 hours of administration [22]. In the event of clinically significant bleeding or major bleeding, warfarin should be held, vitamin K should be administered to aid in normalization of the INR, and fresh frozen plasma (FFP) or prothrombin complex concentrate (PCC) should be transfused for temporary reversal of warfarin's effect. Although FFP remains the most widely used coagulation factor replacement product for urgent and emergent reversal of warfarin [23], studies have shown that PCC is more effective in correcting INR when compared with FFP. A systematic review and metaanalysis of PCC versus FFP for warfarin reversal in patients on warfarin for various indications requiring reversal owing to warfarin-related, clinically relevant bleeding has been performed. This comprehensive study showed that PCC use was associated with a significant decrease in all-cause mortality at 30 days, a greater likelihood of achieving INR normalization, a shorter time to INR correction (mean difference of <6.5 hours), and a lower risk of volume overload, all when compared with the use of FFP [24]. There was no statistically significant difference in the risk of TE or achievement of hemostasis between the 2 groups.

Dabigatran

Dabigatran (Pradaxa) is an oral direct thrombin competitive inhibitor, preventing thrombin from converting fibrinogen to fibrin. Dabigatran has a rapid but predictable anticoagulation effect, reaching peak plasma levels within 1 to 2 hours of ingestion, with a half-life of 12 to 17 hours. In patients with mild to moderate renal insufficiency (creatinine clearance [CrCl] of 30–60 mL/min), the half-life increases to 15 to 18 hours, whereas for those with severe renal insufficiency (CrCl of <30 mL/min), the half-life approaches 24 to 28 hours. Dosing recommendations for the treatment of nonvalvular atrial fibrillation and VTE previously treated with 5 days of parenteral anticoagulation are as follows: 150 mg twice daily for CrCl greater than 30 mL/min and 75 mg twice daily for CrCl between 15 and 30 mL/min [25].

Perioperatively, dabigatran has been shown to have similar rates of thromboembolic events when compared with warfarin with a comparable perioperative bleeding risk. The Randomized Evaluation of Long-Term Anticoagulation Therapy (RE-LY) trial studied periprocedural thromboembolic risk in 4591 patients undergoing elective procedures or surgery and found similar rates of cerebrovascular events, cardiovascular death, and pulmonary embolus between those treated with dabigatran and those treated with warfarin [26]. The RE-COVER II trial reported similar rates of periprocedural bleeding between dabigatran and warfarin, including patients undergoing urgent surgery [27].

Based on its short half-life, dabigatran may be discontinued 2 to 3 days before operative intervention in patients with normal or mildly impaired renal function, and 3 to 4 days before if moderate to severe renal impairment is present. Additionally, dabigatran can be initiated postoperatively, when a patient is safe to be therapeutically anticoagulated. Given its rapid onset of action and short life, bridging therapy is typically not indicated.

Unlike the prothrombin time/INR for warfarin, routine coagulation studies have not been validated for measuring the anticoagulation effect of dabigatran. A prolonged activated partial thromboplastin time likely indicates therapeutic levels of dabigatran; however, a normal activated partial thromboplastin time does not exclude therapeutic dabigatran levels [28].

In patients on dabigatran with clinically relevant or major bleeding, idarucizumab (Praxbind) may be used to reverse the effects of dabigatran. Approved by the FDA in 2015, idarucizumab is a monoclonal antibody that binds dabigatran, which can be used to decrease clinically relevant or major bleeding, or to reverse its anticoagulation effect in patients that may need to undergo emergent surgical intervention. The RE-VERSE AD prospective cohort study showed that idarucizumab completely reversed the anticoagulant effect of dabigatran within minutes [29]. Idarucizumab has a half-life of 47 minutes to 10.3 hours, with a mean clearance time of 6 hours. The recommended dosing is idarucizumab 5 g IV via 2 consecutive 2.5-g infusions, and the dosing does not need to be adjusted for those with renal insufficiency. Common adverse effects include hypokalemia, constipation, hypersensitivity reactions, and thromboembolic events [30].

Rivaroxaban

Rivaroxaban (Xarelto) is an oral direct factor Xa inhibitor, inhibiting the degradation of fibrinogen to fibrin and inactivating platelets. Rivaroxaban is rapidly absorbed and largely albumin bound, reaching peak plasma levels within 2 to 4 hours and with a half-life of 5 to 9 hours. It is metabolized by the liver and excreted predominantly in the urine (66%) and feces (28%). Dosing recommendations for the treatment of nonvalvular atrial fibrillation are as follows: 20 mg once daily with meals for a CrCl of greater than 50 mL/min, and 10 mg once daily with meals for a CrCl between 15 and 50 mL/min. For the treatment of VTE, and to prevent VTE recurrence, rivaroxaban is dosed as 15 mg every 12 hours for 21 days, followed by 20 mg once daily for at least 3 months [31].

Perioperatively, rivaroxaban has been shown to have similar rates of thromboembolic events when compared with warfarin. The ROCKET AF trial compared rivaroxaban with warfarin for the treatment of nonvalvular atrial fibrillation in which patients had temporary interruptions in anticoagulation. The results showed similar thromboembolic risk and similar major bleeding risk between patients experiencing temporary interruptions in anticoagulation with rivaroxaban versus warfarin [32]. The EINSTEIN studies compared the use of rivaroxaban versus LMWH followed by warfarin for the treatment of VTE. The results were significant for similar thromboembolic rates with a decrease in major bleeding events, most noticeably intracranial bleeding [33].

Based on its short half-life, rivaroxaban may be discontinued 48 hours before surgical interventions with a high risk of bleeding, assuming normal renal function, and be restarted postoperatively as soon as hemostasis is ensured. If moderate to severe renal impairment is present, rivaroxaban should be discontinued 72 to 96 hours preoperatively. Given its rapid onset of action and short life, bridging therapy is typically not indicated.

Although rivaroxaban may prolong the prothrombin time and the activated partial thromboplastin time, the most accurate measure of rivaroxaban activity is a calibrated anti-Xa assay, which can exclude clinically significant levels of circulating rivaroxaban [34].

In patients on rivaroxaban with clinically relevant or major bleeding, or needing to undergo an emergent surgical procedure, recombinant coagulation factor Xa (Andexxa) may be used to reverse the effects of rivaroxaban. Approved by the FDA in May of 2018, recombinant coagulation factor Xa is a recombinant coagulation factor Xa shown to reduce anti-factor Xa activity by 97% in those receiving rivaroxaban 20 mg once daily, compared with an 18% decrease in the placebo group. This reversal was noted to take effect within 2 to 5 minutes of an recombinant coagulation factor Xa bolus. This reversal activity persisted for 1 to 2 hours after completion of the infusion, and was associated with restored thrombin generation previously inhibited by treatment with rivaroxaban. No serious or severe adverse events occurred, and no thrombotic events were reported in this randomized, double-blind, placebo-controlled trial [35].

Two dosing regimens for recombinant coagulation factor Xa are approved based on the direct factor Xa inhibitor administered, the dosing, and the time of last dose administered (Table 4). The low-dose regimen consists of an initial IV bolus of 400 mg at 30 mg/min, followed by an infusion of 4 mg/min for up to 120 minutes. The high-dose regimen consists of an initial IV bolus of 800 mg at 30 mg/min, followed by an infusion of 8 mg/min for up to 120 minutes. If a rivaroxaban dose of greater than 10 mg was administered within the last 8 hours, the high-dose regimen should be administered. Otherwise, for rivaroxaban 10 mg or less, the low-dose regimen should be administered [36].

Apixaban

Apixaban (Eliquis) is also an oral direct factor Xa inhibitor and works by the same mechanism as rivaroxaban. It is available as an oral formulary with a

Table 4
Oral anticoagulant summary

Oral anticoagulant		Dosing	Perioperative management	Reversal agent	Reversal dosing
Warfarin					
MOA	VKA, inhibits coagulation factor production	Daily dosing titrated to specific INR goal: INR 2–3 (VTE, atrial fibrillation) INR 2.5–3.5 (prosthetic valve)	Hold 4–5 d preoperatively, check INR Resume immediately postoperatively if hemostasis achieved May require bridging agent if high or very high thromboembolic risk given long onset of action	Minor bleeding or planned surgery: Hold dose(s), vitamin K PO Major bleeding or emergent surgery: PCC or FFP	INR ≥1.5 but <1.9: 1 mg PO INR >1.9 but ≤5.0: 1–2.5 mg PO INR >5.0 but ≤9.0: 2.5–5 mg PO INR >9.0: 2.5–5 mg PO and 2 U FFP 4 units FFP, vitamin K 10 mg IV slow infusion, repeat PRN
Half-life	36–42 h				
Time of onset	3–5 d				
Clearance	Renal				
Dabigatran (Pradaxa)					
MOA	Direct thrombin inhibitor	CrCl >30 mL/min: 150 mg BID CrCl 15–30 mL/min: 75 mg BID	Hold 2–3 d preoperatively if normal renal function, 3–4 d if moderate to severe renal impairment Resume postoperatively once safe to resume therapeutic anticoagulation Bridging only required if patient to remain NPO and moderate to high risk of TE	Idarucizumab (Praxbind) Effect within minutes, therapeutic ~6 h Indicated for major bleeding or emergent surgery	5 mg IV via 2.5 mg IV infusions ×2
Half-life	12–17 h				
Time of onset	1–2 h				
Clearance	Renal				

(continued on next page)

Table 4
(*continued*)

Oral anticoagulant		Dosing	Perioperative management	Reversal agent	Reversal dosing
Rivaroxaban (Xarelto)					
MOA	Direct factor Xa inhibitor	Atrial fibrillation: CrCl >50 mL/min: 20 mg/d CrCl 15–50 mL/min: 10 mg daily VTE: 15 mg BID ×21 d, then 20 mg/d for ≥3 mo	Hold 2 d preoperatively if normal renal function, 3–4 d if moderate to severe renal impairment Resume postoperatively once safe to resume therapeutic anticoagulation Bridging only required if patient to remain NPO and moderate to high risk of TE	Recombinant coagulation factor Xa (Andexxa) Effect within 2–5 min, therapeutic 1–2 h Indicated for major bleeding or emergent surgery	If rivaroxaban 20 mg and taken within last 8 h: 800 mg IV bolus at 30 mg/min, followed by 8 mg/min infusion for up to 120 min If rivaroxaban 10 mg: 400 mg IV bolus at 30 mg/min, followed by 4 mg/min for up to 120 min
Half-life	5–9 h				
Time of onset	2–4 h				
Clearance	66% Renal 28% Fecal				

Apixaban (Eliquis)					
MOA	Direct factor Xa inhibitor	Atrial fibrillation: 5 mg BID 2.5 mg BID if ≥2 of following: >80 years old Cr >1.5 mg/dL Weight <60 kg VTE 10 mg BID ×7 d, then 5 mg BID 2.5 mg BID after 6 mo of treatment for recurrence prophylaxis	Hold 1–2 d preoperatively if normal renal function, 3–4 d if moderate to severe renal impairment Resume postoperatively once safe to resume therapeutic anticoagulation Bridging only required if patient to remain NPO and moderate to high risk of TE	Recombinant coagulation Factor Xa (Andexxa) Effect within 2–5 min, therapeutic 1–2 h Indicated for major bleeding or emergent surgery	If apixaban 10 mg and taken within last 8 h: 800 mg IV bolus at 30 mg/min, followed by 8 mg/min infusion for up to 120 min If apixaban <10 mg: 400 mg IV bolus at 30 mg/min, followed by 4 mg/min for up to 120 min
Half-life	12 h				
Time of onset	3–4 h				
Clearance	27% renal				

Abbreviations: BID, 2 times per day; MOA, mechanism of action; NPO, nil per os; PO, orally; PRN, as needed.

Data from Refs [20–22,25,29–31,35–37].

longer absorption time than that of rivaroxaban, reaching peak plasma levels in 3 to 4 hours with a half-life of 12 hours. Like rivaroxaban, apixaban is metabolized by the liver; unlike rivaroxaban, renal excretion accounts for only 27% of the total drug clearance [37].

For the treatment of nonvalvular atrial fibrillation, 5 mg twice daily dosing has been shown to reduce the risk of ischemic stroke and systemic embolization. However, if the patient has at least 2 of the following characteristics, 2.5 mg twice daily dosing is recommended with the same risk reduction: older than 80 years of age, serum creatinine greater than 1.5 mg/dL, or body weight less than 60 kg [37].

Treatment of VTE is successfully achieved with a 10 mg twice daily dosing for 7 days, followed by 5 mg twice daily dosing for the remainder of the treatment period. Dosing reduction for the aforementioned patient characteristics is not indicated in the treatment of VTE. After a 6-month treatment period, 2.5 mg twice daily dosing can be continued for reduction in the risk of recurrent VTE [37].

Apixaban is also indicated for deep vein thrombosis prophylaxis after hip or knee replacement surgery. Appropriate dosing is as follows: 2.5 mg twice daily for 35 days starting 12 to 24 hours after hip replacement surgery, or 2.5 mg twice daily dosing for 12 days starting 12 to 24 hours after knee replacement surgery [37].

The ARISTOTLE study compared patients with nonvalvular atrial fibrillation treated with apixaban versus warfarin, and found that apixaban was both noninferior and superior to warfarin in thromboembolic risk reduction, with decreased rates of major bleeding events and overall decreased rate of overall mortality [38]. This study excluded patients with end-stage renal disease who are dialysis dependent, a patient population for which many physicians reduce the apixaban dose owing to renal impairment. A retrospective cohort study of 25,523 patients with dialysis-dependent -stage renal disease and atrial fibrillation treated with apixaban or warfarin showed that the standard 5 mg twice daily dosing was associated with a significantly lower risk of thromboembolic events, lower rates of death, and lower risk of major bleeding than both the reduced-dose apixaban and warfarin cohorts [39].

The perioperative management of anticoagulation interruption for patients on apixaban is very similar to that of rivaroxaban owing to its similarly short half-life. Apixaban may be discontinued 24 to 48 hours before surgical interventions with a high risk of bleeding, assuming normal renal function, and be restarted postoperatively as soon as hemostasis is ensured. If moderate to severe renal impairment is present, rivaroxaban should be discontinued 72 to 96 hours preoperatively. Given its rapid onset of action and short life, bridging therapy is typically not indicated. Data from the ARISTOTLE study show that 38% of patients did not stop apixaban before their procedure, and the postprocedure stroke and major bleeding rates were similar to those that did interrupt apixaban therapy. Thus, in low bleeding risk procedures, such as dental extractions and skin lesion excisions, apixaban may be safely continued [40].

Recombinant coagulation factor Xa is also FDA approved for the reversal of apixaban in settings of life-threatening or uncontrolled bleeding. Recombinant coagulation factor Xa was shown to reduce antifactor Xa activity by 92% in those receiving apixaban, similar to the reduction seen in patients taking rivaroxaban [35]. The low-dose and high-dose regimens apply to apixaban as well (see Table 4), with the high-dose regimen reserved only for patients taking more than 5 mg of apixaban per dose with the last administration within 8 hours [36].

FUTURE DIRECTIONS

Although there is convincing evidence to support the use of DOACs as opposed to warfarin for the treatment of VTE and atrial fibrillation, there is a lack of clinical data that directly compare the different DOACs in the perioperative setting. Additionally, the perioperative management of DOACs is largely based on the pharmacokinetics of each agent; however, these recommendations have yet to be validated by clinical trials. The Perioperative Anticoagulant Use for Surgery Evaluation (PAUSE) study is a proposed prospective study designed to develop and assess a standardized protocol for perioperative DOAC management that remains patient-specific [41]. Studies such as the PAUSE study have the potential to remove some of the guess work surgeons use when planning to operate on the increasing number of patients on anticoagulation therapy. And with the recent approval of very high cost reversal agents for many of the DOACs, there is a significant need to validate their efficacy in real-world clinical settings, particularly as the use of these agents become more widely adopted.

SUMMARY

With the advent of DOACs as mainstay anticoagulation therapy for a significant proportion of patients, perioperative anticoagulation management has become an increasingly challenging endeavor for many surgeons. A thorough assessment of the thromboembolic and bleeding risks is critical in navigating these patients safely through the perioperative period. The increasing use of DOACs makes it mandatory for all surgeons to become familiar with the characteristics of each agent. Several DOAC reversal agents are currently available, albeit at a very high cost. Although this article discusses general strategies to help balance the thromboembolic risks associated with interruption in anticoagulation therapy with the risks of bleeding if therapy is continued, there is clearly a need for further studies to help standardize perioperative anticoagulation management that can still be tailored to meet individual patients' needs.

References

[1] January CT, Wann LS, Alpert JS, et al. 2014 AHA/ACC/HRS guideline for the management of patients with atrial fibrillation: a report of the American College of Cardiology/American Heart Association Task Force on practice guidelines and the Heart Rhythm Society. Circulation 2014;130(23):e199–267.

[2] Kearon C, Akl EA, Ornelas J, et al. Antithrombotic therapy for VTE disease. Chest 2016;149(2):315–52.
[3] Douketis JD, Spyropoulos AC, Spencer FA, et al. Perioperative management of antithrombotic therapy: antithrombotic therapy and prevention of thrombosis, 9th ed: American College of Chest Physicians evidence-based clinical practice guidelines. Chest 2012;141(2): e326S–50S.
[4] Lip GY, Nieuwlaat R, Pisters R, et al. Refining clinical risk stratification for predicting stroke and thromboembolism in atrial fibrillation using a novel risk factor-based approach: the Euro Heart Survey on Atrial Fibrillation. Chest 2010;137(2):263–72.
[5] Schulman S, Angerås U, Bergqvist D, et al. Definition of major bleeding in clinical investigations of antihemostatic medicinal products in surgical patients. J Thromb Haemost 2010;8(1):202–4.
[6] Mehran R, Rao SV, Bhatt DL, et al. Standardized bleeding definitions for cardiovascular clinical trials: a consensus report from the Bleeding Academic Research Consortium. Circulation 2011;123(23):2736–47.
[7] Pisters R, Lane DA, Nieuwlaat R, et al. A novel user-friendly score (HAS-BLED) to assess 1-year risk of major bleeding in patients with atrial fibrillation: the Euro Heart Survey. Chest 2010;138(5):1093–100.
[8] Gage BF, Yan Y, Milligan PE, et al. Clinical classification schemes for predicting hemorrhage: results from the National Registry of Atrial Fibrillation (NRAF). Am Heart J 2006;151(3):713–9.
[9] Fang MC, Go AS, Chang Y, et al. A new risk scheme to predict warfarin-associated hemorrhage: the ATRIA (Anticoagulation and Risk Factors in Atrial Fibrillation) Study. J Am Coll Cardiol 2011;58(4):395–401.
[10] Apostolakis S, Lane DA, Guo Y, et al. Performance of the HEMORR2HAGES, ATRIA, and HAS-BLED bleeding risk–prediction scores in patients with atrial fibrillation undergoing anticoagulation: the AMADEUS (evaluating the use of SR34006 compared to warfarin or acenocoumarol in patients with atrial fibrillation) study. J Am Coll Cardiol 2012;60(9):861–7.
[11] Omran HB, Bauersachs R, Rübenacker S, et al. The HAS-BLED score predicts bleedings during bridging of chronic oral anticoagulation. Thromb Haemost 2012;108(07):65–73.
[12] Gorman EW, Perkel D, Dennis D, et al. Validation of the HAS-BLED tool in atrial fibrillation patients receiving rivaroxaban. J Atr Fibrillation 2016;9(2):1461.
[13] Zulkifly H, Lip GYH, Lane DA. Bleeding risk scores in atrial fibrillation and venous thromboembolism. Am J Cardiol 2017;120(7):1139–45.
[14] Hostler DC, Marx ES, Moores LK, et al. Validation of the international medical prevention registry on venous thromboembolism bleeding risk score. Chest 2016;149(2):372–9.
[15] Kearon C, Akl EA, Comerota AJ, et al. Antithrombotic therapy for VTE disease: antithrombotic therapy and prevention of thrombosis, 9th ed: American College of Chest Physicians evidence-based clinical practice guidelines. Chest 2012;141(2, Supplement):e419S–96S.
[16] Douketis JD, Spyropoulos AC, Kaatz S, et al. Perioperative bridging anticoagulation in patients with atrial fibrillation. N Engl J Med 2015;373(9):823–33.
[17] Siegal D, Yudin J, Kaatz S, et al. Periprocedural heparin bridging in patients receiving vitamin K antagonists. Circulation 2012;126(13):1630–9.
[18] Beyer-Westendorf J, Gelbricht V, Förster K, et al. Peri-interventional management of novel oral anticoagulants in daily care: results from the prospective Dresden NOAC registry. Eur Heart J 2014;35(28):1888–96.
[19] Zhu J, Alexander GC, Nazarian S, et al. Trends and variation in oral anticoagulant choice in patients with atrial fibrillation, 2010–2017. Pharmacotherapy 2018;38(9):907–20.
[20] White RH, McKittrick T, Hutchinson R, et al. Temporary discontinuation of warfarin therapy: changes in the international normalized ratio. Ann Intern Med 1995;122(1):40–2.
[21] Ansell J, Hirsh J, Hylek E, et al. Pharmacology and management of the vitamin K antagonists: American College of Chest Physicians evidence-based clinical practice guidelines (8th Edition). Chest 2008;133(6):160S–98S.

[22] Lubetsky A, Yonath H, Olchovsky D, et al. Comparison of oral vs intravenous phytonadione (vitamin k1) in patients with excessive anticoagulation: a prospective randomized controlled study. Arch Intern Med 2003;163(20):2469–73.
[23] Ageno W, Garcia D, Aguilar MI, et al. Prevention and treatment of bleeding complications in patients receiving vitamin K antagonists, part 2: treatment. Am J Hematol 2009;84(9): 584–8.
[24] Chai-Adisaksopha C, Hillis C, Siegal DM, et al. Prothrombin complex concentrates versus fresh frozen plasma for warfarin reversal A systematic review and meta-analysis. Thromb Haemost 2016;116(11):879–90.
[25] **Pradaxa (dabigatran etexilate mesylate)** [package insert]. Ridgefield (CT): Boehringer Ingelheim Pharmaceuticals, Inc.; 2010.
[26] Healey JS, Eikelboom J, Douketis J, et al. Periprocedural bleeding and thromboembolic events with dabigatran compared with warfarin: results from the randomized evaluation of long-term anticoagulation therapy (RE-LY) randomized trial. Circulation 2012;126(3): 343–8.
[27] Schulman S, Carrier M, Lee AY, et al. Perioperative management of dabigatran: a prospective cohort study. Circulation 2015;132(3):167–73.
[28] Samuelson BT, Cuker A. Measurement and reversal of the direct oral anticoagulants. Blood Rev 2017;31(1):77–84.
[29] Pollack CV, Reilly PA, Eikelboom J, et al. Idarucizumab for dabigatran reversal. N Engl J Med 2015;373(6):511–20.
[30] **Praxbind (idarucizumab)** [package insert]. Ridgefield (CT): Boehringer Ingelheim Pharmaceuticals, Inc.; 2015.
[31] **Xarelto (rivaroxaban)** [package insert]. Titusville (NJ): Janssen Pharmaceuticals, Inc.; 2011.
[32] Sherwood MW, Douketis JD, Patel MR, et al. Outcomes of temporary interruption of rivaroxaban compared with warfarin in patients with nonvalvular atrial fibrillation. Circulation 2014;129(18):1850–9.
[33] Investigators TE. Oral rivaroxaban for symptomatic venous thromboembolism. N Engl J Med 2010;363(26):2499–510.
[34] Samama MM, Contant G, Spiro TE, et al. Laboratory assessment of rivaroxaban: a review. Thromb J 2013;11(1):11.
[35] Siegal DM, Curnutte JT, Connolly SJ, et al. Andexanet alfa for the reversal of factor Xa inhibitor activity. N Engl J Med 2015;373(25):2413–24.
[36] **Andexxa (recombinant coagulation factor Xa)** [package insert]. South San Francisco (CA): Portola Pharmaceuticals, Inc.; 2018.
[37] **Eliquis (apixaban)**. Princeton (NJ): Bristol-Myers Squibb Company & Pfizer Inc; 2012.
[38] Granger CB, Alexander JH, McMurray JJ, et al. Apixaban versus warfarin in patients with atrial fibrillation. N Engl J Med 2011;365(11):981–92.
[39] Siontis KC, Zhang X, Eckard A, et al. Outcomes associated with apixaban use in patients with end-stage kidney disease and atrial fibrillation in the United States. Circulation 2018;138(15):1519–29.
[40] Garcia D, Alexander JH, Wallentin L, et al. Management and clinical outcomes in patients treated with apixaban vs warfarin undergoing procedures. Blood 2014;124(25):3692–8.
[41] Douketis JD, Spyropoulos AC, Anderson JM, et al. The perioperative anticoagulant use for surgery evaluation (PAUSE) Study for patients on a direct oral anticoagulant who need an elective surgery or procedure: design and rationale. Thromb Haemost 2017;117(12): 2415–24.

Advances in Surgery 53 (2019) 253–269

ADVANCES IN SURGERY

Status of 5-Year Survivors of the Whipple Procedure for Pancreatic Adenocarcinoma

Winta T. Mehtsun, MD, MPH, Daniel A. Hashimoto, MD, MS, Cristina R. Ferrone, MD*

Department of Surgery, Massachusetts General Hospital, 15 Parkman Street, WAC 460, Boston, MA 02114, USA

Keywords

• Pancreatic cancer • 5-year survivors • Whipple procedures • Neoadjuvant therapy • Adjuvant therapy

Key points

- 5-year survival among pancreatic cancer patients remains dismal at less than 8%.
- Operative resection continues to offer the best chance for long-term survival, yet fewer than 30% of pancreatic cancer patients present early enough to be deemed resectable at diagnosis.
- Few patients are surgical candidates, and even their 5-year survival rate is only 15% to 20%.
- Factors associated with 5-year survival in multivariate analysis include tumor size, tumor grade, lymph node status (number of nodes and ratio), and negative resection margins.

INTRODUCTION

Incidence and Epidemiology of Disease

Despite advances in other solid tumor cancers, pancreatic cancer remains among the most lethal cancer in the United States, with a 5-year survival that is still less than 8% [1]. Although the incidence of other cancers appears to be decreasing, the incidence of pancreatic cancer appears to be on the rise, with an estimated 88,000 new cases annually. Furthermore, projections suggest it will be the second leading cause of cancer-related deaths by 2030 [2].

Disclosure Statement: No financial disclosures.

*Corresponding author. *E-mail address:* cferrone@mgh.harvard.edu

https://doi.org/10.1016/j.yasu.2019.04.012

BRIEF HISTORY OF TREATMENT MODALITIES AND EVOLUTION OF THERAPY

Surgical resection and perioperative mortality/morbidity

Operative resection continues to offer the best chance for long-term survival. Although expansion of multimodal therapy has improved survival in certain cohorts, fewer than 30% of pancreatic cancer patients present early enough to be deemed resectable at diagnosis, both because of the asymptomatic nature of early disease and lack of effective screening tests. Few patients are surgical candidates, yet even their 5-year survival rate is only 15% to 20% [3].

Pancreatic resection has evolved since its first appearance in the early twentieth century ,with advances in technique and perioperative care leading to improvements in perioperative morbidity and mortality (Fig. 1).

Substantial decreases in morbidity and mortality for the Whipple procedure (pancreaticoduodenectomy) began in the 1990s with perioperative mortality in the United States now estimated to be less than 5% [4]. Evidence-based efforts at standardization of perioperative care for Whipple patients contributed to centers of excellence [4–7], while improved understanding of the volume outcome relationship for the Whipple procedure [4–7] has led to relatively unanimous consensus that it should be restricted to high-volume centers [8]. Thus improvement in the perioperative mortality is multifactorial and likely because of the standardization of perioperative care, the development of tertiary care centers with multidisciplinary teams, and the increasing specialization of surgeons [9]. Combined, these efforts have led to the pancreaticoduodenectomy becoming the standard of care for all resectable pancreatic adenocarcinomas, with a mortality rate of less than 3% at high-volume centers [10].

Operative techniques for head of pancreas cancer include the standard pancreaticoduodenectomy (Whipple procedure) and pylorus-preserving pancreaticoduodenectomy. Extended retroperitoneal lymphadenectomy and superior

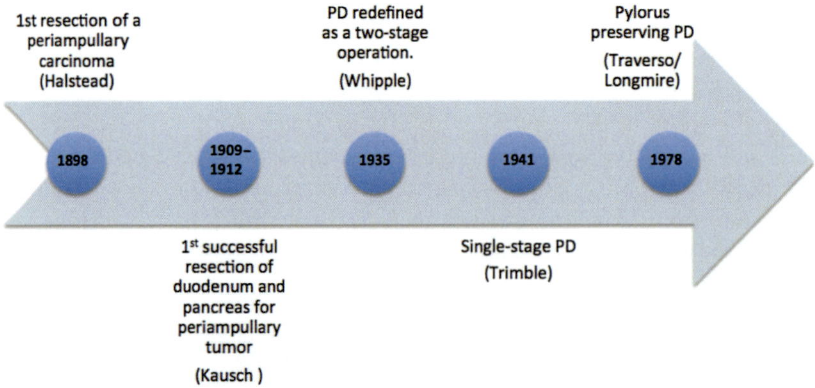

Fig. 1. Evolution of pancreaticoduodenectomy. PD, pancreaticoduodenectomy.

mesenteric vein and/or portal vein resection have recently been evaluated for maximal surgical clearance of disease, yet studies have not reliably confirmed their superiority [11–13].

Leach and colleagues [14] found no survival difference between those patients who require venous resection during pancreaticoduodenectomy for isolated tumor extension to the superior mesenteric vein (SMV) or superior mesenteric portal vein (SMPV) confluence and those who undergo standard pancreaticoduodenectomy.

The type of pancreatic anastomosis has also been examined, including pancreaticojejunostomy versus pancreaticogastrostomy, again without robust evidence supporting one over the other [15–18]. Several institutions have reported their results for laparoscopic or robotic pancreatic resection with comparable results to open resection [19–22]. However, widespread uptake of minimally invasive approaches has still not been achieved because of the complexity of the procedure and the lack of clear benefit.

Although the perioperative mortality for pancreaticoduodenectomy has dropped drastically in recent times, the morbidity rate remains between 30% and 50% [23,24]. Pancreatic fistula continues to be the most serious complication after pancreaticoduodenectomy and occurs in up to 20% of patients, while other major complications include delayed gastric emptying and hemorrhage [23]. A current study using ACS National Surgical Quality Improvement Program (ACS-NSQIP) data found that patients undergoing pancreatic resection are at high risk of complications, Parikh and colleagues [25] found 32% of all resected patients experienced at least 1 complication, and 21% of all complications were considered serious. Using ACS-NSQIP and the National Cancer Data Bank, Merkow and colleagues [26] similarly found that among stage I-III pancreatic adenocarcinoma patients who underwent resection, serious complications were associated with not receiving adjuvant therapy (odds ratio [OR] = 2.20, 95% confidence interval [CI]: 1.73–2.80) and also doubled the likelihood of delaying adjuvant treatment (OR = 2.08, 95% CI: 1.42–3.05). A retrospective institutional study by Ayoma and colleagues also demonstrated that the occurrence of postoperative complications was an independent risk factor for overall survival [27]. The authors anticipate that over the next 2 decades, gains in morbidity will start to mirror those made in mortality, as perioperative care evolves and tertiary care centers with multidisciplinary teams invest more in prevention and early recognition of complications following pancreatic resection.

Neoadjuvant and adjuvant therapy for resectable disease

Both preclinical and clinical data have demonstrated that pancreatic cancer is a systemic disease, and an operation alone will not be a successful strategy for eliminating microscopic disease. Therefore, practice guidelines universally recommend systemic therapy for all stages of pancreatic cancer. This article will limit its summary of therapies to resectable disease, as the focus of this article is on 5-year survivors of the Whipple procedure.

Key adjuvant trials in pancreatic cancer

The survival benefit of adjuvant therapy was established by 3 randomized controlled trials (GITSG [28], RTOG-9704 [29], and CONKO-001 [30]) (Table 1):

- The GITSG trial demonstrated that adjuvant 5-FU-based chemotherapy plus radiotherapy followed by 2 years of 5-FU had a 21-month survival versus 10 months with observation alone ($P = .03$; see Table 1).
- The RTOG-9704 trial compared gemcitabine with fluorouracil before and after fluorouracil-based chemoradiation. In an updated analysis of this trial, the treatment arms did not differ significantly.
- The CONKO-001 trial demonstrated an improvement in survival with 6 months of adjuvant gemcitabine chemotherapy versus observation after surgical resection (median 22.8 months vs 20.2 months; $P = .01$).

Addition of radiation to adjuvant chemotherapy is controversial since it has only demonstrated an improvement in local control, but not overall survival.

- ESPAC-1 trial: 289 patients were randomly (2X2) assigned after resection into 4 different arms: 1) chemoradiotherapy, 2) chemotherapy, 3) chemoradiotherapy followed by chemotherapy, or 4) observation only
- Improvement in survival with adjuvant 5-FU chemotherapy (chemotherapy only and chemoradiotherapy plus chemotherapy groups combined) compared with the observation plus the chemoradiotherapy only groups (median 20.1 months vs 15.5 months; $P=.009$)
- The use of chemoradiation was detrimental according to this study (median survival of 15.9 months for all patients treated in the chemoradiotherapy groups vs 17.9 months in the observation and chemotherapy only groups combined; $P=.05$)
- Trial had limitations with respect to its design and variability in radiation delivery

Table 1
Survival benefit of adjuvant trials

Trial	Patients (N)	Control Arm	Experimental Arm	Median Survival (months)	*P*-value
GITSG (1985) [28]	43	Observation	5-FU plus XRT, followed by 5-FU maintenance therapy	11 vs 21	.03
RTOG-9704 [29]	551	XRT/5-FU + 5- Gemcitabine	XRT/5-FU + 5- Gemcitabine	20 vs 17	.09
CONKO-001 (2013) [30]	368	Observation	Gemcitabine	20.2 vs 22.8	.005
ESPAC-3 [31]	1088	5-FU	Gemcitabine	23 vs 24	.39
ESPAC-4 [32]	730	Gemcitabine	Gemcitabine + capecitabine	25.5 vs 28.0	.032

- Survival benefit associated with bolus 5-FU chemotherapy compared with observation in patients with resected pancreatic cancer

The median survival duration observed with 5-FU chemotherapy in the meta-analysis of the ESPAC-1 and ESPAC-3 data was similar to the median survival associated with gemcitabine treatment in the CONKO-001 study (median 23.2 months vs 22.8 months; see Table 1).

The combination of gemcitabine and capecitabine represents a potential new standard of care following resection for pancreatic ductal adenocarcinoma from the recent results of the ESPAC-4 trial.

NEOADJUVANT THERAPY IN PANCREATIC CANCER

Neoadjuvant therapy is becoming more common for many cancers as better treatments are developed. For cancers that require large operations associated with significant morbidity and mortality, neoadjuvant therapy is especially attractive. By administering neoadjuvant therapy, the biology of the disease can be better understood, and a potentially futile operation can be avoided [33]. Also, because of the significant morbidity of pancreatic resections, up to one-third of patients will not receive adjuvant therapy [33].

The longest-standing neoadjuvant treatment for patients with PDAC is chemoradiotherapy. Photon therapy with 50.4 Gy is utilized to potentially downsize cancers that are deemed borderline or locally advanced in an attempt to get patients to resection [34]. At MD Anderson, Katz and colleagues [35] reported a median overall survival of 23.9 months in 329 patients with PDAC, of whom 91% received neoadjuvant therapy. Neoadjuvant therapy consisted of chemoradiotherapy and isolated chemotherapy. External-beam radiotherapy usually consisted of 50.4 Gy in 28 fractions or 30 Gy in 10 fractions. Concomitant chemotherapy consisted of 5-fluorouracil, paclitaxel, gemcitabine, or capecitabine at radiosensitizing doses. Chemotherapy, in isolation, consisted of gemcitabine alone or in combination. They found that 27% of these patients survived a minimum of 5 years with a median survival of 11 years [35]. Currently Phase III trials comparing neoadjuvant chemotherapy and chemoradiation to upfront resection for resectable PDAC are underway.

Otherwise, the majority of the literature on neoadjuvant therapy consists of observational studies of patients with locally advanced disease [36–40]. A meta-analysis of the efficacy of neoadjuvant therapy (either chemo- or radiotherapy or both) analyzed 111 prospective studies encompassing 4394 patients. Results were notable for a median survival of 22.4 months in patients who underwent neoadjuvant therapy and resection versus 9.5 months for those who underwent therapy, but did not ultimately undergo resection [41].

Currently multiple neoadjuvant studies are underway in both the United States and Europe to assess the efficacy of neoadjuvant therapy utilizing FOLFIRINOX or gemcitabine/abraxane. Patients with metastatic disease demonstrated a significant overall survival advantage in phase III trials [42–44]. Because of the encouraging results in the metastatic setting, patients with locally advanced and borderline resectable disease have also been treated with these regimens. At the Massachusetts General Hospital, 141 locally advanced and borderline resectable patients who received neoadjuvant FOFIRINOX followed by chemoradiation were compared with 110 upfront resectable patients who received no neoadjuvant therapy [45]. Although the operations were longer and the blood loss higher in the neoadjuvant group, the morbidity and mortality were not significantly different between the 2 cohorts. Furthermore, the patients who received neoadjuvant therapy had a higher R0 resection rate and a significantly lower rate of lymph node positivity and perineural invasion, despite being diagnosed at a more advanced stage. The median overall survival of the neoadjuvant group was 37.7 months, which was significantly longer than the 25.1 months for the upfront resectable patients [45].

Improved understanding of and experience with neoadjuvant therapy may help to improve the risk stratification of patients with PDAC, with the goal of optimizing the therapeutic regimen for patients.

FIVE-YEAR SURVIVORS – A SUMMARY OF CURRENT EVIDENCE

Early studies failed to demonstrate any survivors 5 years after Whipple [46,47].

Over the last 30 years, long-term survival following an operation has improved, yet remains dismal; median survival ranges from 13 to 27 months, and 5-year survival ranges from 4% to 27% following resection (Table 2). As highlighted previously, the advent of multimodal therapy, advances in preoperative staging, and the importance of an R0 resection have evolved over this same time period, limiting the application of older studies to the current era of treatment for pancreatic cancer.

INDEPENDENT PREDICTORS OF 5-YEAR SURVIVAL

Patient Factors

Patients undergoing the Whipple procedure for pancreatic adenocarcinoma today are older and have more preoperative comorbidities compared with patients 30 years ago. A population-based study using Surveillance, Epidemiology, and End Results (SEER) Medicare data identified 2461 patients with resected pancreatic adenocarcinoma from 1991 to 2005 and found that the mean age of patients undergoing an operation increased over time (for 1991–1996, mean age 72.1 years vs for 2003–2005, mean age 74.0 years; $P<.001$). Furthermore, only 10.4% (n = 59) of patients undergoing a pancreatic operation from 1991 to 1996 had at least 3 preoperative medical comorbidities, compared with 26.0% (n = 222) of patients undergoing an operation between 2003 and 2005 ($P<.001$) [60]. Despite this trend, most 5-year survival studies have not identified patient factors associated with increased survival. Winter and colleagues identified chronic obstructive pulmonary disease (COPD) as the only patient factor negatively associated with survival on multivariate analysis (hazard ratio [HR]: 2.0, $P=.006$), but this has not been reproduced in other studies. The presence of extensive comorbidities or increased patient age has not correlated with decreased long-term survival following the Whipple

Table 2
Studies examining 5-year survivors of pancreatic adenocarcinoma

Study	Period	Patients	Median Survival (months)	5-year Survival Rate (%)	Univariate Factors Associated with Survival	Multivariate Factors Associated with Survival
Conlon et al, [48] 1996	1983–1989	118	14.3	10.2	• N/A	• N/A
Ahmad et al, [49] 2001	1990–1998	116	16.0	19.0	• No lymph node involvement • Adjuvant chemoradiotherapy	• Adjuvant chemoradi-otherapy
Cleary et al, [50] 2004	1988–1996	123	13.6	14.6	• Tumor size • No jaundice at presentation • No lymph node involvement • Tumor grade • AJCC stage	• AJCC stage • Tumor grade
Winter et al, [10] 2006	1970–2006	1175	18.0	18.0	• No history of DM • No history of COPD • Age <65 y • No blood transfusions • Tumor diameter <3 cm • No lymph node involvement • Negative margins • Well/moderately differentiated tumor • No postoperative pneumonia • No postoperative sepsis • No postoperative bile leak • Adjuvant therapy	• Tumor diameter <3 cm • No lymph node involvement • Negative margins • Well/moderately differentiated tumor • No COPD • No postoperative bile leak • Adjuvant therapy

(*continued on next page*)

Table 2
(*continued*)

Study	Period	Patients	Median Survival (months)	5-year Survival Rate (%)	Univariate Factors Associated with Survival	Multivariate Factors Associated with Survival
Han et al, [51] 2006	1985–1999	123	14.8	12.1	• No lymph node involvement • AJCC stage	• AJCC stage • Resection margin
Howard et al, [52] 2006	1990–2002	226	13.0	4.0	• Age • Tumor size • Tumor differentiation • Negative margin	• Tumor size • Tumor differentiation • Negative margin • No postoperative complications
Cameron et al, [53] 2006	1969–2003	405*	33.0*	18.0	• Not applicable (N/A)	• N/A
Ferrone et al, [54] 2008	1983–2001	618	-	12.1	• N/A	• AJCC stage • Negative margin
Schnelldorfer et al, [55] 2008	1981–2001	357	17	17.4	• Tumor diameter • No lymph node involvement • Number of positive nodes • Preoperative serum albumin • Perioperative blood transfusion	• No lymph node involvement
Katz et al, [35] 2009	1990–2002	329	23.9	27.0%	• Negative margins • No lymph node involvement • No prior attempt at resection	• No lymph node involvement • No prior attempt at resection
Robinson et al, [56] 2012	2002–2009	134	N/A	18.6	• No lymph node involvement • Metastatic to resected lymph node ratio	• Metastatic to lymph node ratio (>15%) • Presence of perineural invasion

Kimura et al, [57] 2014	1988–2008	147	14.4	12.2	• <2 LN metastases • Preoperative serum CA 19-9 < 40 U/mL • No intrapancreatic nerve invasion • R0 resection	• <2 LN metastases • preoperative serum CA19-9 < 40 U/mL • R0 resection
Yamamoto et al, [58] 2015	2000–2008	96	27.1	34.5 (A)	• UICC stage • Preoperative CA19-9 ≤ 200 U/mL • Preoperative DUPAN-2 ≤ 180 U/mL • Tumor size ≤20 mm • R0 resection • No lymph node involvement • No extrapancreatic neural invasion • Absence of portal invasion	• Tumor size ≤20 mm • Negative surgical margins
Lovecek et al, [59] 2016	2000–2011	90	16.9	18.9	• Absence of perineural invasion • Vascular invasion • Stage • No lymph node involvement • No need for transfusion	• Vascular invasion • Postoperative complications

Data from refs. [10,35,48–54,56–59].

procedure. This may be secondary to selection bias inherent in choosing surgical candidates, as these patients may not have been deemed surgical candidates because of their disease profile or overall functional status.

Tumor pathology (tumor size and tumor grade)

Early studies identified tumor size as a prognostic factor for long-term survival after resection of pancreatic cancer [10,50,51,61]. Small tumors (<2 cm) were found to have improved 5-year survival rate (20%–41%) and median survival time (23–38 months) compared with large tumors, which had a 5-year survival rate of 1% to 20% and median survival time of 10 to 17 months [61]. On a multivariate analysis of factors associated with long-term survival of pancreatic adenocarcinoma patients, Han and colleagues [51] identified tumor-related variables including tumor size (HR 5 1.38, P 5 0.03) and tumor differentiation (HR 5 0.76, P 5 0.02) as covariates affecting long-term survival. A study by the Mayo Clinic examined the histopathological and survival characteristics of small ($\leq$2 cm) pancreatic cancers compared with large pancreatic cancers and found that among patients with localized disease (stages I and II), survival was similar regardless of tumor size. However, survival was significantly better in small pancreatic cancers with regional nodal metastasis (stage III) compared with similar stage large pancreatic cancers (5-year survival 44 vs 7%, median survival 58 vs18 months, $P<.001$). Well-differentiated small and large tumors had similar median survivals (76 vs 74 months, p=NS). In multivariate analysis, tumor differentiation, not tumor size, was the only independent factor predicting survival (risk ratio [RR] for moderate vs well-differentiated: 2.6,95% confidence interval [CI] 1.5–4.5, and RR for poorly differentiated vs well-differentiated: 5.0, 95% CI 2.4–10.1) [62]. After neoadjuvant FOLFIRINOX and chemoradiation, Michelakos and colleagues [45] identified resected PDAC tumors greater than 2.5 cm as an independent predictor of decreased overall survival.

Lymph node status

An increasing body of evidence demonstrates the association between lymph node status and long-term survival in resected pancreatic cancer patients [55–57,63–65]. Konstantinidis and colleagues [65] demonstrated node involvement by metastasis or by direct invasion as an equally significant predictor of reduced survival. Also both the number of positive nodes and the lymph node ratio are prognostic factors, with patients with 1 lymph node positive faring better than those with greater than 1 lymph node positive. Katz and colleagues [35] identified negative lymph node status (odds ratio 1.92, P=.02) as significantly associated with 5-year survival on multivariate analysis. Robinson and colleagues examined 134 patients who underwent pancreaticoduodenectomy for pancreatic ductal adenocarcinoma, 78% of whom had T3 disease. For those patients with T3N0 disease, 5-year survival was 71%, whereas those with T3N1 disease had a 5-year survival of 11.5% ($P<.05$). Furthermore, patients with T3N1 disease and a metastatic-to-resected lymph node ratio less than 15% had an overall 5-year survival of 21%, whereas there were no survivors beyond 40 months in patients with a metastatic-to-resected lymph node ratio greater than 15% (P<.01). Other studies have also suggested that the metastatic-to-resected lymph node ratio may be more discriminatory than just the absence or presence of lymph node involvement in determining long-term survival after surgical resection [63,66].

The number of nodes sampled has ramifications for survival. Huebner and colleagues [64] found that patients with less than 11 lymph nodes sampled with pN0 disease had worse survival outcomes compared with those who had greater than 11 nodes sampled, suggesting metastatic nodes were missed because of understaging. The negative survival impact of sampling fewer than 10 to 12 total nodes has also been demonstrated by other population studies [67,68]. Thus, extended lymphadenectomy has been proposed to improve long-term survival. This includes clearance of nodes up to the hepatic hilum and para-aortic nodes from the diaphragmatic hiatus to the level of the inferior mesenteric arteries. However, several studies, including meta-analyses, have failed to demonstrate any convincing survival advantage with this strategy [11,12].

Resection margins

Achieving negative surgical margins (R0) is arguably one of the most consistently reported prognostic factors associated with long-term survival following resection of pancreatic adenocarcinoma [10,51,52,54,69]. Howard and colleagues [52] found that a margin=negative R0 resection (HR = 1.39, P=.03) was associated with increased survival. The authors' own examination of 5-year survivors also found that R0 resections were significantly associated with long-term survival [54]. Their recent analysis found that R0 resections have an improved survival compared with R1 resections, but this survival benefit is lost when the tumor is within 1 mm of the resection margin [69]. Prior studies have shown that patients who undergo a resection with a macroscopically positive margin have survival comparable to that of patients who do not undergo an operation [70,71].

The high incidence of positive margins and intra- and extrapancreatic neural invasion has provoked some institutions to explore extended pancreatic resection together with vascular resection and retroperitoneal lymphadenectomy. However, many recent prospective studies have demonstrated that extended operations tend to increase morbidity and mortality rates without a survival benefit. A systematic review showed no differences in the survival rate between standard and extended operations, with a trend toward increased morbidity in patients undergoing extended operations [72]. Similarly, Farnell and colleagues [11] found that an extended operation was not associated with a survival benefit but did increase the rates of postoperative morbidity.

CA 19-19 levels

CA19-9 levels are known to correlate with burden of pancreatic cancer [73,74]. In the authors' own work, preoperative CA19-9 correlated with stage of disease in 424 consecutive patients with pancreatic adenocarcinoma who underwent resection. A postoperative decrease in CA19-9 and a postoperative CA19-9 value of less than 200 U/mL were strong independent predictors of survival [75]. Kimura and colleagues also found that preoperative CA 19-9 of less than 40 U/mL was associated with increased 5-year survival [57].

SURVEILLANCE OF LONG-TERM SURVIVORS

Similar to short-term survivors, the goal of surveillance is to optimize the detection of local and distant recurrence with the hope of providing patients with therapeutic options that hold the promise of improved quality of life, survival, and/or cure. In addition, surveillance maintains the relationship between providers and patients so that any progression of disease can be more effectively managed through therapy, palliation, or appropriate initiation of hospice [76].

Recommendations by the National Comprehensive Cancer Network include surveillance history and physical examination along with CA19-9 level and an abdominal computed tomography (CT) scan with contrast every 3 to 6 months for the first 2 years, then every 6 to 12 months thereafter. For patients who recur, treatment considerations differ depending on the nature of the recurrence. Local recurrence within the pancreas only may be amenable to repeat resection; however, treatment for local recurrence within the pancreatic bed can range from chemoradiation to different chemotherapy regimens or palliation. No specific guidelines address recurrence in long-term survivors.

QUALITY-OF-LIFE ENDPOINTS

Most quality-of-life studies in pancreatic cancer patients have been limited to time periods prior to the 5-year survival endpoint [77–79]. Recently, however, Fong and colleagues [80] surveyed 305 patients who were alive 5 years after undergoing a Whipple using a validated quality-of-life instrument. Although some patients underwent a Whipple for pancreatic adenocarcinoma, many of the patients underwent a Whipple for intraductal papillary mucinous neoplasm, pancreatic neuroendocrine tumor, or pancreatic cystic disease. They found that long-term survivors demonstrated better global quality of life and physical- and role-functioning scores at 5-year when compared with age- and gender-matched controls.

FUTURE DIRECTIONS

As genomics, proteomics, and data science provide a better understanding of the biology of pancreatic adenocarcinoma, the proportion of 5-year survivors will increase. Early detection of pancreatic cancer is key to improving patient survival, and new diagnostic modalities such as screening of microRNA [81,82], liquid biopsies for proteomic analysis [83] and other biomarkers [84] may provide enhanced screening capabilities for at-risk patients in the future.

To better identify patients who need screening for pancreatic cancer, patient registries and other large-scale clinical databases will play an increasing role in providing the big data necessary to identify predictors of pancreatic cancer. Advances in statistical analysis, including machine learning techniques, may uncover novel genetic or biologic risk factors, elucidate unexpected clinical predictors of pancreatic cancer, or improve the prediction of patient recovery after resection or chemoradiotherapy [85].

The rapid acceleration of technologies across the basic sciences, computer science, and medicine highlights the importance of rigorous academic investigation of pancreatic cancer and its therapies. The continued dedication of patients, clinicians, and scientists in fighting pancreatic cancer will yield important discoveries that can push the 5-year survivor rate to increasing levels.

References

[1] Siegel RL, Miller KD, Jemal A. Cancer statistics, 2017. CA Cancer J Clin 2017;67(1):7–30.
[2] Rahib L, Smith BD, Aizenberg R, et al. Projecting cancer incidence and deaths to 2030: the unexpected burden of thyroid, liver, and pancreas cancers in the United States. Cancer Res 2014;74(11):2913–21.
[3] Sinn M, Bahra M, Liersch T, et al. CONKO-005: adjuvant chemotherapy with gemcitabine plus erlotinib versus gemcitabine alone in patients after R0 resection of pancreatic cancer: a multicenter randomized phase III trial. J Clin Oncol 2017;35(29):3330–7.
[4] Finks JF, Osborne NH, Birkmeyer JD. Trends in hospital volume and operative mortality for high-risk surgery. N Engl J Med 2011;364(22):2128–37.
[5] Reames BN, Ghaferi AA, Birkmeyer JD, et al. Hospital volume and operative mortality in the modern era. Ann Surg 2014;260(2):244–51.
[6] Birkmeyer JD, Siewers AE, Finlayson EV, et al. Hospital volume and surgical mortality in the United States. N Engl J Med 2002;346(15):1128–37.
[7] Buchler MW, Wagner M, Schmied BM, et al. Changes in morbidity after pancreatic resection: toward the end of completion pancreatectomy. Arch Surg 2003;138(12):1310–4 [discussion: 1315].
[8] Birkmeyer JD. Raising the bar for pancreaticoduodenectomy. Ann Surg Oncol 2002;9(9): 826–7.
[9] Pawlik TM, Laheru D, Hruban RH, et al. Evaluating the impact of a single-day multidisciplinary clinic on the management of pancreatic cancer. Ann Surg Oncol 2008;15(8): 2081–8.
[10] Winter JM, Cameron JL, Campbell KA, et al. 1423 pancreaticoduodenectomies for pancreatic cancer: a single-institution experience. J Gastrointest Surg 2006;10(9):1199–210 [discussion: 1210–1].
[11] Farnell MB, Aranha GV, Nimura Y, et al. The role of extended lymphadenectomy for adenocarcinoma of the head of the pancreas: strength of the evidence. J Gastrointest Surg 2008;12(4):651–6.
[12] Farnell MB, Pearson RK, Sarr MG, et al. A prospective randomized trial comparing standard pancreatoduodenectomy with pancreatoduodenectomy with extended lymphadenectomy in resectable pancreatic head adenocarcinoma. Surgery 2005;138(4):618–28 [discussion: 628–30].
[13] Reddy SK, Tyler DS, Pappas TN, et al. Extended resection for pancreatic adenocarcinoma. Oncologist 2007;12(6):654–63.
[14] Leach SD, Lee JE, Charnsangavej C, et al. Survival following pancreaticoduodenectomy with resection of the superior mesenteric-portal vein confluence for adenocarcinoma of the pancreatic head. Br J Surg 1998;85(5):611–7.
[15] McKay A, Mackenzie S, Sutherland FR, et al. Meta-analysis of pancreaticojejunostomy versus pancreaticogastrostomy reconstruction after pancreaticoduodenectomy. Br J Surg 2006;93(8):929–36.

[16] He T, Zhao Y, Chen Q, et al. Pancreaticojejunostomy versus pancreaticogastrostomy after pancreaticoduodenectomy: a systematic review and meta-analysis. Dig Surg 2013;30(1):56–69.
[17] Guerrini GP, Soliani P, D'Amico G, et al. Pancreaticojejunostomy versus pancreaticogastrostomy after pancreaticoduodenectomy: an up-to-date meta-analysis. J Invest Surg 2016;29(3):175–84.
[18] Cheng Y, Briarava M, Lai M, et al. Pancreaticojejunostomy versus pancreaticogastrostomy reconstruction for the prevention of postoperative pancreatic fistula following pancreaticoduodenectomy. Cochrane Database Syst Rev 2017;(9):CD012257.
[19] Adam MA, Thomas S, Youngwirth L, et al. Defining a hospital volume threshold for minimally invasive pancreaticoduodenectomy in the United States. JAMA Surg 2017;152(4): 336–42.
[20] Kendrick ML. Laparoscopic and robotic resection for pancreatic cancer. Cancer J 2012;18(6):571–6.
[21] Kendrick ML, Cusati D. Total laparoscopic pancreaticoduodenectomy: feasibility and outcome in an early experience. Arch Surg 2010;145(1):19–23.
[22] Zureikat AH, Postlewait LM, Liu Y, et al. A multi-institutional comparison of perioperative outcomes of robotic and open pancreaticoduodenectomy. Ann Surg 2016;264(4):640–9.
[23] Lai EC, Lau SH, Lau WY. Measures to prevent pancreatic fistula after pancreatoduodenectomy: a comprehensive review. Arch Surg 2009;144(11):1074–80.
[24] Kagedan DJ, Goyert N, Li Q, et al. The impact of increasing hospital volume on 90-day postoperative outcomes following pancreaticoduodenectomy. J Gastrointest Surg 2017;21(3): 506–15.
[25] Parikh P, Shiloach M, Cohen ME, et al. Pancreatectomy risk calculator: an ACS-NSQIP resource. HPB (Oxford) 2010;12(7):488–97.
[26] Merkow RP, Bilimoria KY, Tomlinson JS, et al. Postoperative complications reduce adjuvant chemotherapy use in resectable pancreatic cancer. Ann Surg 2014;260(2):372–7.
[27] Aoyama T, Oba K, Honda M, et al. Impact of postoperative complications on the colorectal cancer survival and recurrence: analyses of pooled individual patients' data from three large phase III randomized trials. Cancer Med 2017;6(7):1573–80.
[28] Kalser MH, Ellenberg SS. Pancreatic cancer. Adjuvant combined radiation and chemotherapy following curative resection. Arch Surg 1985;120(8):899–903.
[29] Regine WF, Winter KA, Abrams R, et al. Fluorouracil-based chemoradiation with either gemcitabine or fluorouracil chemotherapy after resection of pancreatic adenocarcinoma: 5-year analysis of the U.S. Intergroup/RTOG 9704 phase III trial. Ann Surg Oncol 2011;18(5):1319–26.
[30] Oettle H, Neuhaus P, Hochhaus A, et al. Adjuvant chemotherapy with gemcitabine and long-term outcomes among patients with resected pancreatic cancer: the CONKO-001 randomized trial. JAMA 2013;310:1473–81.
[31] Neoptolemos JP, Stocken DD, Tudur Smith C, et al. Adjuvant 5-fluorouracil and folinic acid vs observation for pancreatic cancer: composite data from the ESPAC-1 and -3(v1) trials. Br J Cancer 2009;100(2):246–50.
[32] Neoptolemos JP, Palmer DH, Ghaneh P, et al. Comparison of adjuvant gemcitabine and capecitabine with gemcitabine monotherapy in patients with resected pancreatic cancer (ESPAC-4): a multicentre, open-label, randomised, phase 3 trial. Lancet 2017;389(10073): 1011–24.
[33] Hoffman JP. Status of neoadjuvant therapy for resectable pancreatic cancer. Surg Oncol Clin N Am 2010;19(2):411–8.
[34] Evans DB, Rich TA, Byrd DR, et al. Preoperative chemoradiation and pancreaticoduodenectomy for adenocarcinoma of the pancreas. Arch Surg 1992;127(11):1335–9.
[35] Katz MH, Wang H, Fleming JB, et al. Long-term survival after multidisciplinary management of resected pancreatic adenocarcinoma. Ann Surg Oncol 2009;16(4):836–47.

[36] Heinrich S, Pestalozzi BC, Schäfer M, et al. Prospective phase II trial of neoadjuvant chemotherapy with gemcitabine and cisplatin for resectable adenocarcinoma of the pancreatic head. J Clin Oncol 2008;26(15):2526–31.
[37] Palmer DH, Stocken DD, Hewitt H, et al. A randomized phase 2 trial of neoadjuvant chemotherapy in resectable pancreatic cancer: gemcitabine alone versus gemcitabine combined with cisplatin. Ann Surg Oncol 2007;14(7):2088–96.
[38] Patel M, Hoffe S, Malafa M, et al. Neoadjuvant GTX Chemotherapy and IMRT-based chemoradiation for borderline resectable pancreatic cancer. J Surg Oncol 2011;104(2):155–61.
[39] Sahora K, Kuehrer I, Eisenhut A, et al. NeoGemOx: gemcitabine and oxaliplatin as neoadjuvant treatment for locally advanced, nonmetastasized pancreatic cancer. Surgery 2011;149(3):311–20.
[40] White RR, Hurwitz HI, Morse MA, et al. Neoadjuvant chemoradiation for localized adenocarcinoma of the pancreas. Ann Surg Oncol 2001;8(10):758–65.
[41] Gillen S, Schuster T, Zum Büschenfelde CM, et al. Preoperative/neoadjuvant therapy in pancreatic cancer: a systematic review and meta-analysis of response and resection percentages. PLoS Med 2010;7(4):e1000267.
[42] Festa V, Andriulli A, Valvano MR, et al. Neoadjuvant chemo-radiotherapy for patients with borderline resectable pancreatic cancer: a meta-analytical evaluation of prospective studies. JOP 2013;14:618–25.
[43] Von Hoff DD, Ervin T, Arena FP, et al. Increased survival in pancreatic cancer with nab-paclitaxel plus gemcitabine. N Engl J Med 2013;369(18):1691–703.
[44] Vaccaro V, Sperduti I, Milella M. FOLFIRINOX versus gemcitabine for metastatic pancreatic cancer. N Engl J Med 2011;365(8):768–9 [author reply: 769].
[45] Michelakos T, Pergolini I, Castillo CF, et al. Predictors of resectability and survival in patients with borderline and locally advanced pancreatic cancer who underwent neoadjuvant treatment with FOLFIRINOX. Ann Surg 2019;269(4):733–40.
[46] Nitecki SS, Sarr MG, Colby TV, et al. Long-term survival after resection for ductal adenocarcinoma of the pancreas. Is it really improving? Ann Surg 1995;221(1):59–66.
[47] Wade TP, el-Ghazzawy AG, Virgo KS, et al. The Whipple resection for cancer in U.S. Department of Veterans Affairs Hospitals. Ann Surg 1995;221(3):241–8.
[48] Conlon KC, Klimstra DS, Brennan MF. Long-term survival after curative resection for pancreatic ductal adenocarcinoma. Clinicopathologic analysis of 5-year survivors. Ann Surg 1996;223(3):273–9.
[49] Ahmad NA, Lewis JD, Ginsberg GG, et al. Long term survival after pancreatic resection for pancreatic adenocarcinoma. Am J Gastroenterol 2001;96(9):2609–15.
[50] Cleary SP, Gryfe R, Guindi M, et al. Prognostic factors in resected pancreatic adenocarcinoma: analysis of actual 5-year survivors. J Am Coll Surg 2004;198:722–31.
[51] Han SS, Jang JY, Kim SW, et al. Analysis of long-term survivors after surgical resection for pancreatic cancer. Pancreas 2006;32(3):271–5.
[52] Howard TJ, Krug JE, Yu J, et al. A margin-negative R0 resection accomplished with minimal postoperative complications is the surgeon's contribution to long-term survival in pancreatic cancer. J Gastrointest Surg 2006;10(10):1338–45 [discussion: 1345–6].
[53] Cameron JL, Riall TS, Coleman J, et al. One thousand consecutive pancreaticoduodenectomies. Ann Surg 2006;244(1):10–5.
[54] Ferrone CR, Brennan MF, Gonen M, et al. Pancreatic adenocarcinoma: the actual 5-year survivors. J Gastrointest Surg 2008;12:701–6.
[55] Schnelldorfer T, Ware AL, Sarr MG, et al. Long-term survival after pancreatoduodenectomy for pancreatic adenocarcinoma: is cure possible? Ann Surg 2008;247:456–62.
[56] Robinson SM, Rahman A, Haugk B, et al. Metastatic lymph node ratio as an important prognostic factor in pancreatic ductal adenocarcinoma. Eur J Surg Oncol 2012;38(4):333–9.

[57] Kimura K, Amano R, Nakata B, et al. Clinical and pathological features of five-year survivors after pancreatectomy for pancreatic adenocarcinoma. World J Surg Oncol 2014;12(1):360.
[58] Yamamoto T, Yagi S, Kinoshita H, et al. Long-term survival after resection of pancreatic cancer: a single-center retrospective analysis. World J Gastroenterol 2015;21(1):262–8.
[59] Lovecek M, Skalicky P, Klos D, et al. Long-term survival after resections for pancreatic ductal adenocarcinoma. Single centre study. Biomed Pap Med Fac Univ Palacky Olomouc Czech Repub 2016;160(2):280–6.
[60] Mayo SC, Gilson MM, Herman JM, et al. Management of patients with pancreatic adenocarcinoma: national trends in patient selection, operative management, and use of adjuvant therapy. J Am Coll Surg 2012;214(1):33–45.
[61] Pantalone D, Ragionieri I, Nesi G. Improved survival in small pancreatic cancer. Dig Surg 2001;18(1):41–6.
[62] Pongprasobchai S, Pannala R, Smyrk TC, et al. Long-term survival and prognostic indicators in small (<or = 2 cm) pancreatic cancer. Pancreatology 2008;8:587–92.
[63] Riediger H, Keck T, Wellner U, et al. The lymph node ratio is the strongest prognostic factor after resection of pancreatic cancer. J Gastrointest Surg 2009;13(7):1337–44.
[64] Huebner M, Kendrick M, Reid-Lombardo KM, et al. Number of lymph nodes evaluated: prognostic value in pancreatic adenocarcinoma. J Gastrointest Surg 2012;16:920–6.
[65] Konstantinidis IT, Deshpande V, Zheng H, et al. Does the mechanism of lymph node invasion affect survival in patients with pancreatic ductal adenocarcinoma? J Gastrointest Surg 2010;14(2):261–7.
[66] Slidell MB, Chang DC, Cameron JL, et al. Impact of total lymph node count and lymph node ratio on staging and survival after pancreatectomy for pancreatic adenocarcinoma: a large, population-based analysis. Ann Surg Oncol 2008;15(1):165–74.
[67] Schwarz RE, Smith DD. Extent of lymph node retrieval and pancreatic cancer survival: information from a large US population database. Ann Surg Oncol 2006;13(9):1189–200.
[68] Hellan M, Sun CL, Artinyan A, et al. The impact of lymph node number on survival in patients with lymph node-negative pancreatic cancer. Pancreas 2008;37(1):19–24.
[69] Konstantinidis IT, Warshaw AL, Allen JN, et al. Pancreatic ductal adenocarcinoma: is there a survival difference for R1 resections versus locally advanced unresectable tumors? What is a "true" R0 resection? Ann Surg 2013;257(4):731–6.
[70] Gillen S, Schuster T, Friess H, et al. Palliative resections versus palliative bypass procedures in pancreatic cancer–a systematic review. Am J Surg 2012;203(4):496–502.
[71] Chandrasegaram MD, Goldstein D, Simes J, et al. Meta-analysis of radical resection rates and margin assessment in pancreatic cancer. Br J Surg 2015;102(12):1459–72.
[72] Michalski CW, Kleeff J, Wente MN, et al. Systematic review and meta-analysis of standard and extended lymphadenectomy in pancreaticoduodenectomy for pancreatic cancer. Br J Surg 2007;94(3):265–73.
[73] Schlieman MG, Ho HS, Bold RJ. Utility of tumor markers in determining resectability of pancreatic cancer. Arch Surg 2003;138(9):951–5 [discussion: 955–6].
[74] Safi F, Schlosser W, Falkenreck S, et al. Prognostic value of CA 19-9 serum course in pancreatic cancer. Hepatogastroenterology 1998;45(19):253–9.
[75] Ferrone CR, Finkelstein DM, Thayer SP, et al. Perioperative CA19-9 levels can predict stage and survival in patients with resectable pancreatic adenocarcinoma. J Clin Oncol 2006;24:2897–902.
[76] Castellanos JA, Merchant NB. Intensity of follow-up after pancreatic cancer resection. Ann Surg Oncol 2014;21(3):747–51.
[77] Cloyd JM, Tran Cao HS, Petzel MQ, et al. Impact of pancreatectomy on long-term patient-reported symptoms and quality of life in recurrence-free survivors of pancreatic and periampullary neoplasms. J Surg Oncol 2017;115(2):144–50.
[78] Huang JJ, Yeo CJ, Sohn TA, et al. Quality of life and outcomes after pancreaticoduodenectomy. Ann Surg 2000;231(6):890–8.

[79] Pezzilli R, Falconi M, Zerbi A, et al. Clinical and patient-reported outcomes after pancreatoduodenectomy for different diseases: a follow-up study. Pancreas 2011;40(6):938–45.
[80] Fong ZV, Alvino DM, Castillo CF, et al. Health-related quality of life and functional outcomes in 5-year survivors after pancreaticoduodenectomy. Ann Surg 2017;266(4):685–92.
[81] Liu J, Gao J, Du Y, et al. Combination of plasma microRNAs with serum CA19-9 for early detection of pancreatic cancer. Int J Cancer 2012;131(3):683–91.
[82] Xu YF, Hannafon BN, Zhao YD, et al. Plasma exosome miR-196a and miR-1246 are potential indicators of localized pancreatic cancer. Oncotarget 2017;8(44):77028–40.
[83] Castillo J, Bernard V, San Lucas FA, et al. Surfaceome profiling enables isolation of cancer-specific exosomal cargo in liquid biopsies from pancreatic cancer patients. Ann Oncol 2017;29(1):223–9.
[84] Mehta KY, Wu HJ, Menon SS, et al. Metabolomic biomarkers of pancreatic cancer: a meta-analysis study. Oncotarget 2017;8(40):68899–915.
[85] Hayward J, Alvarez SA, Ruiz C, et al. Machine learning of clinical performance in a pancreatic cancer database. Artif Intell Med 2010;49(3):187–95.

Advances in Surgery 53 (2019) 271–292

ADVANCES IN SURGERY

Indications for Neoadjuvant Systemic Therapy for Breast Cancer

Kristalyn K. Gallagher, DO, David W. Ollila, MD*

Department of Surgery, Division of Surgical Oncology, The University of North Carolina at Chapel Hill, 170 Manning Drive, CB 7213, 1150 Physicians Office Building, Chapel Hill, NC 27599-7213, USA

Keywords

• Neoadjuvant systemic therapy • Adjuvant systemic therapy • Breast cancer

Key points

- Neoadjuvant and adjuvant systemic therapies offer similar benefits in terms of overall and disease-free survival.
- Neoadjuvant systemic therapy (NST) enables downstaging of the tumor enhancing the surgical treatment options.
- NST reduces the axillary disease burden facilitating less extensive surgery of the axilla.
- Response to NST is a strong prognostic indicator and guides adjuvant treatment planning.
- Certain molecular subtypes of breast cancer respond better to NST, reflecting the need for careful selection of patients who can benefit the most from NST.

INTRODUCTION

Neoadjuvant systemic therapy (NST) was first used in patients with unresectable, advanced, or inflammatory breast cancer with the goal of shrinking the primary tumor, before the planned oncologic resection [1–3]. More recently, NST has been used to convert some patients presenting with stage II–III breast cancer deemed to require a mastectomy to candidates for breast-conserving therapy (BCT) by downsizing the volume of disease [4,5]. Decreasing the

Disclosure Statement: Neither author has any financial disclosures for this article.

*Corresponding author. *E-mail address:* david_ollila@med.unc.edu

https://doi.org/10.1016/j.yasu.2019.04.013

size of a primary breast cancer is often used to justify administration of systemic therapy in the neoadjuvant rather than the adjuvant setting, especially in patients in whom the need for adjuvant therapy is not in question. The main goals of NST are to reduce mortality from breast cancer, to improve surgical options, and to acquire early information on response of the tumor [6].

This article provides an overview of the landmark NST trials in patients with operable breast cancer, discusses the goals for NST, and provides an update on NST by tumor phenotype. Throughout this overview, the authors discuss the research possibilities NST provides and the future directions this may lead.

LANDMARK NEOADJUVANT SYSTEMIC THERAPY TRIALS

The first description of NST (initially referred to as primary chemotherapy) in patients with operable breast cancer was by Jacquillat and colleagues [7,8] in 1983. These pioneers in NST treated 143 stage I–III patients with polychemotherapy and reported a clinical complete response (cCR) in 30% of patients. This initial phase 2 trial spawned several prospective, randomized phase 3 clinical trials.

The first North American NST trial in patients with operable breast cancer was the National Surgical Adjuvant Breast and Bowel Project (NSABP) B-18 trial, a phase 3 trial designed to evaluate differences in neoadjuvant and adjuvant chemotherapy [9]. Between 1988 and 1993, 1523 patients with operable breast cancer were randomized to receive either neoadjuvant or adjuvant adriamycin and cyclophosphamide (AC). In the neoadjuvant group, the overall response rate (ORR) was 80%; the cCR rate was 36%, and the pathologic complete response (pCR) rate was 13%. For the entire cohort, more patients treated neoadjuvantly (67.8%) underwent successful BCT as compared with those treated adjuvantly (59.8%). Among the cohort of patients with tumors larger than 5 cm, 22% underwent breast conservation compared with 8% in the adjuvant therapy group. However, more importantly, with a median follow-up of 5 years [9] and 9 years [10], there was no difference in the disease-free survival (DFS) and overall survival (OS) between the 2 groups [9].

In Europe, the European Organization for Research and Treatment of Cancer conducted trial 10902 [11] in 698 patients with operable breast cancer using neoadjuvant or adjuvant fluorouracil, epirubicin, and cyclophosphamide. Patients receiving neoadjuvant therapy had a 49% ORR, 7% cCR, and 1.7% pCR rate. With median follow-up of 10 years, there is no difference in OS, DFS, or locoregional recurrences [11,12].

The NSABP-B27 trial was designed to evaluate the effect of adding docetaxel (T) to AC in both a neoadjuvant and an adjuvant setting. Between 1995 and 2000, 2411 patients were randomized to 3 arms, including (1) preoperative AC followed by surgery, (2) preoperative AC followed by T and then surgery, and (3) AC followed by surgery followed by T. The addition of T preoperatively to AC significantly increased the proportion of patients having a pCR compared with preoperative AC alone (26% vs 13%). There was no significant difference in OS or DFS between treatment arms [13].

Collectively, these 3 anthracycline-based NST trials demonstrated the order of therapy had no impact on OS or DFS and was safe for patients with operable breast cancer. Furthermore, these 2 trials set the stage for all subsequent NST trials. Preoperative chemotherapy has facilitated the increased use of BCT secondary to tumor downsizing without any increase in locoregional recurrence rates, establishing the safety and efficacy of NST. These clinical trials have set the benchmark for increased use of NST in patients with operable breast cancer.

GOALS OF NEOADJUVANT SYSTEMIC THERAPY

Impact on local-regional therapy

Multiple, prospective, randomized trials have demonstrated the use of NST to convert patients determined to need a mastectomy at presentation into candidates for BCT. However, multiple factors contribute to the candidacy of the patient for BCT, and it is imperative to be cognizant of other factors that may decrease the feasibility/success of BCT in patients, such as ratio of tumor size to native breast size, extent of microcalcifications multicentric tumors, lobular histology, and the ability of the patient to tolerate radiation therapy [14].

When discussing the surgical management for breast cancer, an important consideration is the tumor size to native breast size. Thus, an established benefit of NST is to potentially decrease the size of the index cancer and reduce the extent of surgery required to achieve tumor-free surgical margins. Patients with operable tumors may choose NST to facilitate adequate tumor resection with BCT, with the goal of obtaining negative margins, potentially removing less tissue, and simultaneously providing an improved cosmetic result. Another consideration in tumor to breast size is the extent of suspicious malignant-appearing microcalcifications. Radiographically, NST reduces the size of spiculated masses, but does very little to malignant-appearing microcalcifications. Because of the possibility of residual disease, these malignant-appearing microcalcifications must be removed at the time of surgery. Thus, the patient may or may not be an ideal BCT candidate depending on the extent of microcalcification to breast ratio.

Multicentric, synchronous ipsilateral breast cancers have been associated with increased risk of locoregional recurrence with BCT, and mastectomy is recommended for these patients [15]. Lobular histology is associated with larger underlying breast cancers, and for women with lobular histology and dense breast tissue, MRI has been shown to be effective in helping to delineate the extent of disease. Given these considerations, some patients with lobular pathologic condition may not be eligible for BCT and may require mastectomy, reiterating the necessity of NST in this subgroup. Lobular carcinomas typically have a poor response to chemotherapy when compared with ductal carcinomas. Mathieu and colleagues [16] reported the poor chemosensitivity is secondary to the immunohistochemical profile, making them unacceptable BCT candidates following neoadjuvant chemotherapy. Most lobular carcinomas are strongly estrogen receptor/progesterone receptor (ER/PR) positive, and neoadjuvant endocrine therapy has been described to be more effective in these patients than chemotherapy. Dixon and colleagues [17] evaluated 40 patients with infiltrating lobular carcinoma who were not considered BCT candidates and treated them with 3 months of neoadjuvant letrozole. They report the rate of successful BCT in 81% of patients following neoadjuvant endocrine therapy.

The ability to undergo adjuvant radiation is an important consideration for women undergoing BCT. NSABP-B06 randomized 1851 women to total mastectomy, BCT, or BCT followed by radiation therapy. Patients who received BCT and adjuvant radiation had an loco-regional response of 14.3% versus 39.2% in women undergoing BCT without radiation [18]. There are few contraindications to adjuvant radiation, but include prior breast/chest radiation, pregnancy, and shoulder mobility (patients must be able to lie flat with the arm abducted). Relative contraindications include scleroderma and systemic lupus erythematosus. Because of the significant reduction in LRR, patients who cannot tolerate radiation or who have limited access to radiation facilities are poor candidates for BCT.

Becoming candidates for BCT and actually attempting/achieving tumor-free surgical margins has not been rigorously investigated. In both CALGB 40601 (human epidermal growth factor receptor-2^+, $HER2^+$) [19] and CALGB 40603 (triple-negative breast cancer, TNBC) [20], the treating surgeons were asked to assess whether a patient was a BCT candidate before and after NST. In CALGB 40601, 43% of patients converted from BCT ineligible to BCT eligible. When BCT was actually attempted, tumor-free surgical margins were achieved 80% of the time. Similarly, in CALGB 40603 (TNBC) [20], 42% of patients converted from BCT ineligible to BCT eligible. When BCT was attempted, tumor-free surgical margins were achieved in 93% of patients. Clearly, more research is necessary to determine which patients have truly been converted from BCT ineligible to BCT eligible with NST, but these 2 trials demonstrate that BCT can successfully be achieved in patients who get a good radiographic response to NST.

As the pCR rate to NST increases, omitting surgical resection of the primary breast cancer becomes a provocative, intellectual question. Does a woman with a pCR benefit from a partial mastectomy of the primary site? Several groups [21] have investigated the predictive value of a core biopsy or vacuum-assisted core biopsy (VACB) to determine pCR. Collectively, it appears VACB has a better negative-predictive value, much lower false-negative rate (FNR; <5%) than a core biopsy in patients with a radiographic complete response. A current national, clinical trial NRG BR005 (NCT03188393) is evaluating the negative-predictive value and FNR of performing VACB of primary breast site followed by standard of care partial mastectomy to evaluate if patients with a radiologic complete response may eventually be able to avoid surgical resection. The trial is currently accruing, and it is slated to close in the first quarter of 2019.

Neoadjuvant systemic therapy and the management of the axilla

Despite the first prospective, randomized NST trial, NSABP B-18, being published 30 years ago, the management of the axilla in these patients remains highly controversial. Historically, the traditional management of the axilla in these patients has been an axillary lymph node dissection (ALND). However, NST has been shown to have a significant role in reducing the axillary disease burden in patients with breast cancer with nodal involvement [22]. Thus, the timing and the method for nodal staging in patients planned for NST have been subjects of much debate. Two national, prospective NST trials demonstrate the management of the axillae in these patients is very heterogeneous [23]. In this section, a balanced discussion of the issues will be presented, trying to focus on prospective trial results, not single-institution treatment algorithms or biases.

The accurate assessment of the axillary lymph nodes for regional nodal metastases plays a crucial role in determining the extent of the disease before the use of NST. Given the low sensitivity of physical examination alone for detecting nodal metastases, it is important to evaluate the axilla accurately with noninvasive or minimally invasive approaches, before NST. Of the various imaging modalities (ultrasound, US, MRI, PET), axillary ultrasound (AUS) [15] has been widely adopted because of efficiency, reliability, and relative simplicity of the procedure. AUS can identify radiologically abnormal/enlarged lymph nodes, and then a US-guided fine-needle aspiration or core-needle biopsy can be performed.

For patients who present with clinically and radiographically negative axilla (cN0), performing a sentinel node (SN) biopsy before NST allows for accurate nodal staging negating any potential chemotherapy downstaging of the axillary nodes. Three large trials evaluated the SN identification rate and FNR to determine the feasibility of performing SN after NST. The first SENTINA (SENTinel NeoAdjuvant) study [24] was a European prospective multicenter study between 2009 and 2012 randomizing 1737 patients undergoing NST to the 4 following arms:

A. cN0 had upfront (-NST) SN that was pN0.
B. cN0 had upfront SN that was pN1, then post-NST SN + ALND.
C. cN1 or cN2 went to NST, and if converted to ycN0, had SN + ALND.
D. cN1 or cN2 went to NST and remained ycN1, had ALND only.

Comparing patients with cNO (arm A) with patients who converted to ycN0 (arm C), the investigators demonstrated a successful SN identification rate of 99.1% in patients cN0 (arm A) as compared with an 80.1% identification rate in patients who were ycN0 (Arm C). For the ycN0 group, the FNR was 24.3% if only 1 LN was removed, 18.5% if 2 LN were removed. In arm B, for patients undergoing a second SN, the identification rate was only 60.8% and FNR was 51.6%. The data strongly suggests SN biopsy is most accurate before NST. The disadvantage to this approach is the potential loss of opportunity to spare an ALND, especially in patients who actually achieve a pCR in the axillary nodes.

Performing an SN biopsy after NST provides a chance for nodal downstaging from the NST. If a patient converts from node positive to node negative, she could potentially be spared the added morbidity of ALND. A post hoc analysis of NSABP B-27 (described in detail earlier in the article) demonstrated SN biopsy after NST to be fairly successful, with an identification rate of 85% and a FNR of 9% [25]. Building on the findings of NSAPB B-27, the American College of Surgeons Oncology Group (ACOSOG) 1071 [26] carried out a prospective, phase 2 trial between 2009 and 2011 designed to evaluate the FNR of SN biopsy after NST in women with pathologically positive axillae. The trial evaluated 701 women with pathologic axillary nodes N1–N2 proven by fine-needle aspirate or core biopsy. All patients underwent SN biopsy followed by ALND. The FNR for a patient with cN1 disease was 12.6%, which was higher than the prespecified threshold of 10%. A post hoc subset analysis suggests that the FNR may be lowered by removing more than 2 SN, and by using dual-agent mapping.

The SN FNAC (Sentinel Node biopsy Following NeoAdjuvant Chemotherapy) [27] was a Canadian prospective multicenter trial from 2009 to 2012 with a similar design to ACOSOG 1071. This trial was a smaller patient cohort with 153 patients accrued. The FNR threshold was 10%, which was similar in other trials. They found that the SN identification rate after NST in cN1–2 was 87.6% and FNR was 8.4% when ypN0(i+) was considered a positive node. If ypN0(i+) was considered a negative node, the FNR increased to 13.3%.

Immunostains are not recommended to be routinely performed on SNs, except for patients with invasive lobular cancer [28]. Thus, collectively, all 3 trials demonstrate a FNR exceeding 10% when performing SN *after* NST. Investigators are continuing to look for ways to spare patients an unnecessary axillary dissection.

Post hoc analysis of ACOSOG 1071 suggested that removal of the axillary node, which had been biopsied and clipped, may be more accurate than an SN biopsy. Building on this finding, Caudle and colleagues [29] performed a prospective, single-institution trial evaluating if selective removal of the previous biopsy-proven positive clipped node, targeted axillary dissection (TAD) in addition to SN more accurately reflected the status of the remaining axillary nodes. They found that the previous clipped node was not removed during the SN biopsy in 23% of patients, and SN biopsy alone had a FNR of 10.1%. By identifying and removing the clipped node in addition to SN, the FNR was reduced to 2%. Although promising, TAD still needs to be replicated in other centers, and a prospective, multi-institutional trial is warranted. Clearly, more research/data are necessary so that women who do have a pCR in axillary nodes can be spared the morbidity of an ALND. The tumor status of the axilla after NST is a critical piece of prognostic information, and diagnostic accuracy is paramount.

Response to neoadjuvant systemic therapy as a prognostic indicator

The direct observation of the clinical and pathologic response to NST provides important information about the tumor biology and prognosis and further guides treatment planning. The assessment of response to NST portends the ability to modify treatment approach based on initial response, which may be particularly important for early identification of nonresponsive tumors. Earlier studies suggested pCR as a surrogate for long-term outcomes, such as DFS, event-free survival (EFS), and OS [13,30]. It has been shown that patients who achieve a pCR have the greatest survival advantage, albeit the proportion of patients achieving a pCR is low [13,31]. However, the definition of pCR and its role in long-term outcomes varied significantly between the earlier trials, making the applicability of these findings to clinical practice challenging. To conclusively evaluate the evidence for the correlation between response to NST and long-term outcomes, the Food and Drug Administration established an international working group known as Collaborative Trials in Neoadjuvant Breast Cancer that conducted a pooled meta-analysis of the eligible clinical trials for neoadjuvant therapy [32]. The results of the analysis demonstrated a longer EFS and OS in patients with a pCR than in those with residual invasive cancer, establishing unequivocally the response to NST as a powerful individualized prognostic factor (Fig. 1). The study also showed a higher frequency of pCR in those with aggressive tumor biology (eg, hormone receptor-negative [HR$^-$] disease) than those with low-grade HR-positive disease reiterating the particular importance of NST in more aggressive disease subtypes.

PATIENT AND DRUG REGIMEN SELECTION FOR NEOADJUVANT SYSTEMIC THERAPY

The extent and type of NST recommended for an individual patient depend on the cancer biology, factors such as stage, grade, expression of ER and PR, and HER2 status. Although NST does not improve OS and DFS when compared with adjuvant therapy, it is an attractive approach to enhance surgical options and increase breast conservation [5,6]. The International Consensus Expert

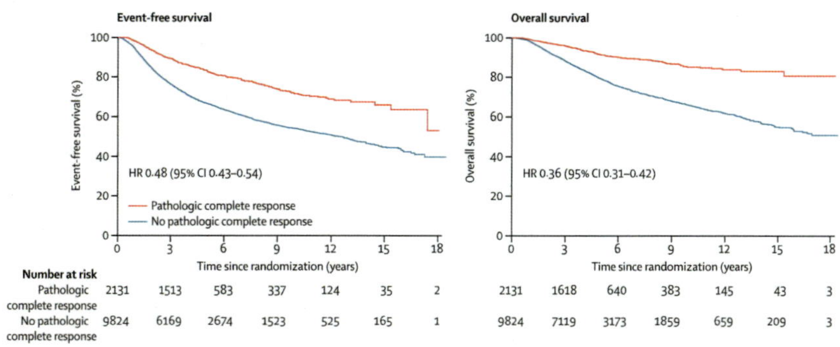

Fig. 1. Association of EFS and OS with pathologic complete response. CI, confidence interval; HR, hazard ratio. (*From* Cortazar P, Zhang L, Untch M, et al. Pathological complete response and long-term clinical benefit in breast cancer: The CTNeoBC pooled analysis. The Lancet. 2014;384(9938):166; with permission.)

Panel currently recommends consideration of NST for any patient in whom adjuvant chemotherapy is indicated [6]. However, the decision to choose NST over adjuvant approach requires a careful consideration of individual patient factors and preferences. The following reviews NST regimens by phenotype, including cytotoxic, targeted therapy, and neoadjuvant endocrine regimens.

Breast cancer is a clinically, histologically, and transcriptionally heterogeneous disease with prognostically significant subtypes. Certain subtypes have a better pathologic response to NST, reflecting a greater potential for curative intent even in some of the most aggressive phenotypes of breast cancer. Multiple, large randomized trials in the last decade have focused on characterizing the pathologic response of different subtypes with multiple preoperative chemotherapeutic agents (Table 1). The findings of the recent GeparQuinto, GBG-44 trial by Untch and colleagues [33] demonstrate substantially higher rates of pCR in Luminal-B/HER2-negative, HER2-positive nonluminal and TNBC with trastuzumab and chemotherapy combination. However, this response was not observed in the Luminal A and Luminal-B/HER2-positive patients. Similarly, the GeparSixto, GB-6 study showed a significant increase in the proportion of TNBC patients depicting pCR with the addition of carboplatin to the regime of neoadjuvant taxane, an anthracycline and targeted therapy reflecting the importance of molecular characterization of the tumor before selecting preoperative chemotherapeutic agents [34] (see Table 1).

Human epidermal growth factor receptor-2 overexpressing patients

For the HER2 overexpressing phenotype, several prospective, randomized clinical trials have been performed examining single-agent versus dual-agent HER2-directed therapy. In the NeoALTTO trial [35], NST paclitaxel was given with either single-agent HER2-directed therapy trastuzumab or lapatinib (a tyrosine kinase inhibitor) or both HER2-directed agents. It demonstrated a statistically higher pCR rate ($P = .0001$) in patients who received both agents (51.3%) as compared with single agents (24.7%, 29.5%). With a median follow-up of 3.8 years, there was no OS or DFS among the 3 groups, but the OS and DFS were significantly better in those who achieved pCR than those who not achieve pCR [36] (Table 2). Cancer and Leukemia Group B (CALGB) 40601 had a similar trial design with NST paclitaxel given with either single-agent (trastuzumab or lapatinib) or both HER2-directed therapies, but different findings. The single-agent lapatinib arm was closed early. The pCR in the dual-agent arm was higher (56%) versus single agent (46%), but this was not statistically significant ($P = .13$). Dual HER2-agent blockade with lapatinib does not seem to be the answer, but other HER2-directed agents have been investigated.

In the NeoSphere trial [37], the addition of pertuzumab (monoclonal antibody against the dimerization domain of HER2) to trastuzumab with or without T showed a dramatic increase in the rates of pCR (45.8%) as compared with single-agent HER2-directed therapy (29%, 24%) [37,38]. Five-year progression-free survival is the highest in the dual-agent HER2-directed therapy

Table 1
Important randomized clinical trials evaluating various chemotherapeutic drugs/regimens

Trial	Number of patients enrolled (n)	Neoadjuvant regimen evaluated	Median follow-up (mo)	Results/conclusions
Buzdar et al, [24] 2007	42	Paclitaxel + 4 cycles of FEC with OR without trastuzumab	36	• pCR rate substantially higher in patients treated with chemotherapy plus trastuzumab vs chemotherapy alone (66.7% vs 25%)
NeoALTTO Trial (2008–2010) (NCT00553358) [25]	455	Trastuzumab/lapatinib/ trastuzumab + lapatinib with paclitaxel followed by adjuvant FEC + same anti-HER2 therapy (all $HER2^+$ tumors)	45	• Proportion of patients achieving pCR significantly higher in combination group (51.3%) vs trastuzumab alone (29.5%) • No difference in DFS or OS among groups
GeparTrio Trial (2002–2005) [26]	2072	Two cycles of TAC followed by 4/6 cycles of TAC in early responders	62	• DFS and OS longer in TAC × 8 cycles group • DFS and OS longer in HR^+ tumors after response guided NST
GeparQuattro Trial (2006–2009) [27] (NCT00288002)	1509	Four cycles of EC followed by 4 cycles of T (EC-T)/T plus capcetabine (EC-TX)/T followed by capcetabine (EX-T-X) (with trastuzumab for $HER2^+$ tumors)	65	• Trastuzumab with anthracycline-taxane–based chemotherapy significantly higher pCR than reference group (31.7% vs 15.7%) • No difference in DFS and OS among $HER2^+$ and $HER2^-$ cohorts • OS after progression better in $HER2^+$ patients treated with anti-HER2 vs $HER2^-$ treated with chemotherapy alone

(*continued on next page*)

Table 1
(*continued*)

Trial	Number of patients enrolled (n)	Neoadjuvant regimen evaluated	Median follow-up (mo)	Results/conclusions
NOAH Trial (Neoadjuvant Herceptin in Patients With HER2-Positive Locally Advanced Breast Cancer) [28]	235	Trastuzumab plus anthracycline-taxane–based chemotherapy/ chemotherapy alone (All $HER2^+$ tumors)	65	• pCR rate in trastuzumab group higher (38%) vs chemotherapy-only group (19%) • Significant association between pCR and OS, DFS • EFS significantly higher (58%) in trastuzumab group at 5.4 y vs chemotherapy-only group (43%)
NeoSphere Trial [29]	417	Trastuzumab + T/ trastuzumab + pertuzumab + T/ trastuzumab + pertuzumab/ pertuzumab + T with 3 cycles of FEC in all groups	60	• Highest 5-y PFS in group receiving trastuzumab + pertuzumab + T (86%) • Highest 5-y DFS in group receiving trastuzumab + pertuzumab + T (84%)
GeparQuinto Trial [30] (NCT00567554)	1948	Epirubicin + cyclophosphamide + T with OR without bevacizumab	NA	• Significantly higher rates of pCR in triple-negative patients with added bevacizumab (39.3% vs 27.9%) • No significant difference in pCR rates with addition of bevacizumab to HR+ patients

Abbreviations: FEC, fluorouracil, epirubicin, cyclophosphamide; NA, not applicable; PFS, progression-free survival; TAC, T, doxorubicin, cyclophosphamide.

Table 2
Recent/ongoing clinical trials evaluating HER2 over expressing tumors

Trial	Number of patients (n)	Regimen/agent	Preliminary findings
CALGB 40601 [40]	305	Paclitaxel + trastuzumab OR paclitaxel + trastuzumab + lapatinib	• No significant differences in pCR rates with or without addition of lapatinib • Toxicity rates were significantly higher on lapatinib arm
EMILIA Trial [37] (NCT00829166)	991	Trastuzumab emtansine (T-DM1) vs capecitabine + lapatinib	• Significantly prolonged PFS and OS and less toxicity with T-DM1 than capecitabine + lapatinib
MARIANNE Study [38]	1095	Trastuzumab emtansine (T-DM1) + pertuzumab vs trastuzumab + taxane vs T-DM1 alone	• T-DM1 and T-DM1 plus pertuzumab showed noninferior PFS with better tolerability than trastuzumab + taxane
ADAPT trial [39][a]	134	Trastuzumab + pertuzumab with (T+P+Pac) OR without paclitaxel (T+P)	• pCR rate substantially higher in T+P+Pac arm (89.2% vs 36.3%)
KRISTINE (or TRIO-021) [40][b] (NCT02131064)	444	T + carboplatin with trastuzumab + pertuzumab (TCHP) vs T-DM1 + pertuzumab (KP)	• pCR rates higher in the TCHP group than in KP group (55.7% vs 44.4%) • More women in the TCHP group underwent breast conserving surgery than in KP group (52.6% vs 41.7%)

Neoadjuvant and Personalized Adaptive Novel Agents to Treat Breast Cancer.
[a]Adjuvant Dynamic Marker-Adjusted Personalized Therapy Trial Optimizing Risk Assessment and Therapy Response Prediction in Early Breast Cancer.
[b]A Study Comparing Kadcyla Plus Perjeta Treatment to Chemotherapy Combined With Herceptin Plus Perjeta in Patients With HER2-Positive Breast Cancer; NCT02131064.

[39]. Similarly, the KRISTINE trial [38] randomized patients to trastuzumab emtansine and pertuzumab versus T, carboplatin, trastuzumab, and pertuzumab with the primary endpoint pCR. The trastuzumab plus pertuzumab arm had the higher pCR rate (55.7% vs 44.4%, $P = .016$).

Collectively, these HER2 NST trials suggest the highest pCR rate is seen when trastuzumab and pertuzumab are combined with chemotherapy. It remains to be seen whether this improved pCR rate translates into an improved OS and DFS (see Table 2).

Triple-negative patients

TNBC, characterized by the lack of ER, PR, and HER2, has no currently available targeted agents. The standard NST regimen remains polychemotherapy. Approximately one-third of TNBC patients will achieve a pCR to NST with anthracycline and taxane [41].

TNBC, currently the most aggressive form of breast cancer, has long evaded targeted therapy. In GeparSixto [34], the TNBC patients were randomized to polychemotherapy ± carboplatin. The addition of carboplatin significantly increased the pCR rate (53.2% vs 36.9%, $P = .005$). CALGB 40603 (ALLIANCE) [42] performed a randomized phase 2 NST trial to evaluate this impact of carboplatin and/or bevacizumab to standard polychemotherapy. The addition of carboplatin significantly increased the pCR rate breast/axilla (54% vs 41%, $P = .0029$). Recent results from the CALGB 40603 and the GeparSixto trials show significantly improved pCR rates with the addition of neoadjuvant carboplatin [34,42]. Including the results of another polychemotherapy ± bevacizumab (BEATRICE), the addition of neoadjuvant bevacizumab does not improve the proportion of patients achieving pCR and may increase the likelihood of adverse events [42–44]. Despite these encouraging results, whether this improvement in pCR rates translates into improved OS and DFS for patients remains questionable. This yet unproven correlation highlights the need for careful selection of chemotherapeutic agents based on the patient's tumor characteristics and utilization of established evidence for subtype specific therapy (Table 3).

Hormone receptor–positive, human epidermal growth factor receptor-2 –negative patients

The patients with $HR^+/HER2^-$ disease, also classified as luminal subtype A or B on gene-expression profiling, are usually slow-growing, low-grade tumors with a good overall prognosis [47]. However, the rate of pCR to NST in $HR^+/HER2^-$ patients is strikingly low, with pCR rates varying from 2% to 10% [6,48]. Significantly improved response rates are observed with the use of neoadjuvant endocrine therapy in this tumor subtype (fully discussed later in this article). Whether there is a benefit of concurrent administration of neoadjuvant cytotoxic chemotherapy and endocrine therapy remains questionable. Some data suggest a benefit of combination letrozole and cyclophosphamide over letrozole alone (response rate of 89.2% vs 72.8%) in elderly HR^+ patients [49] A randomized phase 2 clinical trial conducted by Sugiu and colleagues [45]

Table 3
Therapeutic regimens evaluated/under evaluation for triple-negative breast cancer

Trial	Number of patients (n)	Regimen/agent	Results/conclusions
CALGB 40603 Trial Impact of the Addition of Carboplatin and/or Bevacizumab to Neoadjuvant Once-per-Week Paclitaxel Followed by Dose-Dense Doxorubicin and Cyclophosphamide on Pathologic Complete Response Rates in Stage II to III Triple-Negative Breast Cancer [36]	443	Paclitaxel followed by doxorubicin + cyclophosphamide with OR without cisplatin and/or bevacizumab	• Addition of carboplatin significantly increased the pCR rates as compared with those did not receive carboplatin (60% vs 46%) • Addition of bevacizumab significantly increased the pCR rates as compared with those did not receive carboplatin (59% vs 48%) • Patients receiving both carboplatin and bevacizumab had a pCR of 67%
GeparSixto GBG 66 [31] (NCT01426880)	588	Paclitaxel + doxorubicin + trastuzumab ($HER2^+$ tumors only) + bevacizumab (triple negative tumors only) with OR without carboplatin	• Significant increase in pCR rates in triple-negative disease with addition of carboplatin (53.2% vs 36.9%) • No benefit observed in terms of pCR in $HER2^+$ tumors with addition of carboplatin (32.8% vs 36.8%)
BEATRICE Trial Adjuvant bevacizumab-containing therapy in triple-negative breast cancer [45] (NCT00528567)	2591	Anthracycline and/or taxane with OR without bevacizumab	• No difference in 3-y DFS in patients receiving bevacizumab than those who did not (83.7% vs 82.7%)
Eastern Cooperative Oncology Group E5103 Trial [46]	4994	Doxorubicin + cyclophosphamide followed by paclitaxel alone OR with concurrent bevacizumab OR with sequential bevacizumab	• No difference in 4-y DFS or OS with addition of bevacizumab to standard chemotherapy

(*continued on next page*)

Table 3
(*continued*)

Trial	Number of patients (n)	Regimen/agent	Results/conclusions
A Co-Clinical Trial in Triple Negative Breast Cancer Patients with Genoproteomic Discovery (NCT02124902)	70 (anticipated)	T + carboplatin	Anticipated completion June 2018 Primary outcome of interest: –pCR rates
A Randomized, Double-Blind, Phase III Clinical Trial of Neoadjuvant Chemotherapy With Atezolizumab or Placebo in Patients With Triple-Negative Breast Cancer Followed by Adjuvant Continuation of Atezolizumab or Placebo (NCT03281954)	1520 (anticipated)	Paclitaxel + carboplatin, followed by doxorubicin/epirubicin and cyclophosphamide with OR without atezolizumab	Anticipated completion June 2024 Primary outcome of interest: pCR rates and EFS
CADENCE: Carboplatin and Docetaxel in Neoadjuvant Treatment of ER-Negative, HER2-Negative Breast Cancer: A Co-Clinical Trial with Genoproteomic Discovery (NCT02547987)	44 (anticipated)	T + carboplatin	Anticipated completion September 2020

A Phase II Randomized Controlled Trial of Genomically Directed Therapy After Preoperative Chemotherapy in Patients With Triple Negative Breast Cancer: Hoosier Oncology Group BRE12-158 (NCT02101385)	136 (anticipated)	Experimental Arm A (genomically directed monotherapy) or Control Arm B (standard therapy) Actionable pathways/agents • PIK3CA, PTEN: Everolimus • TOP2A: Doxorubicin • PARP1, BRCA1: Cisplatin and olaparib • VEGFA: Bevacizumab • TYMP: Capecitabine • SSTR2: Octreotide • MGMT: Temozolomide • MYC: Paclitaxel • EGFR: Cetuximab • COX2: Celecoxib • hENT: Gemcitabine • MET: Crizotinib	Anticipated completion December 2021 Primary outcome of interest: Impact of genomic characterization of tumor and effect on disease progression/treatment response by targeted therapy
A Randomized, Double-Blind, Phase III Clinical Trial of Neoadjuvant Chemotherapy With Atezolizumab or Placebo in Patients With Triple-Negative Breast Cancer Followed by Adjuvant Continuation of Atezolizumab or Placebo (NCT03281954)	1520	Paclitaxel + carboplatin, followed by doxorubicin/epirubicin and cyclophosphamide with OR without atezolizumab	Anticipated completion June 2024 Primary outcome of interest: pCR rates and EFS

showed no difference in pCR rates in HR^+ patients administered concurrent chemotherapy and endocrine therapy as compared with chemotherapy alone. However, the reduction in tumor size was significantly greater in the concurrent group. This conflicting body of evidence reflects the need of further studies to evaluate the role of concurrent endocrine and chemotherapy in the management of HR^+/$HER2^-$ patient population (Table 4).

Neoadjuvant endocrine therapy

Given the success of adjuvant antiestrogen therapy for patients who are ER^+, there has been a considerable interest in leveraging the effect of endocrine therapy directed against HRs in the neoadjuvant setting.

Neoadjuvant letrozole trial

In a double-blind phase 3 randomized trial, postmenopausal women with large ER^+ and/or PR^+ breast cancers who required mastectomy or were locally advanced and inoperable were randomized to receive letrozole or tamoxifen for 4 months as primary treatment [55]. Objective response rates by clinical examination and imaging favored the letrozole-treated patients (60% vs 41%; $P = .004$). There was a higher rate of breast-conserving surgery in the letrozole group (48%) than in the tamoxifen group (36%) ($P = .036$).

Neoadjuvant anastrozole trials

There have been 2 large randomized studies comparing anastrozole with tamoxifen in postmenopausal women with HR^+ breast cancer.

In the IMmediate Preoperative Arimidex, Tamoxifen or Combined with Tamoxifen (IMPACT) trial, patients were randomized to receive anastrozole or tamoxifen or both in combination for 3 months before surgery [56]. The primary end point was objective clinical response measured by calipers, with US measurement. There was no significant difference in objective response between the 3 treatments as measured by calipers and US. After 3 months, for patients initially assessed as requiring mastectomy, significantly more were deemed suitable for breast-conserving surgery in the anastrozole arm (46%) than tamoxifen arm (22%) ($P = .03$), but not all patients accepted this recommendation (actual BCT rates, $P =$ not significant).

In the PROACT (PReOperarive Arimidex Compared with Tamoxifen) trial [57], patients were randomized to receive either anastrozole or tamoxifen for 3 months. The primary end point was objective tumor response measured by US scan, and caliper measurement was a secondary end point. No significant difference in objective response was seen between treatment arms. There was, however, a significantly higher objective response in favor of anastrozole in those patients initially assessed as requiring mastectomy (36.6% vs 24.2% on US, $P = .03$; and 48.6% vs 35.8% with calipers, $P = .04$).

A combined analysis of these 2 studies compared ORR and surgery and failed to show any significant difference in objective response or breast-conserving rates between tamoxifen and anastrozole [58]. There was, however, a significant improvement in ORR in favor of anastrozole in the subgroup of

Table 4
Clinical trials evaluating neoadjuvant systemic therapy regimens for hormone receptor–positive breast cancer

Trial	Number of patients enrolled (n)	Neoadjuvant regimen evaluated	Results/conclusions
STAGE Trial [46] (NCT00605267)	204	Goserelin + anastrozole OR goserelin + tamoxifen	• Response rates higher in anastrozole group than those in the tamoxifen group (70.4% vs 50.5%)
Semiglazov et al, [50] 2007	121	Anastrozole/exemestane OR doxorubicin + paclitaxel	• No significant difference in clinical response/ pCR rates between the endocrine arm and chemotherapy arm • Higher toxicity in the chemotherapy arm
METEOR Trial [51] (NCT01589367)	208 (anticipated)	Letrozole + metformin or letrozole + placebo	• *Currently ongoing* (primary outcome of interest: clinical response rate)
Baselga et al, [52] 2009 (NCT00107016)	270	Letrozole + everolimus OR letrozole + placebo	• Clinical response rate higher in combination arm than that in letrozole alone (68.1% vs 59.1%) • Reduction of Ki-67 levels occurred in a higher proportion of patients in the combination arm than letrozole alone (57% vs 30%)
GEICAM/2006–03 Trial [53]	95	Chemotherapy (CT) (epirubicin + cyclophosphamide + T) OR hormonotherapy (HT)(exemestane [+ goserelin in premenopausal patients])	• Overall higher clinical response rate in the CT arm than HT arm (66% vs 48%) • No significant difference between the 2 arms in patients with low Ki-67 levels (CT: 63%, HT: 58%) • Better response rates with CT in those with high Ki-67 levels than HT (67% vs 42%)
NEOCENT Trial [54] (NCT00963729)	44	CT (fluorouracil + epirubicin + cyclophosphamide followed by T) OR letrozole alone	• Highest 5-y PFS in group receiving trastuzumab + pertuzumab + T (86%) • Highest 5-y DFS in group receiving trastuzumab + pertuzumab + T (84%)

patients who were considered to require mastectomy or be inoperable at the outset (47% vs 35%; P = .026) and on US response (36% vs 26%; P= .048). Collectively, these data suggest anastrozole is superior to tamoxifen in patients' tumors that are large and require mastectomy or are inoperable or locally advanced at diagnosis.

The response to the endocrine agents has been shown to correlate with the level of ER expression. Among the endocrine therapy agents, aromatase inhibitors are more effective than tamoxifen in facilitating BCT, as shown by Eiermann and colleagues [55], and the IMPACT trial [56]. Subsequently, the ACOSOG Z1031 trial was a randomized phase 2 trial in 377 women with clinical stage II to II ER-positive breast cancer randomized to 1 of 3 commonly used AIs (letrozole, anastrozole, and exemestane) administered in the neoadjuvant setting [59]. The results of the trial demonstrated significantly improved surgical outcomes especially in patients with Luminal-A subtype of breast cancer. The rate of conversion to BCT was similar among all 3 agents; however, the suppression of circulating estradiol was observed to be highest in patients taking letrozole. Currently, 2 large prospective trials are underway to assess the effect of endocrine therapy agents in the neoadjuvant setting on long-term clinical outcomes (ALTERNATE Trial, NCT01953588; FACE Trial, NCT00248170).

SUMMARY

NST remains the cornerstone for management of large inoperable breast tumors and for inflammatory breast cancer. The use of NST in patients with operable breast cancer has increased substantially the last 2 decades leading to increased BCT rates with equivalent OS and DFS when compared with patients treated with adjuvant therapy. The drastic improvements in the understanding of the tumor biology and recent advances in molecular analysis have facilitated rapid, accurate, molecular subtyping of the tumor and development of efficacious targeted systemic agents, particularly in HER2 overexpressing patients. The pCR rate has increased, but corresponding OS has not yet increased. The challenge remains to translate this wealth of knowledge to the clinic, facilitating the use of NST tailored to the molecular signature of the individual patient.

References

[1] Sorace RA, Bagley CS, Lichter AS, et al. The management of nonmetastatic locally advanced breast cancer using primary induction chemotherapy with hormonal synchronization followed by radiation therapy with or without debulking surgery. World J Surg 1985;9(5):775–85.

[2] Perloff M, Lesnick GJ. Chemotherapy before and after mastectomy in stage III breast cancer. Arch Surg 1982;117(7):879–81.

[3] Schick P, Goodstein J, Moor J, et al. Preoperative chemotherapy followed by mastectomy for locally advanced breast cancer. J Surg Oncol 1983;22(4):278–82.

[4] Barry PA, Schiavon G. Primary systemic treatment in the management of operable breast cancer: best surgical approach for diagnosis, biological evaluation, and research. J Natl Cancer Inst Monogr 2015;2015(51):4–8.

[5] Mauri D, Pavlidis N, Ioannidis JP. Neoadjuvant versus adjuvant systemic treatment in breast cancer: a meta-analysis. J Natl Cancer Inst 2005;97(3):188–94.
[6] Kaufmann M, von Minckwitz G, Bear HD, et al. Recommendations from an international expert panel on the use of neoadjuvant (primary) systemic treatment of operable breast cancer: new perspectives 2006. Ann Oncol 2007;18(12):1927–34.
[7] Jacquillat C, Baillet F, Blondon J, et al. Preliminary results of "neoadjuvant" chemotherapy in initial management of breast cancer (BC). Proc ASCO 1983;2:112.
[8] Jacquillat Cl, Weil M, Auclerc G, et al. Neoadjuvant chemotherapy in the conservative management of breast cancers: study of 143 patients. Recent Results Cancer Res 1986;103: 113–9.
[9] Fisher B, Bryant J, Wolmark N, et al. Effect of preoperative chemotherapy on the outcome of women with operable breast cancer. J Clin Oncol 1998;16(8):2672–85.
[10] Wolmark N, Wang J, Mamounas E, et al. Preoperative chemotherapy in patients with operable breast cancer: nine-year results from National Surgical Adjuvant Breast and Bowel Project B-18. J Natl Cancer Inst Monogr 2001;(30):96–102.
[11] van der Hage JA, van de Velde CJ, Julien JP, et al. Preoperative chemotherapy in primary operable breast cancer: results from the European Organization for Research and Treatment of Cancer trial 10902. J Clin Oncol 2001;19(22):4224–37.
[12] van Nes JG, Putter H, Julien JP, et al. Preoperative chemotherapy is safe in early breast cancer, even after 10 years of follow-up; clinical and translational results from the EORTC trial 10902. Breast Cancer Res Treat 2009;115(1):101–13.
[13] Rastogi P, Anderson SJ, Bear HD, et al. Preoperative chemotherapy: updates of National Surgical Adjuvant Breast and Bowel Project Protocols B-18 and B-27. J Clin Oncol 2008;26(5):778–85.
[14] Newman LA, Buzdar AU, Singletary SE, et al. A prospective trial of preoperative chemotherapy in resectable breast cancer: predictors of breast-conservation therapy feasibility. Ann Surg Oncol 2002;9(3):228–34.
[15] Henry-Tillman R, Glover-Collins K, Preston M, et al. The SAVE review: sonographic analysis versus excision for axillary staging in breast cancer. J Am Coll Surg 2015;220(4):560–7.
[16] Mathieu MC, Rouzier R, Llombart-Cussac A, et al. The poor responsiveness of infiltrating lobular breast carcinomas to neoadjuvant chemotherapy can be explained by their biological profile. Eur J Cancer 2004;40(3):342–51.
[17] Dixon JM, Mamman U, Thomas J. Accuracy of intraoperative frozen-section analysis of axillary nodes. Edinburgh Breast Unit team. Br J Surg 1999;86(3):392–5.
[18] Fisher B, Anderson S, Bryant J, et al. Twenty-year follow-up of a randomized trial comparing total mastectomy, lumpectomy, and lumpectomy plus irradiation for the treatment of invasive breast cancer. N Engl J Med 2002;347(16):1233–41.
[19] Golshan M, Cirrincione CT, Sikov WM, et al. Impact of neoadjuvant therapy on eligibility for and frequency of breast conservation in stage II-III HER2-positive breast cancer: surgical results of CALGB 40601 (Alliance). Breast Cancer Res Treat 2016;160(2):297–304.
[20] Golshan M, Cirrincione CT, Sikov WM, et al. Impact of neoadjuvant chemotherapy in stage II-III triple negative breast cancer on eligibility for breast-conserving surgery and breast conservation rates: surgical results from CALGB 40603 (Alliance). Ann Surg 2015;262(3): 434–9 [discussion: 438–9].
[21] Kuerer HM, Vrancken Peeters M, Rea DW, et al. Nonoperative management for invasive breast cancer after neoadjuvant systemic therapy: conceptual basis and fundamental international feasibility clinical trials. Ann Surg Oncol 2017;24(10):2855–62.
[22] Kuerer HM, Sahin AA, Hunt KK, et al. Incidence and impact of documented eradication of breast cancer axillary lymph node metastases before surgery in patients treated with neoadjuvant chemotherapy. Ann Surg 1999;230(1):72–8.
[23] Ollila DW, Cirrincione CT, Berry DA, et al. Axillary management of stage II/III breast cancer in patients treated with neoadjuvant systemic therapy: results of CALGB 40601 (HER2-positive) and CALGB 40603 (triple-negative). J Am Coll Surg 2017;224(4):688–94.

[24] Kuehn T, Bauerfeind I, Fehm T, et al. Sentinel-lymph-node biopsy in patients with breast cancer before and after neoadjuvant chemotherapy (SENTINA): a prospective, multicentre cohort study. Lancet Oncol 2013;14(7):609–18.
[25] Mamounas EP, Brown A, Anderson S, et al. Sentinel node biopsy after neoadjuvant chemotherapy in breast cancer: results from National Surgical Adjuvant Breast and Bowel Project Protocol B-27. J Clin Oncol 2005;23(12):2694–702.
[26] Boughey JC, Suman VJ, Mittendorf EA, et al. Sentinel lymph node surgery after neoadjuvant chemotherapy in patients with node-positive breast cancer: the ACOSOG Z1071 (Alliance) clinical trial. JAMA 2013;310(14):1455–61.
[27] Boileau JF, Poirier B, Basik M, et al. Sentinel node biopsy after neoadjuvant chemotherapy in biopsy-proven node-positive breast cancer: the SN FNAC study. J Clin Oncol 2015;33(3): 258–64.
[28] Patel A, D'Alfonso T, Cheng E, et al. Sentinel lymph nodes in classic invasive lobular carcinoma of the breast: cytokeratin immunostain ensures detection, and precise determination of extent, of involvement. Am J Surg Pathol 2017;41(11):1499–505.
[29] Caudle AS, Yang WT, Krishnamurthy S, et al. Improved axillary evaluation following neoadjuvant therapy for patients with node-positive breast cancer using selective evaluation of clipped nodes: implementation of targeted axillary dissection. J Clin Oncol 2016;34(10):1072–8.
[30] Smith IC, Heys SD, Hutcheon AW, et al. Neoadjuvant chemotherapy in breast cancer: significantly enhanced response with docetaxel. J Clin Oncol 2002;20(6):1456–66.
[31] Eltahir A, Heys SD, Hutcheon AW, et al. Treatment of large and locally advanced breast cancers using neoadjuvant chemotherapy. Am J Surg 1998;175(2):127–32.
[32] Cortazar P, Zhang L, Untch M, et al. Pathological complete response and long-term clinical benefit in breast cancer: the CTNeoBC pooled analysis. Lancet 2014;384(9938):164–72.
[33] Untch M, Loibl S, Bischoff J, et al. Lapatinib versus trastuzumab in combination with neoadjuvant anthracycline-taxane-based chemotherapy (GeparQuinto, GBG 44): a randomised phase 3 trial. Lancet Oncol 2012;13(2):135–44.
[34] von Minckwitz G, Schneeweiss A, Loibl S, et al. Neoadjuvant carboplatin in patients with triple-negative and HER2-positive early breast cancer (GeparSixto; GBG 66): a randomised phase 2 trial. Lancet Oncol 2014;15(7):747–56.
[35] Baselga J, Bradbury I, Eidtmann H, et al. Lapatinib with trastuzumab for HER2-positive early breast cancer (NeoALTTO): a randomised, open-label, multicentre, phase 3 trial. Lancet 2012;379(9816):633–40.
[36] de Azambuja E, Holmes AP, Piccart-Gebhart M, et al. Lapatinib with trastuzumab for HER2-positive early breast cancer (NeoALTTO): survival outcomes of a randomised, open-label, multicentre, phase 3 trial and their association with pathological complete response. Lancet Oncol 2014;15(10):1137–46.
[37] Gianni L, Pienkowski T, Im YH, et al. Efficacy and safety of neoadjuvant pertuzumab and trastuzumab in women with locally advanced, inflammatory, or early HER2-positive breast cancer (NeoSphere): a randomised multicentre, open-label, phase 2 trial. Lancet Oncol 2012;13(1):25–32.
[38] Hurvitz SA, Martin M, Symmans WF, et al. Neoadjuvant trastuzumab, pertuzumab, and chemotherapy versus trastuzumab emtansine plus pertuzumab in patients with HER2-positive breast cancer (KRISTINE): a randomised, open-label, multicentre, phase 3 trial. Lancet Oncol 2018;19(1):115–26.
[39] Gianni L, Pienkowski T, Im YH, et al. 5-year analysis of neoadjuvant pertuzumab and trastuzumab in patients with locally advanced, inflammatory, or early-stage HER2-positive breast cancer (NeoSphere): a multicentre, open-label, phase 2 randomised trial. Lancet Oncol 2016;17(6):791–800.
[40] Carey LA, Berry DA, Ollila DW, et al. Clinical and translational results of CALGB 40601: a neoadjuvant phase III trial of weekly paclitaxel and trastuzumab with or without lapatinib for

HER2-positive breast cancer. Journal of the Proceedings of the American Society of Clinical Oncology 2013;31:500, (abstr).
[41] Liedtke C, Mazouni C, Hess KR, et al. Response to neoadjuvant therapy and long-term survival in patients with triple-negative breast cancer. J Clin Oncol 2008;26(8):1275–81.
[42] Sikov WM, Berry DA, Perou CM, et al. Impact of the addition of carboplatin and/or bevacizumab to neoadjuvant once-per-week paclitaxel followed by dose-dense doxorubicin and cyclophosphamide on pathologic complete response rates in stage II to III triple-negative breast cancer: CALGB 40603 (Alliance). J Clin Oncol 2015;33(1):13–21.
[43] Cameron D, Brown J, Dent R, et al. Adjuvant bevacizumab-containing therapy in triple-negative breast cancer (BEATRICE): primary results of a randomised, phase 3 trial. Lancet Oncol 2013;14(10):933–42.
[44] Miller K, O'Neill AM, Dang CT, et al. Bevacizumab (Bv) in the adjuvant treatment of HER2-negative breast cancer: final results from Eastern Cooperative Oncology Group E5103. J Clin Oncol 2014;32(15_suppl):500.
[45] Sugiu K, Iwamoto T, Kelly CM, et al. Neoadjuvant chemotherapy with or without concurrent hormone therapy in estrogen receptor-positive breast cancer: NACED-randomized multicenter phase II trial. Acta Med Okayama 2015;69(5):291–9.
[46] Masuda N, Sagara Y, Kinoshita T, et al. Neoadjuvant anastrozole versus tamoxifen in patients receiving goserelin for premenopausal breast cancer (STAGE): a double-blind, randomised phase 3 trial. Lancet Oncol 2012;13(4):345–52.
[47] Sorlie T, Perou CM, Tibshirani R, et al. Gene expression patterns of breast carcinomas distinguish tumor subclasses with clinical implications. Proc Natl Acad Sci U S A 2001;98(19):10869–74.
[48] Colleoni M, Viale G, Zahrieh D, et al. Chemotherapy is more effective in patients with breast cancer not expressing steroid hormone receptors: a study of preoperative treatment. Clin Cancer Res 2004;10(19):6622–8.
[49] Bottini A, Generali D, Brizzi MP, et al. Randomized phase II trial of letrozole and letrozole plus low-dose metronomic oral cyclophosphamide as primary systemic treatment in elderly breast cancer patients. J Clin Oncol 2006;24(22):3623–8.
[50] Semiglazov VF, Semiglazov VV, Dashyan GA, et al. Phase 2 randomized trial of primary endocrine therapy versus chemotherapy in postmenopausal patients with estrogen receptor-positive breast cancer. Cancer 2007;110(2):244–54.
[51] Kim J, Lim W, Kim EK, et al. Phase II randomized trial of neoadjuvant metformin plus letrozole versus placebo plus letrozole for estrogen receptor positive postmenopausal breast cancer (METEOR). BMC Cancer 2014;14:170.
[52] Baselga J, Semiglazov V, van Dam P, et al. Phase II randomized study of neoadjuvant everolimus plus letrozole compared with placebo plus letrozole in patients with estrogen receptor-positive breast cancer. J Clin Oncol 2009;27(16):2630–7.
[53] Alba E, Calvo L, Albanell J, et al. Chemotherapy (CT) and hormonotherapy (HT) as neoadjuvant treatment in luminal breast cancer patients: results from the GEICAM/2006-03, a multicenter, randomized, phase-II study. Ann Oncol 2012;23(12):3069–74.
[54] Palmieri C, Cleator S, Kilburn LS, et al. NEOCENT: a randomised feasibility and translational study comparing neoadjuvant endocrine therapy with chemotherapy in ER-rich postmenopausal primary breast cancer. Breast Cancer Res Treat 2014;148(3):581–90.
[55] Eiermann W, Paepke S, Appfelstaedt J, et al. Preoperative treatment of postmenopausal breast cancer patients with letrozole: a randomized double-blind multicenter study. Ann Oncol 2001;12(11):1527–32.
[56] Smith IE, Dowsett M, Ebbs SR, et al. Neoadjuvant treatment of postmenopausal breast cancer with anastrozole, tamoxifen, or both in combination: the Immediate Preoperative Anastrozole, Tamoxifen, or Combined with Tamoxifen (IMPACT) multicenter double-blind randomized trial. J Clin Oncol 2005;23(22):5108–16.
[57] Cataliotti L, Buzdar AU, Noguchi S, et al. Comparison of anastrozole versus tamoxifen as preoperative therapy in postmenopausal women with hormone receptor-positive breast

cancer: the Pre-Operative "Arimidex" Compared to Tamoxifen (PROACT) trial. Cancer 2006;106(10):2095–103.
[58] Smith IE. Anastrozole versus tamoxifen as preoperative therapy for oestrogen receptor-positive breast cancer in postmenopausal women:combined analysis of the IMPACT and PROACT trials. 4th European Breast Cancer Conference. Hamburg, Germany, March 17, 2004.
[59] Ellis MJ, Suman VJ, Hoog J, et al. Randomized phase II neoadjuvant comparison between letrozole, anastrozole, and exemestane for postmenopausal women with estrogen receptor-rich stage 2 to 3 breast cancer: clinical and biomarker outcomes and predictive value of the baseline PAM50-based intrinsic subtype–ACOSOG Z1031. J Clin Oncol 2011;29(17):2342–9.

Advances in Surgery 53 (2019) 293–303

ADVANCES IN SURGERY

ELSEVIER
MOSBY

Watchful Waiting for Inguinal Hernia

Alexander D. Schroeder, MD, Dustin J. Tubre, MD, Robert J. Fitzgibbons Jr, MD*

Department of Surgery, Creighton University School of Medicine, CHI Health Creighton University-Bergan Mercy Education Building, 7710 Mercy Road, Suite 501, Omaha, NE 68124, USA

Keywords

• Inguinal hernia • Watchful waiting • Routine repair • Herniorrhaphy

Key points

- Inguinal herniorrhaphy is one of the most common surgeries performed worldwide.
- Recent evidence from 3 randomized controlled trials suggests that routine repair of all inguinal hernias at diagnosis is not necessary in asymptomatic or minimally symptomatic men.
- Patients with symptoms caused by their hernias benefit from operative therapy to eliminate pain.
- A strategy of watchful waiting for patients with minimally symptomatic hernias has been shown to be safe; however, patients should be counseled that the crossover rate to surgery approaches 75% by 10 years.
- These data should not be extrapolated to women, as the natural history is different from men, and watchful waiting should not be routinely recommended.

INTRODUCTION

Inguinal hernia is one of the most common afflictions known to humans. The lifetime risk of developing an inguinal hernia is estimated at 27% for men and 3% for woman [1]. In the United States, the annual incidence of an inguinal hernia is 315 per 100,000, and the annual incidence of an inguinal herniorrhaphy is

Disclosure Statement: The authors report no conflicts of interest and have nothing to declare.

The North American Trial was funded by the Agency for Healthcare Research and Quality grant RO1 HS 09860. One of the Authors (RJF) was the principal investigator. Clinical Trials Registration: ClinicalTrials.gov Identifier: NCT00263250.

*Corresponding author. *E-mail address:* fitzjr@creighton.edu

https://doi.org/10.1016/j.yasu.2019.04.014
0065-3411/19/

217 per 100,000 [2,3]. As many as 20 million inguinal herniorrhaphies are performed annually worldwide [4]. These numbers make the socioeconomic consequences of the most appropriate treatment strategy important to health policy makers. Given this high incidence, the most cost-effective strategy that provides a maximum risk-benefit ratio for patients is essential.

Until recently, standard surgical dictum has been to repair all inguinal hernias at diagnosis to prevent the serious complications of bowel obstruction and strangulation, usually referred to as hernia accidents. This is because of the large difference in mortality and morbidity rates between emergent versus elective inguinal hernia repairs. Based on a meta-analysis of multiple studies, a hernia accident results in a mean mortality of 4.0% (range 0% to 22.2%) compared with 0.2% (range 0% to 1.8%) with elective hernia repair [5]. Because modern inguinal herniorrhaphy techniques are safe, effective, and can be performed under local anesthesia for high-risk patients, the logical recommendation is routine repair at diagnosis; but these studies for the most part did not stratify patients according to symptoms.

Recent randomized controlled trails that did stratify for symptoms have challenged this concept for asymptomatic or minimally symptomatic patients with inguinal hernias showing that a strategy of planned nonoperation or "watchful waiting" is safe for this subgroup of patients with a low incidence of hernia accident. With approximately one-third of men with inguinal hernias being either asymptomatic or minimally symptomatic, a very large number of hernia repairs may be unnecessary [6]. Another consideration is that complication rates may not be as favorable as previously believed by many surgeons. The long-term complication of post herniorrhaphy groin pain occurs in 6% to 8% of patients, and has now emerged as the single most pressing issue facing inguinal hernia surgeons [7]. It is an obvious disservice to successfully repair a minimally symptomatic hernia, only to leave a patient with chronic pain; and although recurrence is less with modern techniques of repair, it is still a relevant consideration. Short-term complications are possible, including hematoma or seroma (8%–22%), urinary dysfunction, and early pain [8]. Surgical site infections occur in 1% to 3% of patients [9]. Laparoscopic accidents, such as enterotomies, are rare, but potentially catastrophic.

In this article, the authors examine the available evidence regarding nonoperative treatment or "watchful waiting" of inguinal hernias. The goal is to develop evidence-based recommendations to provide patients with inguinal hernia the treatment strategy that will maximize benefit while minimizing potential risks.

NATURAL HISTORY OF AN INGUINAL HERNIA

The natural history of an untreated inguinal hernia is surprisingly difficult to determine for a condition with such a large prevalence. The problem is the difficulty in finding whole populations in which hernia repairs are not routinely performed. Two studies have reported a yearly risk of a hernia accident at 0.0037 and 0.0038, and have historically been used as a basis to justify repair [10]. The first was from a truss clinic in Paris in the late eighteenth century.

This was at a time before Bassini's operation had become widely accepted and therefore routine repair was rarely performed. The second group came from Cali, Colombia, and was the result of an aggressive 1-year (1965–1966) government initiative, the purpose of which was to accurately examine a stratified, randomized sample of its civilian population, looking at common conditions such as inguinal hernia. Using the formula (1 − [1 − p]e), where p is the probability of an accident per hernia patient per year which is the average of the 2 studies (0.00375) and e from actuarial life tables from the respective years, one can calculate the probability of a hernia accident. Table 1 shows the lifetime probability of a hernia accident for an 18-year-old and a 72-year-old. The difference in the 1980 and 2001 data reflects the fact that the 2001 patients are living longer and thus have more years at risk [11]. The desire to obtain prospective, up-to-date data was the incentive for the development of 3 randomized controlled trials that have served to substantially change the way surgeons approach their patients with inguinal hernia (see Table 1).

THE NORTH AMERICAN TRIAL (2006)

Participants in the North American trial, conducted by Fitzgibbons and colleagues [12], were randomized to "watchful waiting" or conventional Lichtenstein herniorrhaphy. After informed consent, 720 men aged 18 years and older with inguinal hernias that were asymptomatic or minimally symptomatic were recruited. The trial was coordinated at 5 locations across North America, and the initial results were published with a minimum follow-up of 2 years. The physical component score (a 36-item Short Form survey) measured pain that interfered with normal activities and physical function and showed similar results between the 2 groups. The rate of crossover to surgery at 2 years was 23%, with "increased pain" as the most common reason for crossover. The 2 groups were similar at baseline with respect to age, American Society of Anesthesiology classification, preexisting conditions, hernia type, and hernia characteristics. No statistically significant differences were found between the groups regarding operative time, complications, recurrence rates, and satisfaction with the results of the operation. Patients who reported higher baseline pain during activity or "unpleasantness" at the start of the trial were more likely to cross over from the watchful waiting group to the surgery group. These characteristics have helped clinicians council patients who are more likely to require an inguinal herniorrhaphy eventually. Patients who crossed over did report an increase in pain after the operation, but by the 2-year follow-up, it was not

Table 1
Lifetime risk of a hernia accident for an untreated inguinal hernia

	Overall		Male patients	
Age, y	1980	2001	1980	2001
18	1 in 5.18	1 in 4.95	1 in 5.49	1 in 5.15
72	1 in 22.72	1 in 20.41	1 in 27.03	1 in 22.73

significantly higher than that in the group managed conservatively. At 2 years, only 1 patient (0.3%) experienced an acute hernia incarceration that was without strangulation. By the end of the trial, with a maximum follow-up of 4.5 years, another patient had an acute incarceration with bowel obstruction, resulting in a hernia accident rate of 1.8 per 1000 patient-years. The conclusion from the trial was that observation was an acceptable treatment option for men with minimally symptomatic inguinal hernias. A long-term follow-up Kaplan-Meier analysis demonstrated a total crossover rate of 68%, mainly due to pain at 10 years [4]. There were only a total of 3 acute hernias requiring operation.

UNITED KINGDOM TRIAL (2006)

Another randomized controlled trial conducted in a single center in Glasgow, United Kingdom, also investigated watchful waiting for minimally symptomatic men with inguinal hernias [13]. The study recruited 160 men older than 55 years, with 80 men in each arm, and followed them at 6 months, 1 year, and then annually afterward. Pain was assessed using the visual analogue scale score, and the Short Form-36 was used to measure the general health status. The 2 groups had a similar baseline health status. At 1 year, no significant differences were found between the groups for pain at rest, pain with movement, or the use of analgesia. The surgical repair group did have significant improvement in their perceived quality of life. Twenty-three patients (29%) in the watchful waiting group crossed over to surgery, with "increasing pain" and "hernia enlargement" as the most common reasons. Three patients had an acute presentation: 1 with hernia incarceration and 2 with cardiovascular events after crossover to surgery from the watchful waiting group. The degree of hernia protrusion was the only variable identified on the Cox proportional hazards regression model that predicted crossover to surgery. Long-term follow-up at 7.5 years showed a total crossover rate of 72% [14]. Reasons for patients seeking surgical repair of their hernia were pain (72%), quality of life (13%), and an increase in hernia size (11%).

NETHERLANDS TRIAL (2018)

Most recently, results from another randomized controlled trial were published in January 2018 that again sought to shed more light on this controversy [15]. This was a noninferiority trial designed to determine the noninferiority of watchful waiting to elective repair in men aged 50 years and older with mildly symptomatic or asymptomatic inguinal hernias. Recruits were men older than 50 years with asymptomatic or minimally symptomatic inguinal hernias. The same pain scale scoring system was used as in the North American trial. After randomization and final exclusions, 234 patients were assigned to the elective repair group and 262 into the watchful waiting group. Of the 262 patients assigned to watchful waiting, 99 crossed over to elective hernia repair and 163 were treated without surgery. Follow-up physical examinations were performed at 3, 12, 24, and 36 months. The primary endpoint was the difference between the 2 groups in pain/discomfort scores, calculated as a mean of the 4 follow-up visits. Secondary endpoints included health-related change in quality-of-life measures from baseline; 3, 12, 24, and 36-month intervals; overall crossover rate; and event-free survival between the 2 groups. The result of the primary endpoint (mean of the pain/discomfort scores measured at follow-up visits over a 24-month period) was 0.35 (95% confidence interval [CI] 0.28–0.41) in the elective group and 0.58 (95% CI 0.52–0.64) in the watchful waiting group for a difference of 0.23 (95% CI 0.32–0.14). In this noninferiority trial, the widths of these 95% CIs indicated that a difference of means greater than 0.20 in favor of elective repair cannot be excluded. Thus, the data could not rule out a relevant difference in favor of elective repair. Secondary endpoints, such as measures of quality of life and mean changes over time compared with baseline, were not found to reach clinical significance, although there was a slight statistically significant favor for the elective repair group. Of the 262 patients assigned to watchful waiting, 99 (37.8%) crossed over to surgery by 3 years, most often because of worsening hernia-related pain. Of these crossover patients, 2.3% underwent urgent operation, and 1 patient had bowel strangulation. No patients required a bowel resection. The 3-year event-free survival in the elective repair and watching waiting groups were 80.9% and 77.2%, respectively. The 3-year cumulative incidence of patients with 1 or more events was 17.5% (41 of 234) in the elective repair and 20.6% (54 of 262) in the watchful waiting group. In the elective repair group, these events consisted of 25 cases of moderate-severe pain, 1 hernia complication, 1 ischemic orchitis, and 20 recurrent hernias. In the watchful waiting group, 69 patients reported moderate-severe pain, 7 hernia complications in 6 patients, and 7 recurrent hernias. The 3-year cumulative death rates were 3.0% and 3.1% in the repair and watchful waiting group, respectively, with none of these deaths related to hernias. There was no difference in perioperative complication rates between the elective repair group and the crossover patients who underwent surgery. The investigators concluded that although the results of the primary endpoint could not rule out a relevant difference in favor of elective repair, "in view of all other findings" their results justified watchful waiting as a reasonable alternative to surgery in male patients aged 50 years and older.

COMPARISON AMONG THE 3 TRIALS

There are some important differences among the 3 randomized controlled trials (Table 2) and the subsequent long-term follow-up studies from the first 2 studies (Table 3). The North American and Netherlands hernia trials were multicenter trials that included both academic and community medical centers [12,15], whereas the UK trial was conducted in a single academic center [13]. The inclusion criterion for age was broader in the North American hernia trial compared with both the UK and Netherlands trials. The median ages and age span among the trials varied greatly, as well as the framework of the medical system, as a large portion of those in the North American study had private insurance and were predominantly white. The definition of an asymptomatic hernia was different in the 3 trials. In the UK trial, only patients with a visible

Table 2
Comparison of 3 watchful waiting randomized controlled trials

Variable	North American trial	UK trial	Netherlands trial
Patient number	720	160	496
Age	>18 (mean 58)	>55 (mean 70)	>50 (mean 65)
Size	Any	Visible bulge	Any
Reducibility	Not required	Required	Not required

swelling on standing were included, whereas 40% of the patients in the North American hernia trial had only a cough impulse. The Netherlands trial used only physical examination with optional ultrasonography confirmation. There was no difference in pain between the 2 groups at 1 year in the UK trial or at

Table 3
Comparison of crossover rates and long-term follow-up

	North American trial, short-term	North American trial, long-term	UK trial, short-term	UK trial, long-term	Netherlands trial, short-term
Follow-up, y	Mean 3.2 (range 2–4.5)	Maximum 11.5	Median 1.6	Median 7.5 (range 6.2–8.2)	3
Crossover rate	23% at 2 y 32% at 4.5 y	68% at 10 y	29%	54% at 5 y 72% at 7.5 y	38%
Hernia accident rate in watchful waiting group	0.6% (n = 2)	1.2% (n = 3)	1.3% (n = 1)	2.5% (n = 2)	2.3% (n = 6)
Reasons for crossover	Pain (47.1%) Some degree of pain and discomfort (86%)	Pain (54%) Tired of having the hernia (3.3%) Incarceration (2.4%) Advised by doctor to have it repaired (4.1) Employer wanted hernia repaired (0.8%) Other (8.1) Combination of reasons (30.9%)	Pain (48%) Increase in size (35%) Affecting work or leisure activities (13%)	Pain (72%) Quality of life (13%) Increase in size (11%)	Pain (91%) Cosmetic reasons (1%) Unknown (2%)

2 years for the North American hernia trial. The Netherlands trial showed patients had less pain at 3 months in the watchful waiting group; however, at 12 months and afterward, the patients in the elective hernia group had less pain. The Netherlands trial has yet to produce long-term follow-up results and offers only 3-year cumulative data. On long-term follow-up, the number of patients who died in the UK hernia trial watchful waiting group was higher (23%) than in the North American hernia trial watchful waiting group (3.5%). This finding was presumed to be related to the fact that only older patients were included in the UK hernia trial. However, in the Netherlands trial, which also enrolled only older patients, the death rate was much lower at 3.1% (all unrelated to hernias). Patients in the UK trial were seen at 6 months, 12 months, and 5 years in a research clinic or were sent mail questionnaires. Patients in the Netherlands trial had physical examinations at 3, 12, 24, and 36 months. The patients in the North American hernia trial were personally followed by study nurses and examined by independent surgeons at prescribed intervals to ensure objectivity during the 5 years of the original study. Long-term follow-up was yearly by mail questionnaire or by e-mail and telephone encounters if they did not respond to the mail questionnaire. A criticism of the long-term follow-up data from the North American trial was that it was only 65.7% complete. This was caused in part by the inability to obtain institutional review board approval at one of the sites (McGill) for a secondary follow-up study. Also contributing to this might have been the wide geographic distribution of patients in the North American hernia trial, which made it more difficult for the investigators to physically examine patients in a clinic. There are some relevant findings that are consistent in all 3 trials. The hernia accident rate was very low and comparable in all 3 studies. These trials all support that the potential future risk of a hernia accident should not be considered an indication for surgery. Pain was the main reason for crossover in all 3 studies. The median time to crossover was longest in the North American hernia trial (7.3 years). The reason for this could be because a large number of patients had only a cough impulse initially at the time of randomization, whereas patients in the UK trial were required to have a visible bulge. The rate of crossover to surgery was high in all 3 studies. Kaplan-Meyer estimates disclosed a 72% crossover rate in the UK trial at 7.5 years, and in the North American hernia trial, 68% at 10 years. The Netherlands trial crossover rate of 37.8% at 3 years can be assumed to be following a similar trendline. The UK trial group concluded that there was little point in waiting because most patients will require an operation in the future. The North American hernia trial investigators, however, were more cautious and thought that the results may not necessarily imply routine surgery for all asymptomatic inguinal hernias. The Netherlands trial investigators concluded that although they could not rule out a relevant difference in favor of elective repair based on their primary endpoint analyses of the mean pain score over a 24-month period, the overall results including secondary endpoints justified waiting as a reasonable alternative. Investigators

from all 3 studies cited the recruitment process as a limiting factor, as patients in all 3 trials presented to the surgery clinic after referral, mostly from primary care physicians (PCPs). The investigators speculated that applying conclusions based on referred patients to the general population may not be appropriate, assuming the PCP had enough concern to refer them.

A meta-analysis published in 2018 by Gong and Li [16], compares the results of 8 watchful waiting randomized controlled trials, including the 3 trials discussed previously, encompassing a total of 1303 patients. The study found significantly less pain with movement in the operation group ($P<.01$) at a minimum follow-up of 12 months; however, there was no significant differences in the physical component score (as measured by the Short Form-36 Version 2 health-related quality-of-life survey), mortality, surgical complications, or postoperative hernia recurrence. Crossover from watchful waiting to operation was consistent across all studies and confirmed that most patients will have had an operation by 10 years. Pain was the most common reason for the crossover. Because of the overall low rate of acute hernia–related adverse events, the investigators concluded that for asymptomatic or minimally symptomatic inguinal hernias, watchful waiting is a relatively safe and acceptable option in the short-term; however, watchful waiting would rather delay, than avoid a surgical repair in most patients (see Tables 2 and 3).

ECONOMIC IMPACT

In the United States, surgical repair of inguinal hernias accounted for more than $48 billion in 2005 health care expenditures. Stroupe and colleagues [17] looked at the cost-effectiveness of the strategy of watchful waiting on patients involved in the North American hernia trial. To measure the effectiveness of the procedure, they used quality-adjusted life-years (QALY), which incorporates health-related quality of life and medical outcomes into a single measure. By 2 years, the average cost for patients with tension-free repair (TFR) was approximately $1800 higher than for the watchful waiting group. When looked at in terms of QALYs, the average cost per additional QALY unit per patient for TFR patients was $59,065. It is generally agreed that for a procedure to qualify for public funding, a cost per QALY should be $50,000 or greater. The investigators concluded that at 2 years, both watchful waiting and immediate surgery for inguinal hernias are reasonable approaches from the viewpoint of cost-effectiveness. Of significance, this cost analysis was done at 2 years follow-up, by which time 23% of the watchful waiting patients had decided to cross over to receive surgery for various reasons, mostly pain. By 10 years of observation, however, the crossover rate nearly triples. As such, the conclusion/results cannot be considered valid at 10 years. Although the initial data are insightful, additional work must be done to evaluate a more long-term cost analysis. Currently, there are insufficient data to say whether watchful waiting or surgical management strategies are more cost-effective.

INGUINAL HERNIA IN WOMEN

Groin hernia repair is much less likely in women compared with men, with a ratio of roughly 1 to 9 [18]. Although femoral hernias are more common in women than men, inguinal hernia repairs (mainly indirect) still outnumber femoral hernia repairs by a ratio of 5 to 1. The natural history of an untreated groin hernia in women is clearly different from men; thus, recommendations for treatment must be different. Indeed, in the 3 large randomized trials discussed in this article, women were excluded because it was thought that it was unethical to include them. The variations in pelvic anatomy and Hesselbach triangle in women and men decreases a woman's overall chance of having a groin hernia, but ultimately increases a woman's chance of developing femoral hernias. The current recommendation for women is that all should have their hernias repaired at diagnosis, because the incidence of hernia accident is much higher than in men. Koch and colleagues [19] analyzed data from the Swedish Hernia Register between 1992 and 2003 for women undergoing surgery for groin hernias and identified 6895 patients aged 15 years or older. The investigators compared their outcomes with 83,753 men in the same registry. Analysis of their data found that women were more likely to undergo an emergency operation and were more likely to develop a recurrent femoral hernia when compared with men with groin hernias. Because femoral hernias are more dangerous than inguinal, with a much higher incidence of a hernia accident thought to be related to the rigid nature of the femoral canal, it is not surprising that there is an increased incidence of emergent surgery in women. The higher incidence of femoral recurrence in women can be explained by the fact that the most common herniorrhaphy for all groin hernias is the Lichtenstein tension-free hernia repair. In this procedure, the inferior edge of the prosthesis is sewn to the inguinal ligament; thus, the femoral space is not addressed. Because it is not always possible to differentiate inguinal from femoral hernias by physical examination and because concomitant femoral hernias occur, an operation that corrects defects in the direct, indirect, and femoral spaces (the myopectineal orifice) is preferred. It is not surprising that preperitoneal herniorrhaphies, such as the laparoscopic hernia repairs, yield better results in women than the open Lichtenstein repair used commonly in men. However, the Lichtenstein operation can be modified by suturing the inferior edge of the prosthesis to the Cooper ligament instead of the inguinal ligament medially with a transition stich just medial to the femoral vein, which closes the femoral canal.

GUIDELINES FOR TREATMENT OF INGUINAL HERNIA IN MEN

The European Hernia Society (EHS) guidelines were updated with Level 1 studies in 2014 [20] and include the following statement and recommendation:

> Watchful waiting is safe and an acceptable option for men with minimally symptomatic or asymptomatic inguinal hernias. It is very likely (70% chance) that, in time, the symptoms will increase leading to surgical intervention. (Level 1B)

It is recommended in minimally symptomatic or asymptomatic inguinal hernia in men to consider a watchful waiting strategy, especially when older or in the presence of major comorbidity. (Grade B)

More recently, the HerniaSurge Group (made up of the EHS plus international experts) published international guidelines for the management of inguinal hernias [18]. This includes the following statement:

Although most patients will develop symptoms and need surgery, watchful waiting for minimal or asymptomatic inguinal hernias is safe since the risk of hernia complications is low. Management decision is made between the surgeon and patient. (High grade)

SUMMARY

Traditionally it has been recommended to repair all inguinal hernias at diagnosis to prevent the complications of strangulation or bowel obstruction. Three randomized controlled trials comparing a strategy of watchful waiting versus routine repair for asymptomatic or minimally symptomatic men have questioned this, because the chance of one of these complications in this subgroup of patients is extremely low, and the morbidity and mortality for the rare emergently needed repair is not excessive. There appears to be no penalty for delaying surgery, as the surgical complication rates in the long-term crossover patients was the same as those randomized to surgery initially. However, in long-term follow-up, most of the patients were found to have crossed over to surgery, usually because of increasing symptoms. Men older than 65 years cross over at a considerably higher rate than younger men. Although watchful waiting for an asymptomatic or minimally symptomatic inguinal hernia is a safe strategy for men, patients should be counseled that they are probably just delaying surgery rather than avoiding it.

References

[1] Primatesta P, Goldacre MJ. Inguinal hernia repair: incidence of elective and emergency surgery, readmission and mortality. Int J Epidemiol 1996;25:835–9.

[2] Ruhl CE, Everhart JE. Risk factors for inguinal hernia among adults in the US population. Am J Epidemiol 2007;165:1154–61.

[3] Zendejas B, Ramirez T, Jones T, et al. Incidence of inguinal hernia repairs in Olmsted County, MN. Ann Surg 2013;257:520–6.

[4] Fitzgibbons RJ, Ramanan B, Arya S, et al. Long-term results of a randomized controlled trial of a nonoperative strategy (watchful waiting) for men with minimally symptomatic inguinal hernias. Ann Surg 2013;258:508–15.

[5] INCA Trialists Collaboration. Operation compared with watchful waiting in elderly male inguinal hernia patients: a review and data analysis. J Am Coll Surg 2011;212:251–9.e4.

[6] Hair A, Paterson C, Wright D, et al. What effect does the duration of an inguinal hernia have on patient symptoms? J Am Coll Surg 2001;193:125–9.

[7] Chen DC, Hiatt JR, Amid PK. Operative management of refractory neuropathic inguinodynia by a laparoscopic retroperitoneal approach. JAMA Surg 2013;148:962.

[8] Simons MP, Aufenacker T, Bay-Nielsen M, et al. European Hernia Society guidelines on the treatment of inguinal hernia in adult patients. Hernia 2009;13:343–403.

[9] Tubre DJ, Schroeder AD, Estes J, et al. Surgical site infection: the "Achilles heel" of all types of abdominal wall hernia reconstruction. Hernia 2018;22:1003–13.
[10] Neuhauser D. Elective inguinal herniorrhaphy versus truss in the elderly. In: Bunker JP, Barnes BA, MF, editors. Costs, risks, and benefits of surgery. New York: Oxford University Press; 1977. p. 223–39.
[11] Turaga K, Fitzgibbons RJ, Puri V. Inguinal hernias: should we repair? Surg Clin North Am 2008;88:127–38.
[12] Fitzgibbons RJ, Giobbie-Hurder A, Gibbs JO, et al. Watchful waiting vs repair of inguinal hernia in minimally symptomatic men. JAMA 2006;295:285.
[13] O'Dwyer PJ, Norrie J, Alani A, et al. Observation or operation for patients with an asymptomatic inguinal hernia. Ann Surg 2006;244:167–73.
[14] Chung L, Norrie J, O'Dwyer PJ. Long-term follow-up of patients with a painless inguinal hernia from a randomized clinical trial. Br J Surg 2011;98:596–9.
[15] de Goede B, Wijsmuller AR, van Ramshorst GH, et al. Watchful waiting versus surgery of mildly symptomatic or asymptomatic inguinal hernia in men aged 50 years and older: a randomized controlled trial. Ann Surg 2018;267:42–9.
[16] Gong W, Li J. Operation versus watchful waiting in asymptomatic or minimally symptomatic inguinal hernias: the meta-analysis results of randomized controlled trials. Int J Surg 2018;52:120–5.
[17] Stroupe KT, Manheim LM, Luo P, et al. Tension-free repair versus watchful waiting for men with asymptomatic or minimally symptomatic inguinal hernias: a cost-effectiveness analysis. J Am Coll Surg 2006;203:458–68.
[18] HerniaSurge Group. International guidelines for groin hernia management. Hernia 2018;22:1–165.
[19] Koch A, Edwards A, Haapaniemi S, et al. Prospective evaluation of 6895 groin hernia repairs in women. Br J Surg 2005;92:1553–8.
[20] Miserez M, Peeters E, Aufenacker T, et al. Update with level 1 studies of the European Hernia Society guidelines on the treatment of inguinal hernia in adult patients. Hernia 2014;18: 151–63.

Advances in Surgery 53 (2019) 305–325

ADVANCES IN SURGERY

The Opioid Crisis

The Surgeon's Role

Ross F. Goldberg, MD[a,b,*]

[a]Department of Surgery, Maricopa Integrated Health System, 2601 East Roosevelt Street, Hogan Building, Phoenix, AZ 85008, USA; [b]Creighton University School of Medicine - Phoenix, Phoenix, AZ, USA

Keywords

• Opioid epidemic • Health care policy and advocacy • Prescription limitations • Continuing medical education • Enhanced recovery after surgery

Key points

- The opioid epidemic has become a significant public health care crisis in the United States.
- Surgeon overprescribing has played a role in the development of this epidemic, and new evidence-based practices have been implemented to curtail such overprescribing, including the creation of the enhanced recovery after surgery pathways and new multimodal pain management strategies.
- Federal and state legislation has been enacted addressing prescription limitations, new regulations regarding the ability to prescribe, and continuing medical education to better understand pain management options.

INTRODUCTION

Recently, there has been increased awareness and scrutiny of the prescribing habits of physicians and surgeons regarding opioids given the ever-growing presence of opioid abuse and addiction across the United States, culminating in the US government declaring the opioid epidemic a public health emergency on October 16, 2017. The reasons for this epidemic status with opioids are complex. Data have shown that prescribing habits of physicians have played a role, with overprescribing leading to addiction, misuse, opioid dispersion into the community, and potential transformation into illicit drug or heroin use and abuse.

Disclosure Statement: The author has nothing to disclose.

*Department of Surgery, Maricopa Integrated Health System, 2601 East Roosevelt Street, Hogan Building, Phoenix, AZ 85008. *E-mail address:* Ross_Goldberg@dmgaz.org

https://doi.org/10.1016/j.yasu.2019.04.015
0065-3411/19/

The surgeon's role in this epidemic is complicated. In this profession, surgeons cause acute pain when operating or when treating a trauma or burn patient, and there needs to be a balance between managing a patient's pain and overprescribing to try and obliterate the pain. Further challenging the issue is that recent studies have shown that anywhere between 1% and 13% of opioid-naïve surgical patients developed opioid dependence after a surgical encounter [1–5].

Recent interventions, both in the medical world and through legislation and regulation, has led to a reduction in opioid prescriptions by 8% and prescription opioid overdose deaths by 12% [6,7]. All of this work though has not seemed to affect the escalation of opioid overdosing occurring in the United States, with 64,000 people dying from drug overdoses in 2016. More than 42,000 of those deaths were due to opioids; this is a 20% increase from the total of 52,000 drug overdose deaths from the year before [7–9]. The greatest contributor to these overdoses is related to illegally manufactured fentanyl, accounting for 20,000 deaths, followed by heroin at 15,000 deaths, and prescription drugs for less than 15,000 [7].

The medical community has met this epidemic head on, trying to find ways to minimize the reliance on opioid use while still adequately controlling patients' pain. As with any disease process, there is not a single fix for all patients, and the solution does not solely rest in the medical literature. This article reviews the situations that have led to this current state and discusses areas in which surgeons can be involved to address the opioid epidemic.

TIMELINE OF OPIOID ANALGESIC USE

During the 1980s, there was a movement underway to address the perceived undertreatment of postoperative and cancer pain with opioids, culminating in the 1986 Cancer Pain Monograph produced by the World Health Organization [7,10]. This led to the examination of opioid use outside of the oncology field during the 1990s, with opioids becoming the primary modality of chronic noncancer pain treatment in the United States [7,11]. All of this led to the famous pain as the fifth vital sign campaign in 1995, which was launched by the American Pain Society in an attempt to standardize the evaluation and treatment of pain symptoms [7,12]. In 1999, the Veterans Health Administration adopted the pain as the fifth vital sign initiative, increasing support for the concept [7,13]. This was further engrained by the published standards for pain management in 2000 by The Joint Commission (TJC), accentuating the need for quantitative assessments of pain as recommended by the Institute of Medicine. Meanwhile, the Federation of State Medical Boards and the US Drug Enforcement Agency (DEA) issued statements leading to less regulatory scrutiny of opioid prescribing habits [7,14,15].

These changes, loosening regulations while mandating standards for pain management, led to a series of unintended consequences, the largest being a heavy reliance on opioid medication to remedy what was considered inadequate pain control [7]. Patients came to expect that they should have no pain at all. Coupled with this new expectation, changes in the reimbursement patterns with regard to physician and hospital quality ratings started to occur at this time. One such change was with the Centers for Medicare and Medicaid Services' Hospital Consumer Assessment of Healthcare Providers and Systems (HCAHPS) survey, implemented in October 2006, seeking the perspective of recently discharged patients on the details of their hospital experience [16]. The original 32-item survey had 3 questions dedicated to how well a patient's pain was managed during their hospital stay [16,17]. These survey results were available to the public, allowing patients to compare hospitals. These results also became linked with CMS payments through the Value-Based Purchasing program [16]. Hospital administrators were concerned that if they ignored the TJC standards and the HCAHPS survey results they were potentially jeopardizing their federal health care funds, which led to some hospitals investing into opioid therapy, leading to better satisfaction rates from their patients [7,18].

Exacerbating this was that during this time the pharmaceutical companies were heavily pushing the use of opioids, presenting it as a humane treatment option for pain management [7]. The medicolegal pressures grew as well, culminating in litigation for undertreating pain, labeling it as inhumane [7,19]. The new paradigm in medical education was to rely on opioids for pain treatment because of all these changes. This also led to the creation of new extended-release formulations of opioids that were frequently prescribed because, ironically, it was presumed there was a lower likelihood of abuse, when in fact they were heavily abused.

A final piece was the limitations on how to prescribe opioids. Although there was less regulatory scrutiny of prescribing habits, patients were still required to obtain a handwritten prescription from physicians to obtain Schedule II substances [16]. These could not be sent electronically or via fax to pharmacies. This included the commonly used opioids

- Morphine
- Oxycodone
- Hydromorphone
- Methadone
- Hydrocodone [16].

This required patients to physically return to their physician's office to obtain a refill, which was a potential inconvenience to both patient and physician, especially given that some patients were traveling great distances to seek care at tertiary and quaternary care hospitals [16]. To avoid some of these inconveniences, there was the potential for some opioid prescriptions to be for more than necessary just in case there were issues with pain management when the patients returned home [16].

THE SURGEON AND OVERPRESCRIBING

As previously mentioned, it is reasonable for surgeons to treat the acute pain they cause. The issue arises with what is considered appropriate postoperative opioid prescribing because that is poorly defined [16]. The Centers for Disease Control and Prevention (CDC) created guidelines for opioid use in the chronic pain patient [20]; however, there are no guidelines for the acute or postoperative pain patient [16]. This has led to such variability that that there has been found to be a 3-fold to 5-fold difference in prescribing rates in the United States [21]. Studies have shown that surgeons, in particular, account for a large degree of this prescribing variability, with individual surgeons prescribing vastly different amounts for the exact same operation [16,22,23].

Often, the number of pills prescribed exceeds the number of pills used, as evidenced in Table 1, which reviews some of the studies that show the degree of overprescribing occurring with different surgical procedures [16]. Kim and colleagues [28] reported that 66% of opioids went unused after different upper extremity operations [16]. A similar study in general surgery operations, by

Table 1
Results of surgical fields evaluating their postoperative opioid use

Study	Specialty	Number of subjects	Opioid use	Opioid disposal details
Maughan et al, [24] 2016	Dental	74	54% of all pills unused	NR
Harris et al, [25] 2013	Dermatology	72	86% had any pills leftover	53% of patients with leftovers kept
Hill et al, [22] 2017	General Surgery	127	71% of all pills were used	74% of patients with leftovers kept
Bartels et al, [26] 2016	Gynecology	30	53% used 0–5 pills 83% used < half of prescription	77% of patients with leftovers kept
Rodgers et al, [27] 2012	Orthopedics	250	45% used 0–5 pills 77% had any pills leftover	NR
Kim et al, [28] 2016	Orthopedics	1416	66% of all pills unused	Only 5.3% received instructions on disposal
Kumar et al, [29] 2017	Orthopedics	81	37% of all pills unused	75% of patients with leftovers kept
Bartels et al, [26] 2016	Thoracic	31	45% used 0–5 pills 71% had any pills leftover	73% of patients with leftovers kept
Bates et al, [30] 2011	Urology	275	67% had any pills leftover 42% of all pills were unused	91% of patients with leftovers kept

From Theisen K, Jacobs B, Macleod L, Davies B. The United States opioid epidemic: a review of the surgeon's contribution to it and health policy initiatives. BJU Int. 2018; 122(5): 756. Epub 2018 Jul 26; with permission.

Hill and colleagues [22], found 71% of all opioids were unused [16]. A study of dental procedures showed opioids went unused 54% of the time [24], whereas other data showed that 45% of patients undergoing thoracic operations and 54% of patients undergoing cesarean sections only required 0 to 5 opioid pills in the postoperative period [16,26]. When reviewing all these data, it was suggested that surgeons may have served as contributors for opioid overprescribing [16,31].

Between 1997 and 2002, extended-release oxycodone (OxyContin) prescriptions increased from 670,000 to 6.2 million, with overall opioid consumption skyrocketing in the 2000s from 49,946 kg in 2000 to the peak at 165,525 kg in 2012 [7,32,33]. Surgeons had a role to play in this prescription increase. In 2012, a study from the Information Medical Statistics (IMS) Health's National Prescription Audit showed that surgeons accounted for 28.3 million (9.8%) of 289 million opioid prescriptions dispensed [34,35]. In 2015 there were enough prescription opioids dispensed to medicate every adult in the United States with 5 mg of hydrocodone every 4 hours for 3 weeks [16,36]. When compared with the rest of the world, the United States prescribes greater than 50 times more opioids [16,37].

RESULTS OF OVERPRESCRIBING

When these changes regarding opioid practices went into effect, it seemed that there was some success in regard to better pain control, coupled with the thought that opioids had a low addictive potential [38]; however, a short time later, concerns began to arise concerning the amount of treating with opioids. In the past 15 years there has been a quadrupling of prescription opioids sales and mortality in both men and women, as reported by the CDC in their National Vital Statistics System [7,39]. Adding to the concerns has been that, up to now, there has been no level I evidence for the long-term safety of the effect of opioid therapy in treating chronic pain and improving overall function [7]. Instead, there has been an increase in chronic opioid use, and the physical and psychological issues that arise from chronic opioid use, abuse, and addiction.

The evidence has shown that even a single prescription in an opioid-naïve patient can lead to long-term use [2,16,40–42]. A population-based study from Toronto, Canada, evaluated the risk of long-term opioid use in opioid-naïve elderly patients undergoing short-stay surgeries, including varicose vein stripping, laparoscopic cholecystectomy, cataract surgery, and transurethral resection of the prostate, and found that 7.7% of the patients who filled an opioid prescription at the time of surgery were still using prescription opioids 1 year later [2,16]. Another study looked at the risk in opioid-naïve adults undergoing 13 minor and major operations, and found that 6% of opioid-naïve adults who received an opioid prescription perioperatively were still using opioids 3 to 6 months later, and that the rate of use was similar between minor and major operations [16,40]. Similar long-term opioid use rates, ranging from 3.1% to 8.2%, were found in the opioid-naïve population after undergoing an operation [41,42], supporting the finding that a subset of patients who are exposed to a single opioid prescription are at risk of addiction and long-term use [16].

The evidence even goes as far as to suggest that just a single day's prescription of opioids can result in chronic use [16]. Shah and Marin [43] studied 1.3 million opioid-naïve adults who were discharged from the hospital with a new opioid prescription after medical and surgical admissions. They calculated the rate of opioid use 1 and 3 years after initial prescription, finding that a single day's prescription led to a rate of persistent opioid use at 1 year of 6%, increasing to 13.5% for prescriptions that were for at least 7 days [16,43].

The other issue that arises with overprescribing is the unused excess medications; they are rarely discarded and often stored insecurely [16,22,26]. There is a risk of these pills then being dispersed into a community, which can lead to further misuse and abuse [16]. A survey of adults in the United States who abuse prescription opioids found that 50% obtained their pills from a friend or relative for free, whereas another 15% bought or stole from a friend or relative [16,44]. This is further exacerbated because 1 in 5 adults in the United States admit to sharing their prescription opioids with others [16,45]. The abuse of prescription opioids has the potential to serve as a first step to other illicit drug use because 40% to 80% of heroin users admit to abusing prescription opioids before initiating heroin [16,46,47]. Overprescribing cannot be deemed as the sole cause for these issues but, given all that is now known about the potential for misuse and abuse of opioids, prescribing habits and rates need to be altered.

SOLUTIONS FOR THE SURGEON

There are a variety of ways in which a surgeon can have a positive impact on addressing the current opioid epidemic in the United States. To broadly categorize the avenues available, these can be viewed as the patient care or clinical side, and the health care policy and advocacy side. Each side has a different but equal and important role in addressing the issue.

PATIENT CARE AND CLINICAL SOLUTIONS

Surgeons' understanding of and bias toward pain

It is difficult to fully treat someone's pain without understanding the neuroanatomy of pain itself [48]. One needs to understand tolerance, physical dependence, and addiction to be truly responsible when prescribing opioids. The definition of tolerance is the biophysical modulation of opioid receptors after chronic exposure [48]. With chronic exposure, these receptors require an increase in the amount of activation to get the same result, leading to the need to use increased amounts of narcotics to meet the same level of pain relief [48–50]. Physical dependence is the manifestation of withdrawal symptoms due to cessation of the medication. The most pronounced symptoms of withdrawal include diaphoresis, agitation, tachycardia, vomiting, and diarrhea [48]. Addiction is the term used to describe the behavioral changes that occur, such as seeking out the medication despite personal harm to themselves or others [48,50].

When approaching any pain management plan, one also must consider specific patient populations and the potential effect of narcotic use on select groups; this helps lead to developing individual plans, decreasing amounts when needed, and changing the timing of medications [48]. One such group is the elderly. Owing to changes of pharmacokinetics and pharmacodynamics related to aging and polypharmacy, careful consideration is needed before any prescribing of narcotics to the elderly [48,51]. Patients with cardiac and pulmonary comorbidities are susceptible to increased cardiac and respiratory depression, whereas renal and liver disease can prolong drug clearance and metabolism, leading to longer medication half-life and adverse events [52–55]. In patients who have obstructive sleep apnea, additive central depression, and decreased neuromuscular tone, opioid use can worsen the obstruction and pulmonary complications [48,56,57].

Surgeons also must realize their implicit biases on assessment and treatment of patient pain [58]. Factors that play into a surgeon's bias when it comes to assessing pain include patient-reported symptom severity, judgments regarding the patients' trustworthiness, a surgeon's preconceived notion of how painful a particular procedure should be, prior clinical experience in managing various disease states, and the degree of empathy that a surgeon feels toward any given patient or patient population [58,59]. What further complicates matters is when the patient's report of pain does not seem to match with the objective clinical signs when assessing for pain [58].

There have been attempts to diminish the subjective nature of a patient's pain complaints through visual aids such as the Wong-Baker Faces Pain Rating Scale; surgeons are trained to take these results with some skepticism [58,60]. There is justification behind questioning a patient who states their pain is 10 out of 10 on stimulation while resting comfortably, there have been reports showing a direct correlation between patient appearance and how trustworthy they seem to their surgeon and caregivers [58]. This is further supported by the evidence that shows that pain judgment biases have been shown to be rooted in clinicians' perceptions of patient ethnicity, age, gender, skin color, socioeconomic status, and attractiveness, with many of these same factors influencing the prescribing patterns of analgesic agents [61–63].

Clinician experience seems to mediate implicit attitudes about pain assessment, which is especially relevant regarding to the surgeon's capacity to manage postoperative pain [58]. An inexperienced trainee may underestimate the pain associated with a particular case or overmedicate a complaining patient at night, whereas an experienced clinician may undertreat patients based on past experiences that remind them of patients with drug-seeking behaviors or overtreat to obtain improved patient satisfaction scores [58]. The first step in addressing these issues is acknowledging the existence of these implicit biases and then findings ways to mitigate their impact on the treatment of postoperative pain.

Identifying patients at risks

As previously reported, even a single day's use of opioids has a risk of leading to misuse, abuse, and addiction. Yet it was also shown that this chance of abuse was not uniform across all opioid-naïve patients, so it is important to try and identify potential risks or characteristics that could put a subsection of patients at a higher risk versus others. It has also been found that the incidence of prolonged opioid use after surgery varied depending on preoperative patient characteristics and the type of operation that the patient was undergoing [64]. In a retrospective analysis of 641,941 opioid-naïve patients undergoing an operation and 18,011,137 opioid-naïve nonsurgical patients, the incidence of chronic opioid use among nonsurgical patients was 0.136%, whereas in the surgical patients the highest incidence of chronic opioid use occurred after total knee arthroplasty (1.41%) [65]. After risk-stratifying and controlling for age, gender, and the preoperative medication used (antidepressants, antipsychotics, benzodiazepines), patients undergoing total knee arthroplasty, open cholecystectomy, total hip arthroplasty, simple mastectomy, laparoscopic cholecystectomy, open appendectomy, and cesarean section delivery were at significantly increased risk for chronic opioid use after surgery [64,65]. This study found that risk factors for chronic opioid use after surgery among opioid-naïve patients included male gender, age greater than 50 years, preoperative use of benzodiazepines, preoperative use of antidepressants, depression history, alcohol abuse history, and drug abuse history [64,65]. In a similar retrospective cohort of 36,177 opioid-naïve patients undergoing minor (eg, varicose vein removal, laparoscopic cholecystectomy, laparoscopic appendectomy, hemorrhoidectomy, thyroidectomy, transurethral prostate surgery, parathyroidectomy, and carpal tunnel surgery) or major (eg, ventral incisional hernia repair, colectomy, reflux surgery, bariatric surgery, and hysterectomy) operations, the risk factors identified for new persistent opioid use after surgery included preoperative tobacco use, alcohol and substance abuse disorders, mood disorders, anxiety, and preoperative pain disorders [40,64].

Another important risk factor for postoperative persistent or chronic opioid use is the use of opioids preoperatively [64]. In a national, population-based study of patients who underwent upper extremity operations, opioid use before surgery was associated with longer opioid prescriptions with an increase in the number of refills postoperatively [64,66]. It has also been found that between 64% to 77% of chronic opioid users before surgery continue their chronic opioid use after surgery [64,67,68]. Additional risk factors include lower socioeconomic status; preoperative pain; medical comorbidities, such as pulmonary disease and heart failure; depression; and a history of drug, alcohol, or tobacco abuse [5,65]. Understanding which populations are at greater risk for abuse allows the surgeon to individualize a postoperative pain management plan to minimize risk of abuse while also allowing the surgeon to build a rapport with the patient and strengthen the patient–physician relationship.

Patient education

A surgeon's understanding of their practice area and patient population gives them the chance to determine whom among their patients may seek increased opioid prescriptions versus those who choose to forego narcotic pain management [69]. There is a risk that patients who choose to bypass narcotics for perioperative pain management may have issues with adequate pain control, which can lead to increased length of stay and a higher risk of perioperative morbidity [69,70]. If one can better understand these patients and make an effort to educate them on the concept and issues of pain management, there is an opportunity for improving pain control and overall patient satisfaction [69]. It has been shown that patient education decreases the need for postoperative opioid use and improves patient satisfaction [69,71,72]. Every patient encounter provides an opportunity to educate the patient, and using interdisciplinary strategies that involve the surgeon, pain management specialists, nurses, physical and occupational therapists, ancillary staff, families, and other patient support systems is considered an ideal approach to helping to control patient pain while simultaneously minimizing opioid use [69,73].

Patient education about pain control should begin at the initial clinical evaluation and carry over to the preoperative visit [69]. There is an opportunity for the surgeon to educate the patient about the procedure, the degree and extent of expected perioperative pain, recovery time, and the realistic expectations of pain management in the outpatient setting during their recovery [69,74]. The counseling of patients regarding adequate pain control should be based on patient function, referring to the ability to sleep, ambulate, and eat [69]. One of the most crucial education points is to emphasize that any expectation of a patient's pain being at zero is unrealistic [69,75]. Hill and colleagues [22] suggested that setting patient expectations about the number of opioid pills that they will require and receive is beneficial in reducing the number of pills prescribed postoperatively. The best education for the patient should start with face-to-face personal encounters, supplemented with culturally and linguistically appropriate written, video, and Web-based educational materials [74]. An example of patient-centered material that can be used to help surgeons develop a pain management plan along with the patient is shown in Table 2.

Education should not only occur preoperatively but during the postoperative phase as well. By educating patients about their multimodal pain control plan that includes nonopioid medications often helps in strengthening the rapport between surgeon and patient, as well as define goals for pain management [69,76]. This is the time is to reinforce what was discussed preoperatively, that zero pain is not attainable and pain control should be based on the ability to perform certain activities of daily living in the postoperative setting [69]. This education should also include how and when to take their medication [69].

Education also needs to go beyond just opioid use to focus on proper and safe disposal of excess opioid medications. The US Food and Drug Administration (FDA) recommends disposing of opioid pills at Drug Enforcement Administration–approved collection sites or community-based drug take-back

Table 2
Chart template for educating patients on opioid options

Generic name	Brand name	Route of administration	Common dose	Length of effect
Oxycodone (immediate release)	Oxycodone	Orally	5 mg	4–6 h
Oxycodone or acetaminophen	Percocet		5 mg oxycodone or 325 mg acetaminophen	
Hydrocodone or acetaminophen	Vicodin Lortab Lorcet HD		5 mg hydrocodone or 325 mg acetaminophen	
Hydromorphone	Dilaudid		2 mg	
Hydrocodone	Hycodan		5 mg hydrocodone	
Codeine/ acetaminophen	Tylenol #3			
Morphine	MorphaBond (extended-release) Arymo (extended-release)	Orally	15 mg	12 h
Methadone	Methadose Dolophine		5 mg	8 h
Oxycodone (extended-release)	OxyContin		10 mg	12 h
Fentanyl	Actiq Fentora Abstral Duragesic	Orally, transdermal (skin patch)	No recommended dose	Dependent on route of administration

From Torres M, Eskander M, Held J, et al. The general surgeon's role in enhancing patient education about prescription opioids. Bull Am Coll Surg 2017; 102(8): 15-20; with permission.

programs, flushing them down the toilet, placing them in a sealable plastic bag, or dissolving the pills in water and mixing them with compostable materials (eg, coffee grounds) and placing the mixture in a sealable bag before placing in the trash [69,77]. This education should be part of the written materials the patient receives on discharge, to ensure that they understand the correct way to dispose of these medications.

Another way to help educate patients is providing them with educational tools and information while they wait for the surgeon in the office in the waiting rooms and patient examination rooms. The idea is to make all material easy to read and understand, while maintaining cultural sensitivity to patient populations.

The US Department of Veterans Affairs has had reductions in outpatient prescribing of risky opioid regimens thanks to the implementation of systemwide initiatives, showing that patient education programs that offer easily accessible and useful information for veterans and patients have had positive results and safer opioid use [69,78]. One such initiative was the creation of The Opioid Safety Initiative Toolkit, providing a clear explanation of the path between various options and rating the strength and quality of evidence behind each decision of the path [69]. This toolkit is online and helps both patients and physicians with pain management decisions.

Perioperative pain management protocols

Introducing a multimodal approach to postoperative pain management is another avenue with which surgeons can have an impact on the opioid epidemic, by moving away from sole reliance of opioids and introducing new and innovative approaches to postoperative pain control.

A growing subset of pain management is alternative treatment modalities, focusing on evidence-based nonnarcotic interventions to help supplement the treatment of postoperative pain [74]. One of the recommendations from the American Pain Society is scheduling routine nonopioid analgesics as part of the pharmacologic regimen when treating these postoperative patients [48]. The use of nonsteroidal antiinflammatory drugs (NSAIDs), through cyclooxygenase (COX) inhibition, helps prevent the generation of inflammatory mediators such as prostaglandins, which further increase the propagation of nociceptive pain [48]. Other results have shown that combining Tylenol and NSAIDs results in improvement in postoperative pain control, leading to reduced opioid use [48].

Using different forms of perioperative anesthesia, via regional anesthesia (nerve blockade of peripheral nerves) or neuraxial anesthesia (blockade of central nervous system), has been investigated as a way of potentially reducing the risk of postoperative opioid use. This is believed to be successful due to 1 of 2 mechanisms. The first mechanism works through a theory called preventative analgesia [79–81], using the concept that nerve blockade can prevent the transition from acute to chronic pain by directly blocking transmission of pain impulses during the perioperative period, preventing central sensitization and chronic neuropathic pain [64]. The second mechanism is that nerve blocks are a well-established modality for treating acute postoperative pain, which, when severe, can be predictive of the development into chronic pain [64,82]. Regardless, it still has not been shown if these nerve blockades reduce long-term opioid use, even though there has been some success in the acute postoperative period [64].

The use of an intravenous local anesthetic, such as lidocaine, as a way of reducing postoperative opioid consumption has gained increasing interest [64]. The concept is that, by giving this intravenously, a blockade of the proinflammatory responses to surgery occurs, leading to reduced opioid consumption [64,83–85]. Although a recent review of intravenous lidocaine associated it with a decrease in postoperative opioid requirements for a variety of surgeries (eg, abdominal and thoracic procedures), it showed no benefit with others (eg, total hip arthroplasty) [64,83]. Further research is needed to explore the extent to which this modality could be used to mitigate postoperative opioid use.

All these different treatment modalities help feed into the overall concept of enhanced recovery after surgery (ERAS), developed first for colorectal surgery and since expanded to other surgical procedures, to attempt to decrease postoperative adverse events and length of stay [48]. These protocols were developed to address preoperative, intraoperative, and postoperative variables, such as fluid balance and nutrition, to improve efficiency in recovery. A key point of this program is the limitation of narcotic pain medication in the postoperative period, using multimodal pain management with a heavy reliance on nonnarcotic pain medications. For these protocols to be effectively developed and executed, ERAS analgesic regimens need multidisciplinary communication and care coordination [58]. This collaboration must occur between surgeons and perioperative and floor nurses, along with the anesthesiology team, to deliver analgesics beginning in the preoperative patient holding area [58]. Acetaminophen, COX inhibitors, and gamma-amino butyric acid (GABA) analogues given preoperatively help blunt initial nociception and may play a role in decreasing postoperative pain [58]. These agents also constitute the basis of the multimodal postoperative analgesic regimen used in addition to narcotic agents to reduce the reliance on narcotics [58]. This includes incorporating regional anesthesia (nerve blocks, epidurals) and adjunct agents such as intravenous ketamine and lidocaine [58]. Studies have shown that patients complain of less postoperative pain after having these multimodal regimens used in their favor [58,86–88].

Professional surgical organizations have embraced the concept of ERAS and offer information and programs to their members to help them implement these programs. One example is the American College of Surgeons launching the Improving Surgical Care and Recovery program in collaboration with the Agency for Healthcare Research and Quality and the Johns Hopkins Medicine Armstrong Institute for Patient Safety and Quality, providing multidisciplinary strategies for effective perioperative pain management (http://www.facs.org/quality-programs/iscr) [58,89]. Another organization, the Society of American Gastrointestinal and Endoscopic Surgeons (SAGES), has developed the SMART Enhanced Recovery Program, combining open and mostly minimally invasive surgical approaches with with enhanced recovery care plans, to improve recovery and reduce postoperative narcotic use (http://www.sages.org/smart-enhanced-recovery-program/) [90]. Unfortunately, even with these new provisions put into place, surgeons seem reluctant to change their practices at the time of discharge. A recent study out of the University of California, Los Angeles, found that there was no difference in opioid prescribing at the time of discharge when they compared pre-ERAS with post-ERAS implementation at their institution [16,91]. Without changing postdischarge practices, it will be hard to assess the maximal benefit these ERAS pathways can have.

Other groups are working on gathering real-time data on opioid prescribing habits to combat the issues of overprescribing and opioid abuse. They are then using and publishing these data to help guide fellow surgeons to use fewer narcotics while still maintaining adequate postoperative pain control, working with this new multimodality approach. One such group is the Michigan Opioid

Prescription Engagement Network (OPEN), led by 22 physicians devoted to improving patient care in Michigan, representing all major hospitals and surgical specialties, and funded by Blue Cross and Blue Shield of Michigan (http://michigan-open.org/) [31,92]. Part of this ongoing work has culminated in the online publication of recommended opioid prescribing guidelines for several common operations, listing all common narcotic modalities down to the pill number, which is constantly updated based on new evidence-based data (https://opioidprescribing.info/) [31,93].

Clinician education about opioid management

It is acknowledged that most health care professionals have not received an adequate amount of education regarding pain management during their training [58,94]. This has been further supported when practice patterns have been examined after the introduction of pain management education [58]. One study showed that introducing procedure-specific recommendations enabled surgeons to reduce the number of narcotic pills they prescribed by more than 50% and that patients who received opioids were adequately managed with those initial prescriptions in 80% of the 246 cases examined [58,95]. Currently, there are insufficient formal curricula for pain assessment and management, and these lack breadth and standardization, although efforts have been made to improve on this [58].

For the most part, most residents learn their pain management strategies from their attending surgeons, extended to both analgesic selection and dosing for each level of pain severity, with trends toward opioid use [58]. Junior-level resident pain management strategies often encompass the trial and error approach, arbitrarily changing dosing amounts and frequencies based on the reported level of pain the patient is subjectively stating [58]. Patients with preoperative chronic pain or who have symptoms that cannot be controlled with conventional methods are often referred to a pain management specialist during their postoperative recovery period [58].

It is incumbent on the surgeon to develop a deeper and more meaningful understanding of the relationship between patient symptomology, prescribing patterns, educational interventions, and subsequent outcomes [58]. One example is the University of Toronto, Ontario, Canada, which has instituted a multidisciplinary transitional pain service to manage patients who have chronic postoperative pain and also reduce opioid use [58,96]. Although this group did manage to look at the issues regarding overprescribing, there still needs to be development of understanding and mitigating the development of dependent or chronic postoperative pain [58].

HEALTH CARE POLICY AND ADVOCACY

Federal regulation

Although there have been plenty of changes on the clinical side, the legislative and regulatory bodies have also been active in attempting to curtail the spread of the opioid epidemic. The DEA has implemented several opioid-related policy changes to help address the ongoing issues. In October 2014, the DEA rescheduled hydrocodone from a Schedule III to the more restrictive Schedule II substance under the Controlled Substances Act [97]. This move led to prescriptions for hydrocodone decreasing by 22% in the first year after this change was implemented [97,98]. This was followed in October 2016 by the DEA reducing the amount of Schedule II opioid medications that can be manufactured by 25% or more, decreasing the total available supply of these medications [97,99].

Another policy-level intervention that occurred focused on the HCAHPS survey. The 3 questions in the survey related to patient pain control were removed, effective January 2018 [16]. These questions shifted focus from pain control to how well the hospital staff communicates with patients about pain control [16]. This was done to remove the linking of hospital and physician reimbursement with the treatment of a patient's pain, eliminating potential conscious or subconscious opioid prescribing for the sake of maximizing financial return or hospital ratings [16].

In 2012, the FDA responded to the crisis by changing the mandatory labeling for extended-release or long-acting opioids, removing the treatment indication for moderate pain [97,100,101]. Starting in May 2014, the new indication for these medications was for pain "severe enough to require daily, around-the-clock, long-term opioid treatment and for which alternative treatments are inadequate" [97,100]. Other federal interventions were included in the Affordable Care Act, which called for states to develop prescription drug monitoring programs (PDMPs) and increase the funding for substance abuse treatment programs because it was recognized that this issue needed to be addressed from several areas to be successful [97,102].

On July 22, 2016, President Obama signed the Comprehensive Addiction and Recovery Act (CARA), calling for the implementation of incremental steps to combat the opioid epidemic, which expanded access to evidence-based therapies to treat patients who have disorders related to certain opioids, including methadone, buprenorphine, and naltrexone [97,103,104]. This was followed by the signing of the Substance Use Disorder Prevention that Promotes Opioid Recovery and Treatment for Patients and Communities (SUPPORT) Act by President Trump on October 24, 2018. This is designed to assist Medicare in helping states provide coverage and services to people who need substance use disorder treatment, specifically focusing on opioid use disorder, as well as to address law enforcement efforts against illicit drugs and to combat overprescribing of opioids [105–110].

State regulation

Several states have enacted legislation to reduce opioid-related adverse events, with the number of states growing every year. Forty-nine states, plus the District of Columbia and St. Louis County (Missouri) have enacted some form of PDMP regulations, each with specific requirements regarding opioid access and use. Examples of success with this legislative move are New York and

Tennessee, which showed a reduction in patients seeking prescriptions from multiple prescribers by 75% and 36%, respectively [97,111].

Numerous states now require that licensed physicians undergo supplemental opioid prescribing or addiction education for licensure, whereas others require that health care professionals undergo this training if they are responsible for pain management or treating addiction [97,112]. Some states also are now adding medical school teaching requirements to ensure adequate pain management concepts are taught.

Many states now have also added opioid prescription limitations, along with enacting regulations to curtail clinics and prescribers from dispensing these medications from their offices [97]. This started in 2016, with Massachusetts passing the first law in the United States [113]. As of early April 2018, legislation has been enacted in 28 states that had some type of prescription limit, guidance, or requirement related to opioid prescribing [113]. Many of these bills focus on the days of supply; others also included dosage limits, putting exceptions in for certain subsets of patients and not including chronic pain treatments. In the future, more legislation is likely to be enacted to address the ongoing issues.

Surgeon and physician involvement

Numerous medical and surgical organizations are actively engaged with both federal and state legislators, along with regulatory bodies, to ensure that safe practices are implemented and ensuring that these do not hinder the ability of surgeons and physicians to take care of their patients in a comprehensive fashion. Using evidence-based resources to help guide their positions, these groups lobby state and federal officials and provide background and information to help construct reasonable policies that protect patients. Many organizations are developing policies and guidelines with the common goal to diminish the opioid epidemic, including the American Medical Association, which has a Task Force to Reduce Opioid Abuse, using evidence-based strategies to combat the opioid epidemic [97].

Many of the ultimate changes that occurred in the previously mentioned enacted legislation occurred with the input and guidance of surgeons, among other stakeholders. The future direction of this epidemic depends on the efforts of the individual surgeons, advocating for evidence-based legislation that addresses opioid use, not just as individuals but also through their respective state and national professional organizations.

SUMMARY

The opioid epidemic began after an effort to relive pain and over the years has evolved into the current complex health problem. Opioid-related deaths now exceed liver cancer or prostate cancer deaths in the United States [97]. There is still hope that, although the issue with opioid misuse still exists in many ways, through changes in practices, education, and advocacy, the medical community can help remedy the epidemic while still adequately caring for patients.

This requires all surgeons to be involved on numerous fronts, maintaining an understanding of evidence-based practices and incorporating them into their own surgical practice, while cultivating educational opportunities for both the surgeon and the patient, and continuing to advocate for evidence-based legislation to help protect patients but not inhibit the ability to appropriately treat them. The only way for this to be accomplished is if all surgeons participate and work together to implement these changes for the better.

References

[1] Gavin K. Fighting the opioid epidemic. Michigan Today; 2016. Available at: http://michigantoday.umich.edu/fighting-the-opioid-epidemic/. Accessed November 4, 2018.

[2] Alam A, Gomes T, Zheng H, et al. Long-term analgesic use after low-risk surgery: a retrospective cohort study. Arch Intern Med 2012;172(5):425–30.

[3] Schoenfeld AJ, Nwosu K, Jiang W, et al. Risk factors for prolonged opioid use following spine surgery, and the association with surgical intensity, among opioid-naïve patients. J Bone Joint Surg Am 2017;99(15):1247–52.

[4] Shah A, Hayes CJ, Martin BC. Factors influencing long-term opioid use among opioid naïve patients: an examination of initial prescription characteristics and pain etiologies. J Pain 2017;18(11):1374–83.

[5] Johnson SP, Chung KC, Zhong L, et al. Risk of prolonged opioid use among opioid-naïve patients following common hand surgery procedures. J Hand Surg Am 2016;41(10):947–57.e3.

[6] Dowell D, Zhang K, Noonan RK, et al. Mandatory provider review and pain clinic laws reduce the amounts of opioids prescribed and overdose death rates. Health Aff (Millwood) 2016;35:1876–83.

[7] Jones MR, Viswanath O, Peck J, et al. A brief history of the opioid epidemic and strategies for pain medicine. Pain Ther 2018;7(1):13–21.

[8] Dowell D, Noonan RK, Houry D. Underlying factors in drug overdose deaths. JAMA 2017;318:2295–6.

[9] US Centers for Disease Control and Prevention. Provisional counts of drug overdose deaths as of August 6, 2017. Available at: https://www.cdc.gov/nchs/data/health_policy/monthly-drug-overdose-death-estimates.pdf. Accessed November 4, 2018.

[10] WHO. Cancer pain relief. Geneva (Switzerland): WHO; 1986.

[11] Stein C. Opioid treatment of chronic nonmalignant pain. Anesth Analg 1997;84(4):912–4.

[12] Campbell JN. APS 1995 presidential address. Pain Forum 1996;1(5):85–8.

[13] Mularski RA, White-Chu F, Overbay D, et al. Measuring pain as the 5th vital sign does not improve quality of pain management. J Gen Intern Med 2006;21(6):607–12.

[14] Baker DW. History of The Joint Commission's pain standards: lessons for today's prescription opioid epidemic. JAMA 2017;317(11):1117–8.

[15] Joranson DE, Gilson AM, Dahl JL, et al. Pain management, controlled substances, and state medical board policy: a decade of change. J Pain Symptom Manage 2002;23(2):138–47.

[16] Theisen K, Jacobs B, Macleod L, et al. The United States opioid epidemic: a review of the surgeon's contribution to it and health policy initiatives. BJU Int 2018;122(5):754–9.

[17] Centers for Medicare & Medicaid Services, Baltimore, MD. Available at: www.hcahpsonline.org. Accessed November 4, 2018.

[18] Fenton JJ, Jerant AF, Bertakis KD, et al. The cost of satisfaction: a national study of patient satisfaction, health care utilization, expenditures, and mortality. Arch Intern Med 2012;172(5):405–11.

[19] Tucker KL. Medico-legal case report and commentary: inadequate pain management in the context of terminal cancer. The case of Lester Tomlinson. Pain Med 2004;5:214–28.

[20] Dowell D, Haegerich TM, Chou R. CDC guideline for prescribing opioids for chronic pain – United States, 2016. MMWR Morb Mortal Wkly Rep 2016;65:1–49.
[21] Paulozzi LJ, Hockenberry JM. Vital signs: variation among States in prescribing of opioid pain relievers and benzodiazepines – United States, 2012. MMWR Morb Mortal Wkly Rep 2014;63:563–8.
[22] Hill MV, Stucke RS, Barth RJ. Wide variation and excessive dosage of opioid prescriptions for common general surgical procedures. Ann Surg 2017;265:709–14.
[23] Scully RE, Jiang W, Lipsitz S, et al. Defining optimal length of opioid pain medication prescription after common surgical procedures. JAMA Surg 2018;153:37–43.
[24] Maughan BC, Shofer FS, Wanner KJ, et al. Unused opioid analgesics and drug disposal following outpatient dental surgery: a randomized control trial. Drug Alcohol Depend 2016;68:328–34.
[25] Harris K, Larsen B, Calder S, et al. Opioid pain medication use after dermatologic surgery: a prospective observational study of 212 dermatologic surgery patients. JAMA Dermatol 2013;149:317–21.
[26] Bartels K, Dingmann C, Bullard KJ, et al. Opioid use and storage patterns by patients after hospital discharge following surgery. PLoS One 2016;11:e0147972.
[27] Rodgers J, Fitzgerald K, Finnerty E. Opioid consumption following outpatient upper extremity surgery. J Hand Surg Am 2012;37:645–50.
[28] Kim N, Abboudi J, Jones C, et al. A prospective evaluation of opioid utilization after upper-extremity surgical procedures: identifying consumption patterns and determining prescribing guidelines. J Bone Joint Surg Am 2016;98:e89.
[29] Kumar K, Dines JS, Allen AA, et al. Unused opioid pills after outpatient shoulder surgeries given current perioperative prescribing habits. Am J Sports Med 2017;45:636–41.
[30] Bates C, Southwick A, Bishoff J. Overprescription of postoperative narcotics: a look at postoperative pain medication delivery, consumption and disposal in urological practice. J Urol 2011;185:551–5.
[31] Waljee JF, Brummett CM, Englesbe MJ. Iatrogenic opioid dependence in the United States: are surgeons the gatekeepers? Ann Surg 2017;265:728–30.
[32] Hwang CS, Chang HY, Alexander GC. Impact of abuse-deterrent OxyContin on prescription opioid utilization. Pharmacoepidemiol Drug Saf 2015;24(2):197–204.
[33] Manchikanti L, Kaye AM, Knezevic N, et al. Responsible, safe, and effective prescription of opioids for chronic non-cancer pain: American Society of Interventional Pain Physicians (ASIPP) guidelines. Pain Physician 2017;20(2S):S3–92.
[34] Levy B, Paulozzi L, Mack KA, et al. Trends in opioid analgesic-prescribing rates by specialty, US, 2007-2012. Am J Prev Med 2015;49:409–13.
[35] Tan WH, Yu J, Feaman S, et al. Opioid medication use in the surgical patient: an assessment of prescribing patterns and use. J Am Coll Surg 2018;227(2):203–11.
[36] Guy GP Jr, Zhang K, Bohn MK, et al. Changes in opioid prescribing in the United States, 2006-2015. MMWR Morb Mortal Wkly Rep 2017;66:697–704.
[37] Tick H, Nielsen A, Pelletier K, et al, The Pain Task Force of the Academic Consortium for Integrative Medicine and Health. Evidence-based nonpharmacologic strategies for comprehensive pain care. a consortium pain task force white paper. Explore (NY) 2018;14(3):177–211.
[38] Porter JH. Addiction rare in patients treated with narcotics. N Engl J Med 1980;302:123.
[39] Centers for Disease Control and Prevention. National vital statistics system mortality data 2015. Available at: http://www.cdc.gov/nchs/deaths.htm. Accessed November 4, 2018.
[40] Brummett CM, Goesling J, Moser S, et al. New persistent opioid use after minor and major surgical procedures in US adults. JAMA Surg 2017;152:e170504.
[41] Goesling J, Zaidi B, Hassett AL, et al. Trends and predictors of opioid use after total knee and total hip arthroplasty. Pain 2016;157:1259–65.

[42] Clarke H, Ko DT, Yun L, et al. Rates and risk factors for prolonged opioid use after major surgery: population based cohort study. BMJ 2014;348:1251.
[43] Shah A, Marin BC. Characteristics of initial prescription episodes and likelihood of long-term opioid use – United States, 2006-2015. MMWR Morb Mortal Wkly Rep 2017;66: 265–9.
[44] Lipari R. How people obtain the prescription pain relievers they misuse. The CBHSQ Report. Rockville (MD): Center for Behavioral Health Statistics and Quality, Substance Abuse and Mental Health Services Administration; 2017.
[45] Kennedy-Hendricks A, McDonald E, McGinty EE, et al. Medication sharing, storage, and disposal practices for opioid medications among US adults. JAMA Intern Med 2016;176: 1027–9.
[46] Pollini RA, Cuevas-Mota J, Metzner M, et al. Problematic use of prescription-type opioids prior to heroin use among young heroin injectors. Subst Abuse Rehabil 2011;2:173–80.
[47] Muhuri PK, Davies MC. Association of nonmedical pain reliever use and initiation of heroin use in the United States. *CBHSQ data review.* SAMHSA; 2013. Available at: http://www.samhsa.gov/data/. Accessed November 4, 2018.
[48] Alimi Y, Economopoulos KP, Smelser W, et al. Postoperative opioid prescriptions: How surgeons can alleviate the opioid crisis. Bull Am Coll Surg 2017;102(8):21–6.
[49] Pathan H, Williams J. Basic opioid pharmacology: an update. Br J Pain 2012;6(1):11–6.
[50] Kosten TR, George TP. The neurobiology of opioid dependence: Implications for treatment. Sci Pract Perspect 2002;1(1):13–20.
[51] Gosch M. Analgesics in geriatric patients. Adverse side effects and interactions. Z Gerontol Geriatr 2015;48(5):483–92.
[52] Richards S, Torre L, Lawther B. Buprenorphine-related complications in elderly hospitalized patients: a case series. Anaesth Intensive Care 2017;45(2):256–61.
[53] Innaurato G, Piguet V, Simonet ML. Analgesia in patients with hepatic impairment. Rev Med Suisse 2015;11(480):1380, 1382–4.
[54] Imani F, Motavaf M, Safari S, et al. The therapeutic use of analgesics in patients with liver cirrhosis: a literature review and evidence-based recommendations. Hepat Mon 2014;14(10):e23539.
[55] Rolke R, Rolke S, Hiddemann S, et al. Update palliative pain therapy. Internist (Berl) 2016;57(10):959–70.
[56] Hassamal S, Miotto K, Wang T, et al. A narrative review: the effects of opioids on sleep disordered breathing in chronic pain patients and methadone maintained patients. Am J Addict 2016;25(6):452–65.
[57] Bluth T, Pelosi P, de Abreu MG. The obese patient undergoing nonbariatric surgery. Curr Opin Anaesthesiol 2016;29(3):421–9.
[58] Flink B, Duggan EM, Neuwirth MG, et al. Surgeons and the opioid epidemic: treatment and education strategies for the practicing surgeon. Bull Am Coll Surg 2017;102(8): 27–31.
[59] Cameron CD, Spring VL, Todd AR. The empathy impulse: a multinomial model of intentional and unintentional empathy for pain. Emotion 2017;17(3):395–411.
[60] Baker CM, Wong DL. Q.U.E.S.T.: a process of pain assessment in children (continuing education credit). Orthop Nurs 1987;6(1):11–21.
[61] Hirsh AT, Hollingshead NA, Ashburn-Nardo L, et al. The interaction of patient race, provider bias, and clinical ambiguity on pain management decisions. J Pain 2015;16(6): 558–68.
[62] Ashton-James CE, Nicholas MK. Appearance of trustworthiness: an implicit source of bias in judgments of patients' pain. Pain 2016;157(8):1583–5.
[63] Sabin JA, Greenwald AG. The influence of implicit bias on treatment recommendations for 4 common pediatric conditions: pain, urinary tract infection, attention deficit hyperactivity disorder, and asthma. Am J Public Health 2012;102(5):988–95.

[64] Hah JM, Bateman BT, Ratliff J, et al. Chronic Opioid use after surgery: implications for perioperative management in the face of the opioid epidemic. Anesth Analg 2017;125(5):1733–40.
[65] Sun EC, Darnall BD, Baker LC, et al. Incidence of and risk factors for chronic opioid use among opioid-naïve patients in the postoperative period. JAMA Intern Med 2016;176(9):1286–93.
[66] Waljee JF, Zhong L, Hou H, et al. The use of opioid analgesics following common upper extremity surgical procedures: a national, population-based study. Plast Reconstr Surg 2016;137(2):355e–64e.
[67] Raebel MA, Newcomer SR, Reifler LM, et al. Chronic use of opioid medications before and after bariatric surgery. JAMA 2013;310(13):1369–76.
[68] Zarling BJ, Yokhana SS, Herzog DT, et al. Preoperative and postoperative opiate use by the arthroplasty patient. J Arthroplasty 2016;31(10):2081–4.
[69] Torres M, Eskander M, Held J, et al. The general surgeon's role in enhancing patient education about prescription opioids. Bull Am Coll Surg 2017;102(8):15–20.
[70] Zuccaro SM, Vellucci R, Sarzi-Puttini P, et al. Barriers to pain management: focus on opioid therapy. Clin Drug Investig 2012;32(Suppl 1):11–9.
[71] Angioli R, Plotti F, Capriglione S, et al. The effects of giving patients verbal or written preoperative information in gynecologic oncology survey: a randomized study and the medical-legal point of view. Eur J Obstet Gynecol Reprod Biol 2014;177:67–71.
[72] Kruzik N. Benefits of preoperative education for adult elective surgery patients. AORN J 2009;90(3):381–7.
[73] Nielsen S, Campbell G, Peacock A, et al. Health service utilization by people living with chronic non-cancer pain: findings from the Pain and Opioids IN Treatment (POINT) study. Aust Health Rev 2015;40(5):490–9.
[74] Chou R, Gordon DB, de Leon-Casasola OA, et al. Management of postoperative pain: a clinical practice guideline from the American Pain Society, the American Society of Regional Anesthesia and Pain Medicine, and the American Society of Anesthesiologists' Committee on Regional Anesthesia, Executive Committee, and Administrative Council. J Pain 2016;17(2):131–57.
[75] Gawande AA. It's time to adopt electronic prescriptions for opioids. Ann Surg 2017;265(4):693–4.
[76] Wilson M, Roll JM, Corbett C, et al. Empowering patients with persistent pain using an Internet-based self-management program. Pain Manag Nurs 2015;16(4):503–14.
[77] Traynor K. Some unused narcotics should go down the drain, FDA says. Am J Health Syst Pharm 2009;66(23):2070–2.
[78] Lin LA, Bohnert ASB, Kerns RD, et al. Impact of the Opioid Safety Initiative on opioid-related prescribing in veterans. Pain 2017;158(5):833–9.
[79] Dahl JB, Moiniche S. Pre-emptive analgesia. Br Med Bull 2004;71:13–27.
[80] Liu SS, Buvanendran A, Rathmell JP, et al. A cross-sectional survey or prevalence and risk factors for persistent postsurgical pain 1 year after total hip and knee replacement. Reg Anesth Pain Med 2012;37(4):415–22.
[81] Vadivelu N, Mitra S, Schermer E, et al. Preventive analgesia for postoperative pain control: a broader concept. Local Reg Anesth 2014;7:17–22.
[82] Kehlet H, Jensen TS, Woolf CJ. Persistent postsurgical pain: risk factors and prevention. Lancet 2006;367(9522):1618–25.
[83] Dunn LK, Durieux ME. Perioperative use of intravenous lidocaine. Anesthesiology 2017;126(4):729–37.
[84] Leliefeld PH, Wessels CM, Leenen LP, et al. The role of neutrophils in immune dysfunction during severe inflammation. Crit Care 2016;20:73.
[85] Hollmann MW, Durieux ME. Local anesthetics and the inflammatory response: a new therapeutic indication? Anesthesiology 2000;93(3):858–75.

[86] Ljungqvist O, Scott M, Fearon KC. Enhanced recovery after surgery: a review. JAMA Surg 2017;152(3):292–8.
[87] Garimella V, Cellini C. Postoperative pain control. Clin Colon Rectal Surg 2013;26(3): 191–6.
[88] Schmidt PC, Ruchell G, Mackey SC, et al. Perioperative gabapentinoids: choice of agent, dose, timing, and effects on chronic postsurgical pain. Anesthesiology 2013;119(5): 1215–21.
[89] American College of Surgeons. AHRQ safety program for improving surgical care and recovery. Available at: http://www.facs.org/quality-programs/iscr. Accessed November 4, 2018.
[90] SAGES SMART enhanced recovery program. Available at: http://www.sages.org/smart-enhanced-recovery-program/. Accessed November 4, 2018.
[91] Brandal D, Lee C, Grogan T, et al. Impact of enhanced recovery after surgery and opioid-free anesthesia on opioid prescriptions at discharge from the hospital: a historical-prospective study. Anesth Analg 2017;125:1784–92.
[92] Michigan opioid prescribing engagement network. Available at: http://michigan-open.org. Accessed November 4, 2018.
[93] Opioid prescribing recommendations for surgery. Available at: https://opioidprescribing.info. Accessed November 4, 2018.
[94] Davis MP, Mehta Z. Opioids and chronic pain: where is the balance? Curr Oncol Rep 2016;18(12):71.
[95] Hill MV, Stucke RS, McMahon ML, et al. An educational intervention decreases opioid prescribing after general surgical operations. Ann Surg 2018;267(3):468–72.
[96] Huang A, Azam A, Segal S, et al. Chronic postsurgical pain and persistent opioid use following surgery: the need for a transitional pain service. Pain Manag 2016;6(5): 435–43.
[97] McNicoll CF, Yorkgitis BK, Sangji NF, et al. Surgical leadership is required to reverse the opioid crisis. Bull Am Coll Surg 2017;102(8):32–40.
[98] Jones CM, Lurie PG, Throckmorton DC. Effect of U.S. Drug Enforcement Administration's rescheduling of hydrocodone combination analgesic products on opioid analgesic prescribing. JAMA Intern Med 2016;176(3):399–402.
[99] Drug Enforcement Administration. DEA reduced amount of opioid controlled substances to be manufactured in 2017. Available at: http://www.dea.gov/divisions/hq/2016/hq100416.shtml. Accessed November 4, 2018.
[100] Barlas S. FDA requires new labeling for some opioids: modest changes walk narrow political line. P T 2013;38(11):644.
[101] Califf RM, Woodcock J, Ostroff S. A proactive response to prescription opioid abuse. N Engl J Med 2016;374(15):1480–5.
[102] Department of Health and Human Services. The affordable care act and the prevention and public health fund report to Congress for FY2012. Available at: http://www.hhs.gov/sites/default/files/open/prevention/fy-2012-aca-pphf-report-to-congress.pdf. Accessed November 4, 2018.
[103] Library of Congress. S. 524. Comprehensive Addiction and Recovery Act of 2016. Available at: http://www.conggress.gov/bill/114th-congress/senate-bill/524/text. Accessed November 4, 2018.
[104] National Alliance for Model State Drug Laws. Substances monitored by PMP. Available at: http://www.namsdl.org/library/8D7261F8-E47D-B6A5-DD0CAFA98FEA4846/. Accessed November 4, 2018.
[105] Library of Congress. HR 6. SUPPORT for Patients and Communities Act of 2018. Available at: http://www.congress.gov/bill/115th-congress/house-bill/6. Accessed November 4, 2018.

[106] Federation of State Medical Boards. Continuing Medical Education: Board by board overview. Available at: http://www.fsmb.org/Media/Default/PDF/FSMB/Advocacy/GR-POL_CME_Overview_by_State.pdf. Accessed November 4, 2018.
[107] Johnson H, Paulozzi L, Porucznik C, et al. Hal Johnson Consulting and Division of Disease Control and Health Promotion, Florida Department of Health. Decline in drug overdose deaths after state policy changes – Florida, 2010-2012. MMWR Morb Mortal Wkly Rep 2014;63(26):569–74.
[108] Liepert AE, Ackerman TL. 2016 state legislative year in review and a look ahead. Bull Am Coll Surg 2016;101(12):35–9.
[109] U.S. Department of Justice. Drug Enforcement Administration. Practitioner's license requirements. Available at: http://www.deadiversion.usdoj.gov/drugreg/reg_apps/pract_state_lic_require.htm. Accessed November 4, 2018.
[110] Massachusetts Medical Society. Fact Sheet: An act relative to substance use treatment, education and prevention. Available at: http://www.massmed.org/Advocay/Key-Issues/Opioid-Abuse/Fact-Sheet–An-Act-Relative-to-Substance-Use-Treatment,-Education-and-Prevention/#.WPDUt2f2aUI. Accessed November 4, 2018.
[111] Centers for Disease Control and Prevention. Opioid overdose: State information: State successes. Available at: http://www.cdc.gov/drugoverdose/policy/successes/html. Accessed November 4, 2018.
[112] CME State Requirements. American College of Surgeons. Available at: https://www.facs.org/education/cme/state-mandates. Accessed November 4, 2018.
[113] National Conference of State Legislatures. Prescribing Policies: States Confront Opioid Overdose Epidemic. Available at: http://www.ncsl.org/research/health/prescribing-policies-states-confront-opioid-overdose-epidemic.aspx. Accessed November 4, 2018.

FSC
www.fsc.org
MIX
Papier | Fördert gute Waldnutzung
FSC® C083411

Kolibri 360 GmbH
Ferdinand-Jühlke-Straße 7
99095 Erfurt, Deutschland
produktsicherheit@kolibri360.de